Mental Health in Historical Perspective

Series Editors
Catharine Coleborne
School of Humanities and Social Science
University of Newcastle
Callaghan, NSW, Australia

Matthew Smith
Centre for the Social History of Health and Healthcare
University of Strathclyde
Glasgow, UK

Covering all historical periods and geographical contexts, the series explores how mental illness has been understood, experienced, diagnosed, treated and contested. It will publish works that engage actively with contemporary debates related to mental health and, as such, will be of interest not only to historians, but also mental health professionals, patients and policy makers. With its focus on mental health, rather than just psychiatry, the series will endeavour to provide more patient-centred histories. Although this has long been an aim of health historians, it has not been realised, and this series aims to change that.

The scope of the series is kept as broad as possible to attract good quality proposals about all aspects of the history of mental health from all periods. The series emphasises interdisciplinary approaches to the field of study, and encourages short titles, longer works, collections, and titles which stretch the boundaries of academic publishing in new ways.

More information about this series at
http://www.palgrave.com/gp/series/14806

Robert Ellis • Sarah Kendal
Steven J. Taylor
Editors

Voices in the History of Madness

Personal and Professional Perspectives on Mental Health and Illness

palgrave
macmillan

Editors
Robert Ellis
School of Arts and Humanities
University of Huddersfield
Huddersfield, UK

Sarah Kendal
School of Healthcare
University of Leeds
Leeds, UK

Steven J. Taylor
School of History
University of Kent
Canterbury, UK

ISSN 2634-6036 ISSN 2634-6044 (electronic)
Mental Health in Historical Perspective
ISBN 978-3-030-69561-3 ISBN 978-3-030-69559-0 (eBook)
https://doi.org/10.1007/978-3-030-69559-0

Cover illustration: agefotostock / Alamy Stock Photo

This Palgrave Macmillan imprint is published by the registered company Springer Nature Switzerland AG.
The registered company address is: Gewerbestrasse 11, 6330 Cham, Switzerland

Acknowledgements

The origins of this volume lay in the Voices of Madness conference, hosted by the Centre for Health Histories at the University of Huddersfield, UK, in September 2016. We would like to express our gratitude for the financial support that we received for that event from the Centre and from the School of Human and Health Sciences.

The aim of the conference was to stimulate new interdisciplinary conversations on the theme of 'voice', and we are grateful for all the contributions to what were a very rich and fruitful two days. In organising the conference, and in editing this collection, we wanted to reflect the breadth of chronologies and methodologies of new research taking place in a range of contexts and locations. Ultimately, we have incorporated contributions that reflect innovative research on four continents, contributed by writers who speak from diverse perspectives. We would like to say thank you to our contributors for their diligence, patience and collegiality.

Thanks are also due to Catharine Coleborne and Tommy Dickinson, whose conference keynotes influenced the discussions leading to this collection. Professor Coleborne generously agreed to add a Coda to this volume. We are grateful to Andrew Clifton for his helpful notes on Chap. 18. At Palgrave Macmillan we want to acknowledge Molly Beck, Maeve Sinnott, Lucy Kidwell and Joe Johnson for their support, as well as series editors Catharine Coleborne and Matthew Smith and their peer reviewers for their helpful and encouraging comments.

Finally, a big thank you to Rob Piggott for his important administrative support at the closing stages of this project and to Vipin Kumar Mani and the team at Springer Nature for their patient and professional handling of the various typesetting and proofing amendments.

Contents

1 Voices in the History of Madness: An Introduction to Personal and Professional Perspectives 1
Robert Ellis, Sarah Kendal, and Steven J. Taylor
Part I Shifting Perspectives in the Industry of Madness 4
Part II Reconstructing Patient Perspectives 8
Part III The Visual and the Material 11
Part IV Mad Studies and Activism 13

Part I Shifting Perspectives in the Industry of Madness 23

2 Accepted and Rejected: Late Nineteenth-Century Application for Admission to the Scottish National Institution for the Education of Imbecile Children 25
Iain Hutchison
Early Ethos and Evolution 27
Selected and Rejected: Outcomes 31
Beyond the Gates of the SNI 38
Conclusions 42

3 Mental Health in the Vernacular: Print and Counter-Hegemonic Approaches to Madness in Colonial Bengal 49
Pradipto Roy
Prelude: Epistemic Challenges in the Concept of Psyche in Modern South Asia 50
The Concept of Madness in Premodern South Asia 51
The World of Print in Colonial Bengal 52
Medical Books in the Vernacular 54
Mental Health in Vernacular Health Periodicals 55
Closing Remarks 64

4 "The Root of All Evil is Inactivity": The Response of French Psychiatrists to New Approaches to Patient Work and Occupation, 1918–1939 71
Jane Freebody
Introduction 71
Historiography 73
Patient Work before 1918 73
The Aftermath of World War I 75
Criticisms of Patient Work 75
"More Active Therapy"—A New Theory Regarding Patient Occupation 78
The Effect of the New Theory on Practice in Asylums 81
Impediments to the Adoption of More Active Therapy 82
Conclusion 88

5 Distant Voices: Treatment of Mentally Ill Children at the Copenhagen University Hospital in Denmark, c. 1935–1976 95
Jennie Sejr Junghans
Introduction 95
Admission 99
Conflicts 101
Diagnostic Tools and Treatment 104
Distant Voices? 107
Concluding Remarks 110

Part II Reconstructing Patient Perspectives 115

6 **Experiences of the Madhouse in England, 1650–1810** 117
Leonard Smith
To the Madhouse 119
In the Madhouse 123
Perceptions of the Proprietor 127
Conclusions 130

7 **"Tells his Story Quite Rationally and Collectedly": Examining the Casebooks of the Grahamstown Lunatic Asylum, 1890–1910, for Cases of Delusion Where Patients Voiced their Life Stories** 137
Rory du Plessis
The Life Stories and Testimonies of Sanity Given by the Patients 139
Cross-examination of a Patient's Personal Account of Restored Sanity 143
Personal Accounts of Institutionalisation 146
Conclusion 149

8 **Dehumanizing Experience, Rehumanizing Self-Awareness: Perception of Violence in Psychiatric Hospitals of Soviet Lithuania** 155
Tomas Vaiseta
Patient View and Medical Gaze 158
The Hidden Power of Medical Discourse: The Externalization of the Self 161
In Alignment with Medical Discourse: Violence as a Result of Disorder 164
Shelter of Medical Discourse: Violence as an Enforcement of Madness 166
Conclusions 168

9 **"I Like My Job because It Will Get Me Out Quicker": Work, Independence, and Disability at Indiana's Central State Hospital (1986–1993)** 173
Emily Beckman, Elizabeth Nelson, and Modupe Labode
Work and Disability 175
Central State Hospital 176

Methodology 178
Results: Patient Goals and Experiences of Work 179
Staff Goals and Policy Changes During the Closure 182

10 "More than Bricks and Mortar": Meaningful Care Practices in the Old State Mental Hospitals 191
Verusca Calabria, Di Bailey, and Graham Bowpitt
Introduction 191
Background 192
Methodology 194
Contested Meanings of Institutional Care 196
Community Psychiatry at the Nottingham Mental Hospitals 197
Fragmentation of Services in Community 200
Experiencing Neglect in Community 204
Conclusion 206
Data Access Statement 208

Part III The Visual and the Material 217

11 Tracking Traces of the Art Extraordinary Collection 219
Cheryl McGeachan
Archives, Voices and Traces 223
Gym Hall, Barlinnie Prison 225
An Unmarked Grave, Sleepyhillock Cemetery 229
Conclusions 232

12 Patient Photographs, Patient Voices: Recovering Patient Experience in the Nineteenth-Century Asylum 237
Katherine Rawling
Introduction 237
The 'Voice' of a Photograph 239
A Picture Tells a Thousand Words? 243
Multiple Voices 253
Conclusion 258

13 A Boundary Between Two Worlds? Community Perceptions of Former Asylums in Lancashire, England 263
Carolyn Gibbeson and Katie Beattie
Introduction 263
An Image of Fear and Isolation 264
Methodology 265
Lancaster Moor and Whittingham Hospitals: A Brief History 266
Memory and Legacy 267
Former Asylums as Heritage 272
Conclusions 275

Part IV Mad Studies and Activism 285

14 Brutal Sanity and Mad Compassion: Tracing the Voice of Dorothea Buck 287
Elena Demke
On Voice and the Obstacles to Voicing Madness 287
Historiography and Framing the Study of the Voice of the Mad 289
Biographical Aspects 290
Towards a Genealogy of Dorothea's Voice 293
Past and Present Intertwined: Researching Literature and Searching for Allies 293
Seeking Allies 295
Voice and Emotional Labour: Dealing with the Challenge of Power Structures 297
Framing in Terms of Contradictions and Paradoxes: Her Memoirs 299
Voicing Mad Wisdom 300
In Conclusion: Emergence of a New Expertise 301

15 Mad Activists and the Left in Ontario, 1970s to 2000 307
Geoffrey Reaume
Introduction: Mad Activists, Identity Politics and the Left 307
Deinstitutionalization in Canada 312
Disability and Mad Movement Activists in Ontario 313
Race, Gender, Sexual Orientation and Ontario's Mad Movement 316
Class, Unions and Mad People's Civil Rights 319
Conclusion 325

16 Knowing Our Own Minds: Transforming the Knowledge Base of Madness and Distress 333
Alison Faulkner
Finding Our Voices: A Brief History 334
Letting Stories Breathe: The Power of Personal Narratives 337
Finding Safe Spaces 338
Experiential Knowledge 341
The Role of Survivor Research 343
The Challenges… 345
Looking to the Future 349
Conclusions 350
References 351

17 Making Public Their Use of History: Reflections on the History of Collective Action by Psychiatric Patients, the Oor Mad History Project and Survivors History Group 359
Mark Gallagher
Introduction 359
The Disappearance of Patient Views and Voices in the History of Medicine 362
A Twentieth-Century Turning Point: From Formal Systems and Functionalist Grids to the Insurrection of Subjugated Knowledges 365
A 'Question of Levels': Doing History from 'A Level Below Which You Cannot Sink' 369
Conclusion: Making Public Use of History Requires Embracing That Sinking Feeling of Difficulty and Conflict 372
References 377

18 *Often, When I Am Using My Voice… It Does Not Go Well*: Perspectives on the Service User Experience 383
Megan Alikhanizadeh, Corey Hartley, Sarah Kendal, Liz Neill, and Gemma Trainor
Introduction 383
The Social and Political Background to Contemporary Models of Mental Health Care 384
The Policy Context 390

Is Social Media the Future for Youth Mental Health Support? 391
Mitigating the Risks of Social Media 392
The Voice of Lived Experience 393
Conclusion 397

19 Coda: Speaking Madness: Word, Image, Action 403
Catharine Coleborne
Making Sense of Madness 406
Word, Image, Action 408

Correction to: Mental Health in the Vernacular: Print and Counter-Hegemonic Approaches to Madness in Colonial Bengal C1
Pradipto Roy

Name Index 413

Place Index 421

Subject Index 425

Notes on Contributors

Megan Alikhanizadeh is involved with local and national projects working alongside young people, currently in the role of MindMate Project Worker, and is an advisor for Common Room North www.commonroom.uk.com. With lived experience of mental illness and accessing services, Megan is extremely passionate about using her insight and empathy to try to help others and improve the situation for young people's mental health, and also amplifying unheard voices in an uncensored way, enabling professionals and services to better support young people, and generally reducing stigma through education and awareness of the realities of mental illness.

Di Bailey is Professor of Mental Health and Academic Director of Research and Innovation in the School of Social Sciences at Nottingham Trent University, UK. Di has extensive experience in mental health practice. She has particular research expertise in participatory-action-research, systematic reviews, evaluation research. Di was Calabria's PhD supervisor.

Katie Beattie is a graduate of the BSc Real Estate course at Sheffield Hallam.

Emily Beckman is Director and Assistant Professor of Medical Humanities and Health Studies in the School of Liberal Arts at Indiana University-Purdue University, Indianapolis (IUPUI), and co-Director of the Scholarly Concentration in Medical Humanities at the Indiana University School of Medicine.

Graham Bowpitt is Associate Professor in Social Policy in the School of Social Sciences at Nottingham Trent University, UK. Graham has a specialist interest in social exclusion, policy process, comparative social policy, theoretical social policy and the development of social work. Graham was Calabria's PhD supervisor.

Verusca Calabria is an Early Career Research Fellow in the department of Social Work, School of Social Sciences, Nottingham Trent University, UK. Calabria is an interdisciplinary qualitative researcher and an experienced oral history practitioner. Her research expertise includes psychosocial approaches to mental health, oral history, participatory-action-research and service user involvement.

Catharine Coleborne is Professor of History at the University of Newcastle, Australia. She is the author of *Why Talk About Madness?* (Palgrave, 2020), and is currently researching and writing about the histories of mental health, narratives of madness, and post-institutional care in the twentieth century.

Elena Demke is a historian, currently conducting a survivor-led project on the 'meaning of things in experiences of distress, madness and of psychiatric interventions', at MHB Brandenburg. On the occasion of Dorothea Buck's 100th birthday, she co-edited a volume of more than 80 'voices on psychosis as self-discovery'.

Rory du Plessis is a senior lecturer in the School of the Arts at the University of Pretoria (UP), where he teaches Visual Culture Studies. He holds a PhD from the Centre for Ethics and Philosophy of Health Sciences (UP). He is the co-editor of the journal *Image & Text*.

Robert Ellis is Reader in History at the University of Huddersfield and the author of *London and its Asylums: Politics and Madness* (2020). He has published widely on the histories of mental ill-health and learning disability, and has co-produced a range of impact and engagement projects that have emphasised their contemporary relevance.

Alison Faulkner is a survivor researcher with around 30 years' experience of working in mental health research, training and consultancy. She holds a PhD from City, University of London on the role and value of experiential knowledge in mental health research. She has been self-employed since 2002, and has worked for most of the major UK mental health charities, including the National Survivor User Network (NSUN), Mind and

Together for Mental Wellbeing. In the late 1990s, she managed one of the first user-led research programmes in the UK at the Mental Health Foundation: 'Strategies for Living'. In recent years, much of her work has focused on peer support from a survivor perspective, and she works closely with NSUN. Alison has personal experience of mental distress and of using mental health services, including inpatient care, medication, psychotherapy, A&E and crisis services.

Jane Freebody holds a Wellcome Trust-funded PhD in the history of medicine from Oxford Brookes University, February 2020. Her thesis, entitled 'What did they do all day? Patient Work, Psychiatry and Society in England and France, 1918–1939', focuses on the role of work and occupation in English and French mental hospitals.

Mark Gallagher is a historian who completed a PhD on deinstitutionalisation and the history of collective action by psychiatric patients in Scotland, and more recently has been investigating the papers of psychiatrist Dr Ronald Sandison and the history of the use of LSD to treat patients at Powick Hospital.

Carolyn Gibbeson is a senior lecturer in Real Estate and joint Course Leader for the BSc Real Estate programme at Sheffield Hallam University. She worked as a surveyor prior to completing her PhD, titled 'After the Asylum: Place, value and heritage in the redevelopment of historic former asylums', in 2018.

Corey Hartley has worked in special educational needs as a personal and academic tutor for the past few years, alongside working as an early career researcher with particular interests in young people's mental health and mental health services, societal stigmatisation, gender queer marginality and postmodernist feminist literature.

Iain Hutchison is a research affiliate at the Centre for the History of Medicine at the University of Glasgow. He is a fellow of the Royal Historical Society, and a board member of the Disability History Association and of the Scottish Records Association. He is reviews editor for H-Disability.

Jennie Sejr Junghans is a PhD researcher at the European University Institute in Florence (Italy), where she is currently finishing her dissertation on the history of child psychiatry in Denmark and England c. 1900–1960. Her main areas of research are history of psychiatry and medical ethics.

Sarah Kendal is a research fellow at the University of Leeds. She practised as a mental health nurse in the UK for over two decades before moving into research and education. Her interests focus on improving young people's mental health outcomes and promoting public engagement in mental health research and services. She has published widely in the field of mental health.

Modupe Labode is a curator at the National Museum of American History in Washington, DC.

Cheryl McGeachan is a lecturer in Human Geography at the University of Glasgow. Her research specialises in the geographies of mental ill-health in historical and contemporary settings. Recent work includes a collaboration with Glasgow Museums and a range of community partners to work with the Art Extraordinary Collection.

Liz Neill has been working alongside children and young people enabling their voice and influence in the area of mental health for over 20 years—developing useful models of participation and co-production, and campaigning for improvements to mental health services. Her work includes consultancy on local and national programmes including MindMate Leeds, YoungMinds' VIK project, and working on national research studies and other initiatives in relation to lived experience and young people's mental health. Liz is Director at Common Room North www.commonroom.uk.com and a trustee at a local third sector youth information and counselling service in Leeds.

Elizabeth Nelson is an assistant professor in the Medical Humanities and Health Studies Program at Indiana University-Purdue University, Indianapolis (IUPUI), and an adjunct assistant professor of Africana Studies and History. She also coordinates the Indiana Women's Prison History Project.

Katherine Rawling is a lecturer in the History of Science and Medicine at the University of Leeds. She specialises in the history of medical photography and has published with *Social History of Medicine* and *Medical Humanities*. Her first book, *Photography in English Asylums, c.1880–1914: The Institutional Eye*, will be published by Palgrave Macmillan in 2021.

Geoffrey Reaume created the first university credit course in Mad People's History, which he has taught since 2000. He is currently an associate professor in Critical Disability Studies at York University, Toronto, Canada.

Pradipto Roy is a health professional, political enthusiast and social science researcher based in India. His research encompasses mental health, decolonisation, HPSTM, philosophy of mind and history of ideas. This chapter stems from his doctoral work on the history of subcontinental mental health at the NIMHANS, Bengaluru (supported by the Wellcome Trust, London). Presently he is the Andrew W. Mellon Post-Doctoral Fellow at the CSSSC, Kolkata.

Leonard Smith is Honorary Senior Research Fellow in the Institute of Applied Health Research, University of Birmingham. He has published extensively on the history of mental health institutions, including *Private Madhouses in England, 1640–1815: Commercialised Care for the Insane* (Palgrave Macmillan, 2020). He has worked within mental health services since the 1970s.

Steven J. Taylor is Lecturer in the History of Medicine at the University of Kent. His research explores ideas and constructions of childhood health, lay and professional diagnoses, ability and disability, and institutional care. His first monograph, *Child Insanity in England, 1845–1907*, was published by Palgrave Macmillan in 2017. He is currently working on his second monograph that investigates the experience of residential special schooling in the early twentieth-century England.

Gemma Trainor is a senior lecturer in Mental Health at Liverpool John Moores University with over 30 years nursing experience, including 15 years as a nurse consultant at specialist inpatient/outpatient facilities for young people. She is an active researcher and has published regularly on mental health issues affecting young people.

Tomas Vaiseta is an associate professor at Vilnius University, Faculty of History. He published two historical monographs: on Soviet everyday life and ideology *Society of Boredom* (2014) and on the social history of a psychiatric hospital during the Soviet period *Summerhouse* (2018).

List of Figures

Fig. 2.1	Agnes, upon admission to Stirling District Asylum from the SNI, age 24. (Reproduced with permission of NHS Forth Valley Archive, University of Stirling Archives)	38
Fig. 2.2	Hannah while she was a private patient of the Royal Earlswood Asylum. (Reproduced with permission of the Surrey History Centre. Copyright of Surrey History Centre)	41
Fig. 12.1	Photographer unknown, William, admitted 29/11/1905. Newcastle-upon-Tyne City Lunatic Asylum Casebook, males, TWAS HO/SN/13/14. 280. Permission to reproduce from Tyne and Wear Archives and Museums	244
Fig. 12.2	Detail of Figure 12.1. Permission to reproduce from Tyne and Wear Archives and Museums	245
Fig. 12.3	Photographer unknown, Margaret, admitted 29/11/1905. Newcastle-upon-Tyne City Lunatic Asylum Casebook, females, TWAS HO/SN/13/34. 475. Permission to reproduce from Tyne and Wear Archives and Museums	246
Fig. 12.4	Photographer unknown, Matilda, admitted 1/6/1900. Newcastle-upon-Tyne City Lunatic Asylum Casebook, females, TWAS HO/SN/13/36. 322. Permission to reproduce from Tyne and Wear Archives and Museums	247
Fig. 12.5	Photographer unknown, Mary, admitted 17/6/1903. Newcastle-upon-Tyne City Lunatic Asylum Casebook, females, TWAS HO/SN/13/38. 115. Permission to reproduce from Tyne and Wear Archives and Museums	248

Fig. 12.6	Photographer unknown, Louisa, admitted 15/8/1904. Newcastle-upon-Tyne City Lunatic Asylum Casebook, females, TWAS HO/SN/13/38. 442. Permission to reproduce from Tyne and Wear Archives and Museums	249
Fig. 12.7	Constance on first admission, Holloway Sanatorium Casebook No.2, females (certified patients admitted January-September 1889), WMS 5157/5157. 193. Credit: Wellcome Collection	250
Fig. 12.8	Constance on second admission, Holloway Sanatorium Casebook No. 4, females (certified patients admitted July 1890-June 1891), WMS 5157/5158: 249. Credit: Wellcome Collection	251
Fig. 12.9	Photographer unknown, admission page for Rose, Holloway Sanatorium Casebook (certified patients admitted Jun 1885-Jan 1889) Surrey History Centre 3473/3/1. 94. Reproduced by permission of Surrey History Centre	252
Fig. 12.10	Detail of Figure 12.9. Reproduced by permission of Surrey History Centre	253
Fig. 12.11	Photographer unknown, Agnes and attendants (1891), Holloway Sanatorium Casebook No.4, females (certified patients admitted July 1890-June 1891), WMS 5157/5158. 143. Credit: Wellcome Collection	255
Fig. 12.12	Photographer unknown, Constance and attendants, Holloway Sanatorium Casebook No.2, females (certified patients admitted January - September 1889), WMS 5157/5157. 192. Credit: Wellcome Collection	255
Fig. 12.13	Photographer unknown, Frances and attendant, Holloway Sanatorium Casebook No.11, females (certified patients admitted May 1898-May 1899), WMS 5157/5159. 17. Credit: Wellcome Collection	256
Fig. 12.14	Photographer unknown, Ellen, admitted 3/6/1904. Newcastle-upon-Tyne City Lunatic Asylum Casebook, females, TWAS HO.SN/13/38. 382. Permission to reproduce from Tyne and Wear Archives and Museums	256
Fig. 12.15	Photographer unknown, Thomas, June 1903. Holloway Sanatorium Casebook No.11, males. WMS 5157/8160. 338. Credit: Wellcome Collection	257
Fig. 15.1	Campaign Newsletter, 1991	322
Fig. 16.1	Cartoon by Merinda Epstein: the symptom as story	339
Fig. 16.2	The National Survivor User Network	343

CHAPTER 1

Voices in the History of Madness: An Introduction to Personal and Professional Perspectives

Robert Ellis, Sarah Kendal, and Steven J. Taylor

An invitation to
Berrywood Asylum

If you want to earn your living in a humble useless way,
Just drop in at 'Berrywood', they're sure to let you stay,
But before you gain admission you first must qualify,
And my parish Duston, in the twinkling of an eye,
Will put you through your paces, swear you're right clean 'up the pole',
'Square' a nice obliging magistrate, charge a guinea for the whole,
Now when once you've passed the portals, whether you're well or ill,
You can stop and live for ever, they'll never send the bill,
And if you are not noisy and disturb the watchman's rest,
Or upset some kind Attendant who waits upon each guest,

R. Ellis (✉)
School of Arts and Humanities, University of Huddersfield, Huddersfield, UK
e-mail: r.ellis@hud.ac.uk

R. Ellis et al. (eds.), *Voices in the History of Madness*, Mental Health in Historical Perspective,
https://doi.org/10.1007/978-3-030-69559-0_1

> You can live just like an Alderman, all labour you can think,
> Badging 'bacca and such luxuries from the barmy blokes that work.
>
> Poem written by John Hobbs, a patient at the Berrywood Asylum, Northampton, 1906.

On his admission to the English Northamptonshire County Lunatic Asylum, known locally as 'Berrywood', John Hobbs, aged 61, was described as 'incoherent', 'dull', and 'downcast'.[1] When inspected by the asylum's Medical Superintendent he was said to be 'rambling from religion and heresy to Shakespeare and has many hallucinations of hearing'. Further notes contained in his surviving case file are unremarkable, with the attendant who observed him commenting that he 'made himself quite at home' two days after his arrival. Had it not been for the poem that he penned while resident inside the asylum, or its survival in the medical record, Hobbs would most likely be lost amongst the statistics medical notes lying within the leather bound casebooks. We would be blinded to his cunning behaviour in securing free meals and lodging and would not have glimpsed the 'kind' attendants or the 'luxuries' he received while confined.[2] It seems clear, moreover, that Hobbs was determined to defy his description of 'dull' and 'downcast' and from his poetry we are able to directly access the 'voice' of the 'insane' patient. We learn that Hobbs was lucid, with a good understanding of how to take advantage of the welfare system.

The serendipitous survival of this poem reminds us that we very rarely hear the voices of those who have been described, diagnosed, or certified as 'mad' in the past. As Sally Swartz has pointed out, the recording of people's lives in case notes are framed by clinical theories and techniques, which recreate clinical subjects.[3] From its very existence, Hobbs' poem emphasises the absences of voice, the silences, and the 'epistemic violence'[4]

S. Kendal
School of Healthcare, University of Leeds, Leeds, UK
e-mail: s.kendal@leeds.ac.uk

S. J. Taylor
School of History, University of Kent, Canterbury, UK
e-mail: st642@kent.ac.uk

imposed on the broader sweep of people, including those outside of institutions, who can help shed light on these histories.

With this in mind, the aim of this interdisciplinary volume is to bring together new research that broadens our understanding of the multiplicity of voices in the histories of mental ill-health. As Catharine Coleborne recalls in the final chapter, this volume grew out of a conference held at the University of Huddersfield, England, in 2016. It was framed by Roy Porter's call for more emphasis on attempting to understand the experience of people who have lived with, or alongside, mental ill-health and its many consequences. In the chapters that follow, we hear from people who have experienced mental health difficulties, contest the diagnoses imposed upon them, and were on the receiving end of regimens and treatments. Alongside medical notes, we find records of decisions made by hospital administrators and parish officials, each with their own financial and political agendas that speak to wider issues of power and powerlessness. Correspondence with families reminds us that those deemed to be mentally ill were not ciphers; they were living human beings with their own histories, their own people, their own preferences, hopes, successes and losses. The contributions utilise a range of methodologies, drawing on archival materials, oral histories, personal testimonies, artwork, material culture, the built environment, and literature. They provide novel insights into the voices of individuals, institutions, and communities in a variety of chronological and international contexts.

While each chapter adopts its own approach to define, record, and examine 'voices of madness', they are all bound together by key overlapping themes that divide the volume into four parts; these are: Shifting Perspectives in the Industry of Madness; Reconstructing Patient Perspectives; The Visual and the Material; and Mad Studies and Activism. The language of mental ill-health is an important element to consider throughout the volume. In the introduction, for example, we have tended to refer to 'patients', which reflects our own backgrounds, interests and training. As suggested within the following pages, however, the lexicon of psychiatry and mental health changes over time, somewhat aligned with shifting societal sensibilities. Perspectives matter: a 'mental health survivor' may consider that they survived the treatment foisted upon them, and the stigma they faced, rather than any medical condition. Terms including 'inmate', 'patient', 'client', 'service user', 'sufferer', 'survivor', and 'person with lived experience' have fallen in or out of favour in different contexts.[5] Therefore, we have not required our authors to adhere to any list of acceptable terms; they have chosen the phrases and terminology that best suit their own contribution.

Part I Shifting Perspectives in the Industry of Madness

Like an industry, 'madness' creates opportunities, roles and economic activity. For a long time, the most dominant voices in the field were medical ones and, in the early histories of madness, they were largely positive about their impact on the treatment of the insane. The records were written mainly by medical men, and tended to present a longitudinal history of psychiatry as one of shared endeavour in frequently frustrating circumstances. Daniel Hack Tuke is a good example of someone who made a virtue of his ancestors' distrust of the medical profession to, nonetheless, demonstrate their role in the progressive history of psychiatry.[6] In this respect, it is possible to draw a line from the medical journals and treatises of the nineteenth century to the histories written by psychiatrists in the twentieth. Alexander Walk, Honorary Librarian of the Royal College of Psychiatrists and editor of the *Journal of Mental Science*, and German Berrios, Psychiatrist and University Lecturer, as well as the mother and son team of Ida Macalpine and Richard Hunter, all published and collaborated more widely in the production of historical outputs.[7] Walk, for example, was responsible for 'a detailed and valuable revision' of Kathleen Jones's *Mental Health and Social Policy* in its final stages.[8]

Although not all of those early histories had stressed the progressive nature of the histories of mental health care or were straightforwardly 'Whiggish' in tone,[9] Michel Foucault's *Madness and Civilisation* came to represent a significant, and oft-cited step in what would be a revisionist critique of the previously benign interpretations of psychiatry's longer-term history. To this, we can add David Rothman's *The Discovery of the Asylum* (1971), Andrew Scull's *Museums of Madness* (1979), described as 'arguably the most influential monograph on the History of Psychiatry in Britain', and Klaus Doerner's *Madness and the Bourgeoisie* (1981).[10] Rothman had been influenced by Erving Goffman's *Asylums* (1961), which introduced the idea of the mental hospital as a highly regulated 'total institution' that denied its patients any semblance of personality.[11] These revisionist critiques focused on sociological, structural, and economic reasons for the rise of psychiatry and its institutions in France, Germany, the United States, and the United Kingdom.

The shift in tone led to rancorous disagreements about the nature of madness, its histories, definitions, and treatments. Sometimes, those in the psychiatric profession rankled at the claims being made by historians, sociologists, and philosophers,[12] but the battle lines were not drawn on the simple distinctions between 'insiders' and 'outsiders'. David Cooper, a psychiatrist who worked with R.D. Laing, was a key figure in the anti-psychiatry movement, and in 1967 he provided the foreword to the English translation of Foucault's *Madness and Civilisation* (1961).[13] Similarly, Thomas Szasz's *Myth of Mental Illness* (1961) and his later *Manufacture of Madness* (1970) were framed by his work as a practising psychiatrist. As their titles indicated, these works proposed that mental illnesses were contingent on factors such as prevailing social values and socio-economics.

Despite the ongoing crossovers between historical analysis and practitioner perspective, the histories of madness were a niche interest for a long time. In the late twentieth century, Roy Porter wrote of the 'general indifference' of the majority of those within the British psychiatric community, while Scull described the whole field as 'impoverished'.[14] The mushrooming of interest in the field since that time has been facilitated, according to Scull, by an 'invasion of the history of psychiatry by social historians'.[15] *The Anatomy of Madness* volumes, the Squibb Series of *Lectures in the History of Psychiatry*, and the establishment of the *History of Psychiatry* journal in the early 1990s were all vehicles for academic and practitioner voices to be heard in a public, if somewhat limited, academic space.

With an increasing breadth of studies, we are now more likely to recognise the dissonant voices within psychiatry. In the UK, for example, across the period covered by this collection, we might point to other, similar, intra-professional and internecine disputes such as the one between John Monro of the Bethlem Hospital and William Battie of the newer and supposedly more innovative St Luke's, London, which was founded in 1751.[16] In (old) York, in the second decade of the nineteenth century, a public battle between representatives of the York Lunatic Asylum and the Quaker-run Retreat took place in the pages of the local newspaper, the *York Courant*.[17] Similarly, national press coverage of Edward Wakefield's 'discovery' of James Norris and other 'naked and chained' male patients illuminated the darkest recesses of the notorious Bethlem Asylum in London, UK.[18] Later in the nineteenth century, there were professional spats about the use or otherwise of mechanical 'restraint', which by the 1870s had descended into an 'often acrimonious' debate between English and American alienists.[19] In the same period, a scientific understanding of the apparently soft bones of the insane was being used to try to rescue the reputation of allegedly brutish asylum regimes.[20] These are by no means the only examples of disagreement but they are indicative of the professional disputes that spilled out into the public consciousness, via treatises, newspaper articles and, later, television documentaries. The voices we hear in these places emphasise the fact that psychiatry can be controversial, both now and in the past.

As a team of editors we have had to acknowledge and consider how best to honour our responsibilities to the people we write about, and their families, past and present. In the course of developing this volume we embraced tensions between our two research disciplines of mental health history and clinical mental health. We debated moral, legal, and ethical concerns around source attribution between ourselves and with contributors: in a volume about 'voice', does naming a person allow them some dignity and status and enable their voice to be heard in some way; or does it undermine their voice, identity, and rights, and those of their descendants? By anonymising individuals whose voices we are seeking to reveal and examine, are we silencing their views and, again, removing them from a platform to speak out or, on the other hand, are we shielding individuals, and potentially their families, from painful, possibly stigmatising, experiences? Finding a way to move forward that balanced the identity and voice of an individual against their privacy was complex. Editorial meetings alerted us to the shared understandings of the importance of anonymity.[21] Our eventual decision to move a little towards contemporary norms of health and historical research by including forenames and the first letter of the surname, seemed consistent with the values that underpinned the 2016 Voices conference which initiated this volume.

Building on this, the first part of the volume adds to our understanding of the voices of professionals in care and treatment regimens across the nineteenth and twentieth centuries. The relatively privileged status of the professionals, compared with their charges, is aptly reflected in their appearance at the beginning of the volume, albeit emphasising the shifts and changes that were taking place. The volume gradually unfolds on a wider constituency as each chapter seeks to uncover the roles of others, many of whom were claiming to advocate on behalf of vulnerable individuals they had some responsibility for. As Melling et al. observed, 'there is now much more scepticism about the ideological power of psychiatric physicians'[22] and our authors consider wider medical and administrative encounters in specific national and international contexts. Indeed, one may question whether sufficient attention has been paid to the supporting structures of the madness industry, despite some of the more recent contributions examining, for example, the political context of asylums[23] and how this directly affected the treatment of those admitted,[24] and despite the fact that the construct of 'locus of control' has substantial purchase in the theoretical underpinning of mental health therapies.[25]

Iain Hutchison, in Chap. 2, explores the processes of admission of children to the Scottish National Institute [SNI], drawing out from the archives a clear story of financially driven decision-making on the part of the relevant authorities. In central Scotland, the voices of children and families on the matter of institutional care for children during the nineteenth century are all but silent: Hutchison highlights a familiar problem of recovering children's voices, and instead concentrates on the role of administrators and philanthropists in the admissions process. He emphasises the voices of clergymen and parents as well as local doctors and their roles in the supply and demand of institutional space.

Conflicting ideas about the treatment of the insane were also present in medical discourse of British-occupied India in the nineteenth century. As has been shown in Ernst's and Mills' treatments of colonial psychiatry during the Raj, this history is inextricably bound with the story of Empire.[26] Power as a theme inevitably emerges from any examination of mental health history, but in the context of a foreign occupation it is, arguably, the overarching construct. Pradipto Roy develops this theme further in Chap. 3 with an account of how, during the Raj, the voice of the press was instrumental, and subtly subversive, in communicating and shaping ideas about madness. Roy argues that during this period of India's history, ancient ayurvedic medicine and values were at odds with westernised treatments preferred by the foreign ruling class, and the Bengali press was able to circulate material that publicised both the debate and the concerns of indigenous doctors.

In Chap. 4, Jane Freebody offers an important analysis of patient work in inter-war French asylums. Work as a (moral) therapy is a well-covered path in the histories of institutions, yet Freebody makes a significant contribution to advancing knowledge on this topic. Her analysis uncovers tensions between professionals who advocated a more purist approach to therapy, and those who, influenced by both a shift in understanding about the aetiologies of mental illness and also the requirements imposed by post-war re-building, actively encouraged the contributions that patients made to asylum finances. In this respect, her account of the 'More Active

Therapy' adds to our understanding of some of the wider changes that occurred as a result of the First World War, including the rather prosaic, day-to-day demands pertaining to the management of in-patient populations.

Children are again the focus in Chap. 5. Jennie Sejr Junghans draws on an extensive archive of medical records that describes slowly shifting attitudes towards the care of mentally ill children in Denmark. Where such children could not be looked after at home, it had been the practice to admit them to mental hospitals designed for adults, and not adapted to the needs of young people. However, by the 1930s a more enlightened understanding of children's mental health needs resulted in new models of care, including a children's outpatient clinic at the Copenhagen University Hospital which opened in 1935 and operated until 1976. The move toward community models of treatment is a developing theme of the historiography.[27] In the US, the Kennedy administration of the 1960s stimulated a programme of deinstitutionalisation that ultimately led to a widely accepted view that meeting the mental health needs of children required a more holistic approach than could be derived from medicine alone.[28] Similar developments were occurring elsewhere by the twentieth century, with the growing realisation that a child's outward behaviour (a primary concern of adults) reflected their external and their internal worlds, both of which should therefore be of interest.[29] Junghans also finds a greater appetite in children's care settings for trying relatively new therapies of psychoanalysis and psychology, compared with the regimens in adult care settings.

Part II Reconstructing Patient Perspectives

In Part II the contributions turn to what people had to say about their treatment, bringing a range of methodologies to task. As editor Sarah Kendal recalls, 'Many of us who worked in the old psychiatric hospitals in the 1980s remember sitting with elderly patients who had been admitted to an asylum as a teenager, and had spent their lives within its walls. If we got a chance to look at patient notes we might find scrawled comments like "FLK" (funny looking kid) in the margins. Some women had been locked up with a condition called "moral insanity" and few of these long-stay patients had visitors'. Seminal texts such as Plath's 'The Bell Jar',[30] and Gilman's 'The Yellow Wallpaper'[31] come into sharp relief when one met and talked with a living person who could have been the protagonist in such literature.

Despite this, it is apparent that patients were never really absent from the thoughts of their contemporaries. Indeed, many of the intra-professional disagreements about the nature or direction of care co-opted patient voices to support a particular professional or political narrative.[32] Inevitably, the shadow of Porter's call for scholars to think more carefully about the lived experience of mental ill-health looms large over all of the contributions in this volume.[33] With an interest in 'history from below' and the will to understand the impact on, mediation by, and agency of the people on the receiving end of treatment, our understanding of the many voices in the histories of madness has been extended since Porter's call. Space precludes an in-depth literature review here but we can reasonably suggest that historians are now much more aware of the range of actors in the care (or otherwise) of vulnerable individuals, including family,[34] local communities,[35] funding bodies and administrators,[36] attendants, nurses and doctors,[37] as well as patients themselves.[38] Then, there were those who were prepared to go on record to tell their own stories and speak for themselves.[39] This has always been easier for those with the financial wherewithal to self-publish, or the right connections, but the extension of historiographical analyses into the fields of class, gender, and ethnicity means that these are no longer episodes necessarily consigned to the past. The danger here, of course, is that we present a somewhat generous interpretation of History's ability to shine, what might be called, a democratic light on the past. For Foucault, the introduction of patient autobiography in the first half of the nineteenth century became a key factor in the extent to which psychiatry could control and discipline patients.[40] Similarly, as Porter pointed out, there were plenty of examples in the twentieth century and beyond, that speak to journalist Nellie Bly's experience of being told to 'shut up' while undercover in the Blackwell Asylum in New York in 1887.[41] This disinclination to listen to the 'voices of madness' can also be seen in William Sargent's opposition to psychoanalysis, sometimes referred to as a 'talking cure', and in Richard Hunter and Ida Macalpine's exhortation to reorient psychiatry from 'listening to looking'.[42] Sargent was 'perhaps Britain's "most celebrated" mid twentieth-century psychiatrist, whereas Hunter and Macalpine were both "distinguished psychiatrists and historians of psychiatry" reflecting, once again, the silencing power of those in charge of vulnerable individuals.[43]

With these things in mind, the authors in Part II seek to recover the subaltern voices of the patients. Leonard Smith, in Chap. 6, explores the treatment of the mentally ill in London during the late seventeenth and eighteenth centuries. He draws on individual testimonies from published and unpublished texts, articles and letters to describe why, and how, an individual arrived at a madhouse, and what treatments they experienced. This illuminates the power politics inherent in the madness industry and illustrates the co-occurence of some of the period's more entrenched attitudes with more enlightened thinking that was developing at the time.[44] An epistolary approach is also taken by Rory du Plessis (Chap. 7) who brings insights into the history of madness in South Africa from 1890 to 1910. Although few first-hand accounts of experience were found, du Plessis discovers rich stories in correspondence and casebooks that chime with the life of John Hobbs, whose poem opened this chapter. The stories explain how the diagnosis of the 'delusional' could be completely revised on hearing patients' own accounts of their experiences. On the other hand, for some patients, permission to leave the asylum was a matter of agreeing with their diagnosis.

Similarly, Tomas Vaiseta's work (Chap. 8) on Soviet Lithuania explores the lives of mental hospital patients in the twentieth century, at a time when the institutional sector was growing in the USSR. Using the letters of patients, he frames their exposés of violence and the threats of violence within the context of medical discourses. In this respect, parallels can be drawn with the west; but his research showcases not only opposition to the brutalising aspects of 'care' but also the ongoing battle faced by patients in defining themselves as individuals. In Chap. 9, Beckman, Nelson, and Labode use a patient-produced publication from the Indiana Central State Hospital to explore the lived experience of employment and patient independence within a psychiatric institution at the end of the twentieth century. We have seen that the press can be used both as a vehicle for radical therapists and also as a tool for patients to share ideas on self-help and therapy.[45] At the Indiana Central State Hospital, the analysis begins at a time when the institution shifted from offering patients employment in external sheltered workshops to providing supported work within the hospital. The chapter concentrates on patient and supervisor voices, drawing out contrasting expectations of the new employment arrangements.

Further institutional experiences of care are examined by Verusca Calabria, Di Bailey, and Graham Bowpitt (Chap. 10) who use an oral history methodology to explore the complexity of staff/patient relationships in twentieth-century England. In the histories of mental ill-health, the positive representations of former staff, seen earlier in this chapter, can be contrasted with stories of ill-treatment, abuse, and neglect. Bly's *Ten Days in a Mad House* (1887), Barbara Robb's *Sans Everything* (1967) and scandals at Ely Mental Hospital (1967), and Winterbourne View (2011) in the UK are just some of the more well-known examples of the darker side of institutions for vulnerable individuals. By contrast, Calabria et al. build on work to consider the safe spaces lost to the processes of de-institutionalisation.[46] The chapter presents the generally positive interactions that occurred between patients and staff in communities situated in close proximity to mental hospitals. Calabria, Bailey, and Bowpitt reveal how communities of patients developed their own techniques to manage mental health based on experience and fed these into wider discussions about running wards and the hospital more generally.

Part III The Visual and the Material

The penultimate part of the volume moves away from written records and oral testimonies to consider voices in art, material culture, and architecture. Cultural sources have, for a long time, been important considerations of historians of mental ill-health and disability. Sander Gilman wrote of their importance, not only in reflecting treatment regimens but also in shaping public understandings of them.[47] The upheaval of World War I, for example, transformed many widely held ideas (especially in England) about the interconnectivity of mental health and social class, masculinity, patriotism, and religion.[48] The immediate impact of the War in changing attitudes has been challenged recently,[49] but for many, including generations of school children, the poetry of Siegfried Sassoon, Wilfrid Owen and others, remains an enduring and readily accessible insight into its impact.[50]

As Tracey Loughran points out in her overview of Andrew Motion's 'An Equal Voice' 2009 Remembrance Day poem, poetry does not necessarily give voice to the voiceless. Motion had drawn heavily on the voices within *War of Nerves* and its author, Ben Shephard, had questioned just how 'new' the poem was. As Loughran argues, however, it offered an opportunity to bring patient perspectives to new audiences; and this is a theme considered by Cheryl McGeachan.[51] Her exploration of the Art Extraordinary Collections held at Glasgow Museums Resource Centre, Scotland, (Chap. 11) illustrates what can be found when we think about the depth of material and meaning, of art produced in psychiatric institutions. This is made starkly apparent when considering artists made famous by their institutionalisation, such as Richard Dadd, alongside other 'outsider artists' who were anonymised by the naming of collections after the people responsible for bringing them together.[52] As McGeachan puts it: individuals 'paint, sculpt or draw due to a compulsion to express an intense personal vision'. Self-expression occurs through non-verbal or written forms. Friendships, growing up, feuds, enemies, trickery, romance, education, industry, domestic politics, perhaps some family business that relied on the absence of a key individual, were part of the patchwork of life in an institution; but little, if any, of this would appear in formal records. As historians, we may find a material and emotional connection between the voices of mental health contained in creative forms and our sense of the people who have lived within the walls of an institution. Art moves beyond 'traditional bounded walls of the archive'. It promises a new route for listening to their voices and understanding their lives. Reflecting on her student nursing days, editor Sarah Kendal recalls a gentle elderly lady from a large and wealthy family. She had spent most of her adult life accommodated in a suite of rooms within an old mental hospital. During that time, she had occasionally taken a cruise, accompanied by some hospital staff; now she was in a dormitory with the other women (arguably her real family), unvisited, unprivileged, and as far as the staff could tell, forgotten by the outside world. She died on the hospital ward, and many staff went to see her in the hospital mortuary to pay their respects. Did that woman, born into wealth and advantage, ever have a voice?

Trying to answer some of these questions, Katherine Rawling (Chap. 12) builds on a growing interest in photography in the history of medicine. Studies like that of Jane Hamlett and Mark Jackson have revealed how photography has been used as a medium to understand the material culture and diagnostic practices of institutions.[53] Yet, as historians of pauper lunatic asylums often discover, and as John Hobb's experience of Berrywood highlighted, the patient casefiles, or medical notes in modern parlance, could be surprisingly sparse of detail, even for long stay patients. While this is reflective of overcrowding and the curative failure of the institutions, archivists and scholars relying on medical casefiles to understand the lives of the people kept inside these institutions might rue the lost details that would illustrate and illuminate the lives of their subjects. In some asylums, as the nineteenth century progressed, the accessibility of photographic equipment meant that patient photographs were included with casefiles records with increasing regularity. Rawling recognises the limitation of written records and seeks the 'elusive patient voice' through scrutiny of photographs of patients, noting that images contradict the text and can provide competing narratives of lived experience.

Likewise, it is possible to learn about the experience of psychiatric patients through an understanding of their lived surroundings.[54] Perhaps the longest enduring image of mental health in the popular psyche is that of the institutions of madness. These were often huge structures, located at the peripheries of urban areas, that modern day culture often tells us restrained and cruelly treated their helpless residents. Tying into Calabria's earlier chapter, the architecture of madness had its own presence and the impact of asylums on two local communities in the North-West of England is explored by Gibbeson and Beattie in Chap. 13. This contribution focuses on the interactions between former asylum sites and localities, particularly concentrating on their cultural legacies in collective memory.

Part IV Mad Studies and Activism

From the late twentieth century, paradigmatic shifts in the 'industry of madness', sought to place (some) service users at the heart of decision-making processes,[55] driven in part by the shift from institutionalisation to community-based treatment models and partly by a neoliberal—and linguistic—remodelling of individuals from 'inmates' and 'patients' to service users, clients, and consumers.[56] The new language implied increasing agency, but there is a danger in assuming that the rise of community care and the development of service user groups was enabling, without acknowledging the complexities of illness, resistance, dependence, self-belief, stigma, finance, and all the other layers of human activity that impact on an individual's right to self-determination and happiness. The chapters in Part IV offer critical perspectives on the uncertain rise and impact of the mental health service user movement.

There are differing views on where to draw the boundaries between safety, represented by a physical institution that can exert a great deal of control and therefore minimise certain risks; and autonomy, represented by community arrangements where people can more easily make their own judgements about risk. The line is drawn differently in different contexts. For instance, well-funded mental health services may favour a proactive approach, intervening perhaps at the stage when a problem is developing or anticipated, but not yet obvious.[57] Elsewhere, a lack of funding combined with strong views on personal liberty may mean that mental health services are unlikely to see a service user until after a significant problem has occurred. This might be, for example, because they have been brought to a facility against their will by the police or a social worker after an incident in the community. Then there are those affected by a move from one environment where culturally coded behaviour is acceptable to another one where it is not. Potentially vulnerable groups here are migrants[58] but it could equally be something as prosaic as moving from a noisy and spontaneous community into one that strives for quiet and order, such as an in-patient facility. Either way, judgements about appropriate risk, behaviour, autonomy, and safety will vary.[59]

The 'autonomy vs safety' dichotomy is at the heart of much debate in contemporary mental health discourse.[60] Perhaps historians should not accept that the 'truth' of patient experience can be implied, or interpreted, from third-party archives; because when we listen directly to patient voices, we hear new and different ideas. For instance, the chapters in this volume that are authored by people who have used mental health services, suggest that the authors are used to grappling with the slippery concept of '"help" without "control"'. Previous chapters in the volume raise similar themes of ambivalence about mental health care; that is, a tension between needing some support, at times, but not wishing to surrender voice, agency, or human rights. This point is hardly difficult to grasp in the abstract, and would seem strange in the world of physical medicine, yet appears to have baffled certain parts of the establishment for centuries.[61]

Returning to the subject of agency, in Chap. 14, Elena Demke offers a biographical account of the German activist, author, psychiatric patient, and holocaust survivor Dorothea Buck. Living through that turbulent century, Buck documented her experiences in and out of institutions and made sense of her psychosis within that context. Throughout her life she demonstrated what could be achieved through her own agency, with little social status or power. Demke explains Buck's methods of inserting herself into discourse through her writing and activism, through collaborations, conflicts, and analysis of narrative structures. The chapter takes in Buck's reflections on her experiences of the Nazi regime and observations of how post-war Germany responded to its recent history, while developing ideas around madness during the second half of the twentieth century.

The development of networks of survivor groups has been explored in national and international contexts.[62] Geoffrey Reaume (Chap. 15) describes the development of the 'mad movement' in North America and

Canada during the 1970s against a background of wider developments, also known as 'new social movements'. He explores the difficulties and tensions in the relationship between 'mad' activists and the left in late-twentieth century Ontario and examines the importance of ethnicity and gender in this dialogue. A central focus of this chapter is how former mental health service users strived to find a place in the established discourse of the Left, and establish political legitimacy. Alison Faulkner's Chap. 16 shares synergies with Reaume in that it explores the importance of the survivor voice and how it can be ignored and, to an extent, belittled by the medical establishment and academic communities. Her chapter offers an important insight into how the voices of service users become heard and accepted, and the ongoing challenges facing survivors.

Mark Gallagher, in Chap. 17, explores the formation of two groups in the twenty-first century. The 'Survivors History Group' and 'Oor Mad History' were formed in London and Edinburgh respectively, with a view to creating the histories of 'collective action by psychiatric patients'. As a former mental health practitioner and service user, Gallagher places himself at the heart of his analysis of both the historiography of 'voice' and his involvement in the projects. He notes that some patients employed the term 'survivor' because it emphasised their criticisms of systems of care. Others, however, eschewed the term as being too confrontational. Gallagher provides a history of 'mad studies', through the lens of the two projects which '*have presented a challenge to professional historians and others conducting research in the history of psychiatry, including academics and medics based at universities, because they have opened the field of inquiry up to a range of sources and discourses about which most interested scholars had previously been unaware*'. As this volume shows there is still much to be learned and this section further emphasises that those wishing to understand mental health histories should actively be seeking out the voices of those who can speak for themselves.

Continuing these themes, in Chap. 18, Megan Alikhanizadeh, Corey Hartley, Sarah Kendal, Liz Neill and Gemma Trainor offer a nuanced reflection on some of the more intangible constructs of madness from the perspectives of practitioners and young service users in the UK. These accounts necessarily address the issue of power, which Foucault had noted to be central to understanding the phenomenon of how madness is perceived in society.[63] This chapter presents issues relating to youth mental health from the point of view of young people with personal experience of mental illness, and professionals who support them to have a voice. Issues relating to youth mental health are presented and discussed, with the intention of encouraging readers to consider the journey from historical treatments of madness, considered elsewhere in this volume, to the present-day predicaments and opportunities faced by young people with mental health difficulties.

As Catharine Coleborne reminds us in the coda (Chap. 19), there is still much to be learned from inter-disciplinary dialogue and in this final part, the issue of agency is addressed head-on. It reminds us that it does not appear as an automatic right. Giving voice to people does not necessarily give them power. We see that the 'horror' in gothic novels about madness often occurs when the protagonist attains agency—when in Bronte's classic novel, the madwoman in the attic finally influences events to make things happen to other people. And yet even then, she barely speaks; she does not have a literal voice. It was Jean Rhys' 1966 novel over a hundred years later that gave this protagonist a voice and a story of her own.[64] Much of the vast literature around madness in the nineteenth, twentieth and twenty-first centuries contains treatments of the same themes: absence of voice and agency.[65] Many works, such as Kafka's novels from the early twentieth century,[66] or Sylvia Plath's accounts of mental illness,[67] combine this with meditations on anxiety and oppression. In the literary world of mid-twentieth century New York, Dorothy Parker's biting verse reflected that in sex as in madness, voice is an unreliable asset for a woman.[68] If there seems to be a gender bias here, one may heed the social structures that have long directed women to look inwards rather than outwards. It is self-evident that the internal madness depicted by great writers such as Dostoyevsky,[69] Kafka,[70] or Camus[71] reflect the same dreary, stultifying, aimlessness that is familiar to human beings whose circumstances have robbed them of agency. However, the gloom is not unremitting. Increasingly, light, shade, voice and agency co-exist in literary treatments of madness, allowing, for example, a determined protagonist, who is living with dementia, to set off on a path glittering with points of humour.[72] We may take from this, that despite the harrowing historiography contained within these pages, the human spirit is alive and well.

Notes

1. Northamptonshire County Record Office, St Crispin Hospital Casefiles, Male Patient Casebook 12, NCLA/6/2/2/12, pp. 59–60.
2. Historians have debated the nature of life in the asylum in comparison to the poor law workhouse, see: Smith, C. 2006 'Family, Community and the

Victorian Asylum: A Case Study of Northampton General Lunatic Asylum and its Pauper Lunatics', *Family and Community History*, 9:2, pp. 109–124.
3. Swartz, Sally. Can the Clinical Subject Speak? Some thoughts on Subaltern Psychology, 2005 *Theory and Psychology*, 15:4, 505–525. 507–508.
4. Swartz, Sally. Can the Clinical Subject Speak? Some thoughts on Subaltern Psychology, 2005 *Theory and Psychology*, 15:4, 505–525. 507–508.
5. See, for example, Basset, Thurstine and Theo Stickley. 2010. *Voices of Experience: Narratives of Mental Health Survivors*. Chichester: Wiley-Blackwell; Nelson, Geoffrey, Joanna Ochocka, Rich Janzen, John Trainor, Paula Goering, and Jonathan Lomotey. 2007. 'A Longitudinal Study of Mental Health consumer/survivor Initiatives: Part V–Outcomes at 3-year follow-up.' *Journal of Community Psychology* 35 (5): 655–665.
6. Hack Tuke, Daniel. 1882. *Chapters in History of the Insane in the British Isles*. London: Kegan Paul, Trench and Company.
7. Walk A. 1990. Medico-psychologists, Maudsley and The Maudsley, in Murray RM and Turner T (eds), *Lectures on the History of Psychiatry, The Squibb Series*, London: Royal College of Psychiatrists, 12–27. Hunter, Richard and Macalpine, Ida. 1963. *Three Hundred Years of Psychiatry*. Oxford University Press. Hunter, Richard and Macalpine, Ida. 1969. *George III and the Mad Business*. London: Allen Lane. Hunter, Richard and Macalpine, Ida. 1974. *Psychiatry for the Poor. Colney Hatch Asylum–Friern Hospital 1851–1973*. London: Wm Dawson.
8. Jones, Kathleen. 1960, *Mental Health and Social Policy 1845–1959*, London: Routledge and Kegan Paul: vii.
9. Porter suggests that, in hindsight, Macalpine and Hunter 'come off well' when faced with accusations of having committed 'the sin of Whiggery'. Porter R. 1994. Ida Macalpine and Richard Hunter: history between psychoanalysis and psychiatry. In: Micale M and Porter R (eds) Discovering the History of Psychiatry. Oxford: Oxford University Press, 83–94.
10. Doerner's book had been first published in German in 1969. Doerner, K. 1981. *Madmen and the Bourgeoisie: A Social History of Insanity and Psychiatry*. Oxford: Basil Blackwell. Bartlett, P. and Wright, D. 1999. Community Care and its antecedents. In *Outside the Walls of the Asylum. The History of care in the Community 1750–2000*, eds Peter Bartlett and David Wright, 1–18 London: The Athlone Press.
11. Scull, Andrew. 1989. Social Order/mental disorder: Anglo-American Psychiatry in Historical Perspective. Berkeley: university of California Press: 96–97.
12. Hare, Edward. 1983. 'Was Insanity on the Increase?' *British Journal of Psychiatry*, 143: 439–455. Scull, Andrew. 1984. Was Insanity Increasing. A response to Edward Hare. *British Journal of Psychiatry*, 144: 432–436.

13. Foucault, M. 1967. *Madness and civilization: A history of insanity in the Age of Reason*, London: Tavistock Publications; originally *Historie de la Folie á l'âge Classique*, Paris: Plon 1962.
14. Porter, R. 1994. Ida Macalpine and Richard Hunter: History between Psychoanalysis and Psychiatry. In *Discovering the History of Psychiatry*, eds Mark Micale and Roy Porter, 83–94 Oxford University Press: 84. Scull, A. 2006. *The Insanity of Place/The Place of Insanity*, London: Routledge: 4.
15. Scull, Andrew. 2006. The insanity of place/the place of insanity: essays on the history of psychiatry. London: Routledge.
16. Andrews, Jonathan, Briggs, Asa, Porter, Roy, Tucker Penny, and Waddington, Keir. 2013. *The History of Bethlem*. London: Routledge.
17. Digby, A. 1983. Changes in the Asylum: The Case of York, 1777–1815. *The Economic History Review*, *36*:2, 218–239.
18. Scull, Andrew. MacKenzie, Charlotte and Hervey, Nicholas. 1996. *Masters of Bedlam: the Transformation of the Mad-doctoring Trade*. Princeton: Princeton University Press: 30–32.
19. Scull, Andrew. MacKenzie, Charlotte and Hervey, Nicholas. 1996. *Masters of Bedlam: the Transformation of the Mad-doctoring Trade*. Princeton: Princeton University Press. Suzuki, Akihito. 1995. The Politics and Ideology of Non-restraint: The Case of the Hanwell Asylum. *Medical History* 39: 1–17. Tomes, Nancy. 1988. The great restraint controversy: a comparative perspective on Anglo-American psychiatry in the nineteenth century. In *The Anatomy of Madness, Vol III, The Asylum and its Psychiatry*, eds W.F. Bynum, Roy Porter and Michael Shepherd, 191–225 London: Routledge.
20. Wallis, J. 2015. Investigating the body in the Victorian Asylum. London: Palgrave. 113–120.
21. 'Publishing Information About Patients.' BMJ : British Medical Journal 312, no. 7030 (March 2, 1996): 578; Orb, Angelica, Laurel Eisenhauer, and Dianne Wynaden. 'Ethics in Qualitative Research.' *Journal of Nursing Scholarship* 33, no. 1 (January 1, 2001): 93–96.
22. Melling Joseph, Adair Richard and Forsyth Bill. 1997. 'A Proper Lunatic for Two Years': Pauper Lunatic Children in Victorian and Edwardian England. Child Admissions to the Devon County Asylum, 1845–1914. *Journal of Social History*, 31: 2, 371–405: 393.
23. Ellis, R. 2013. 'A constant irritation to the townspeople'? Local, Regional and National Politics and London's County Asylums at Epsom. *Social History of Medicine*, Volume 26, Issue 4, November 2013, Pages 653–671, https://doi.org/10.1093/shm/hkt002.
24. Taylor, Steven J. 2012. "All his ways are those of an idiot': The admission, treatment of and social reaction to two 'idiot' children of the Northampton Pauper Lunatic Asylum, 1877–1883', *Family and Community History*, vol. 15/1, pp. 34–43.

25. Galvin, Benjamin M., Amy E. Randel, Brian J. Collins, and Russell E. Johnson. 2018. 'Changing the Focus of Locus (of Control): A Targeted Review of the Locus of Control Literature and Agenda for Future Research.' *Journal of Organizational Behavior* 39 (7): 820–833.
26. Ernst, Waltraud. 1991. Mad Tales of the Raj: The European Insane in British India 1800–1858, London: Routledge; Mills, James H. Madness, Cannabis, and Colonialism: The 'Native-Only' Lunatic Asylums of British India, 1857–1900. New York: St. Martin's Press.
27. See, for example, Bartlett P and Wright D (eds). 1999 *Outside the Walls of the Asylum: The History of Care in the Community 1750–2000.* London: The Athlone Press. Baur N. 2013 Family influence and psychiatric care: Physical treatments in Devon Mental Hospitals c. 1920 to the 1970s. *Endeavour* 37(3): 172–183. Long V (2011) Often there is a Good Deal to be Done, But Socially Rather Than Medically': The Psychiatric Social Worker as Social Therapist, 1945–70. *Medical History*, 223–239. Pickstone. J 1992 Psychiatry in district general hospitals: History, contingency and local innovations in the early years of the National Health Service. In Pickstone J (ed.) *Medical Innovations in Historical Perspective.* Hampshire: Palgrave, 185–199.
28. Levine, M., 2015. Children come first? A brief history of children's mental health services. *American Journal of Orthopsychiatry*, 85(5), pp. S22–S28.
29. Shuttleworth, Sally. 2010; 2011; 2013; The Mind of the Child: Child Development in Literature, Science and Medicine, 1840–1900. Oxford: Oxford University Press; Sinha, Vinod, Nishant Goyal, and Joyita Sinha. 2018. 'History of Child and Adolescent Psychiatry at Central Institute of Psychiatry: Journey of Erna Hoch Centre for Child and Adolescent Psychiatry.' *Indian Journal of Psychiatry* 60 (6): 264–269; Nelleke Bakker (2010) Before Ritalin: children and neurasthenia in the Netherlands, Paedagogica Historica, 46:3, 383–401; Taylor, Steven J. 2020 'Planning for the Future: State Education and the Shaping of 'Healthy' Minds' in Taylor and Brumby (eds.), *Healthy Minds in the Twentieth Century: In and Beyond the Asylum*, Basingstoke: Palgrave Macmillan, 73–93.
30. Plath, S. 1963. *The Bell Jar.* Heinemann: New Hampshire.
31. Gilman, Charlotte Perkins. 1980. 'The Yellow Wallpaper.' *The Charlotte Perkins Gilman Reader.* Ed & Intro. Ann J. Lane. New York: Pantheon, 3–20.
32. Ellis, R. 2020. *London and its Asylums, 1888–1914.* Politics and Madness. London: Palgrave Macmillan.
33. Porter, Roy. 1985. 'The Patient's View: Doing Medical History from Below', *Theory and Society*, 14:2, 175–198. Porter R. 1987. *Mind forg'd manacles: a history of madness in England from the restoration to the regency.* London: Athlone. Porter R. 1992. The patient in England, c1660–1880.

In: Wear A, ed. *Medicine in society: historical essays.* Cambridge: Cambridge University Press. 91–118. Porter R. 1996 *Social history of madness: stories of the insane.* London: Weidenfeld and Nicolson.

34. van Rosmalen, L., van der Veer, R., & C. P. van der Horst, F. 2020. The nature of love: Harlow, Bowlby and Bettelheim on affectionless mothers. *History of Psychiatry*; Akihito. 2006. *Madness at Home: The Psychiatrist, the Patient, and the Family in England, 1820–1860.* 1st ed. Vol. 13; 13. Berkeley: University of California Press; Taylor, Steven J. 2017 "She was Frightened while Pregnant by a Monkey at the Zoo': Constructing the Mentally Imperfect Child in Nineteenth-Century England', *Social History of Medicine*, 30:4, 748–766; Kumar, R. 1994. 'Postnatal Mental Illness: A Transcultural Perspective.' *Social Psychiatry and Psychiatric Epidemiology* 29 (6): 250–264.
35. Minas, Harry and Milton Lewis. 2017. *Mental Health in Asia and the Pacific: Historical and Cultural Perspectives.* 1st 2017. ed. New York, NY: Springer US.
36. Rogers, Anne. 2014. *A Sociology of Mental Health and Illness.* 5th ed. Maidenhead: Open University Press.
37. McCrae, Niall and Peter Nolan. 2016. *The Story of Nursing in British Mental Hospitals: Echoes from the Corridors.* London & New York: Routledge, Taylor & Francis Group.
38. Thiher, Allen. 1999. *Revels in Madness: Insanity in Medicine and Literature.* Ann Arbor: University of Michigan Press. See also: The Madness and Literature Network, available at: http://www.madnessandliterature.org/index.php.
39. Philanthropos. 1861. A Voice from the Wilderness: Being a Plea for a Lunatic Asylum for the Middle Classes, on Self-supporting Principles. London: John Churchill. Lowe, Louisa. 1883. The Bastilles of England: Or the Lunacy Laws at Work. London: Crockenden & Co.
40. Foucault, Michel. 2008. Psychiatric Power. Lectures at the Collège de France, 1973–1974. Basingstoke: Palgrave Macmillan: 158.
41. Roy Porter's Foreword in Ingram A. 1997. *Voices of Madness*, Stroud: Sutton Publishing, vii. See also Porter, Roy. 2002. *Madness a Brief History*, Oxford: Oxford University Press. Bly, Nellie. 1887. *Ten Days in a Mad House.* New York: Norman L. Munro.
42. Ibid.
43. Ibid.
44. Ingram A. 1997. *Voices of Madness*, Stroud: Sutton Publishing, vii. See also Porter, Roy. 2002. *Madness a Brief History*, Oxford: Oxford University Press.
45. Dunst, Alexander. 2016. All the fits that's news to print. De-institutionalisation and the Anti-Psychiatric movement in the United States, 1970–86. In *De-institutionalisation and After. Post-Was Psychiatry in the Western World.* 57–74.

46. Davies, K. 2007. 'A small corner that's for myself'. Space, Place, and patients' experience of mental health care, 1948–98. In *Madness, Architecture and the Built Environment*, eds Leslie Topp, James E. Moran and Jonathan Andrews, 305–20. London: Routledge.
47. Gilman, S. 1988. Disease and Representation. Gilman, S. 1996. Seeing the Insane.
48. Church, Johanna. 2016. 'Literary Representations of Shell Shock as a Result of World War I in the Works of Virginia Woolf and Ernest Hemingway.' *Peace & Change* 41 (1): 52–63. Jones, Edgar and Simon Wessely. 2005; 2006; *Shell Shock to PTSD: Military Psychiatry from 1900 to the Gulf War*. Vol. no. 47; no. 47; Hove; New York: Psychology Press.
49. Loughran, Tracey. 2017. *Shell-shock and Medical Culture in First World War Britain*, Cambridge University Press.
50. Imperial War Museum staff. 2018. 9 Poets of the First World War. Available at: https://www.iwm.org.uk/history/9-poets-of-the-first-world-war. Norgate, Paul. 1987. 'Shell-Shock and Poetry: Wilfred Owen at Craiglockhart Hospital.' *English (Leicester)* 36 (154): 1–35; For a fictionalised account of the role of Craiglockhart in the treatment of shell shock, see also: Barker, Pat. 2008. *Regeneration*. London: Penguin.
51. Loughran, Tracey. 2012. Shell Shock, Trauma, and the First World War: The Making of a Diagnosis and Its Histories. *Journal of the History of Medicine and Allied Sciences*, 67:1. 94–119.
52. Andrews, Jonathan, Briggs, Asa, Porter, Roy, Tucker Penny, and Waddington, Keir. 2013. *The History of Bethlem*. London: Routledge. Belinda Robson, A History of the Cunningham Dax Collection of 'Psychiatric Art': From Art Therapy to Public Education, *Health and History*, 1:4 (Dec., 1999), pp. 330–346. Anna Ostrowska, The Adamson Collection: illustrations of mental illness or a testament to spontaneous artistic expression?' *Journal of Visual Communication in Medicine*, 2015.
53. Hamlett, J. 2015 *At Home in the Institution: Material Life in Asylums, Lodging Houses and Schools in Victorian and Edwardian England*, Basingstoke: Palgrave Macmillan; Jackson, M. 1995, 'Images of Deviance: Visual Representations of Mental Defectives in Early Twentieth-Century Medical Texts', *The British Journal for the History of Science*, 28:3, 319–337.
54. Andrews, J.; Moran, J. and Topp, L.E. (eds), 2007 *Madness, Architecture and the Built Environment: Psychiatric Spaces in Historical Context*, New York: Routledge.
55. Wallcraft J, Schrank B, Amering M, Wallcraft J, Nettle M. 2009. History, context and language. In: Wallcraft J, Schrank B, Amering M, eds. Handbook of service user involvement in mental health research. Oxford: Wiley-Blackwell: 1–12.

56. Coleborne, Catharine. 2020. Why Talk About Madness? Bringing History into the Conversation. London: Palgrave Macmillan: 53–56.
57. Ontario Hospital Association. 2016. *A Practical Guide to Mental Health and the Law in Ontario*. Ontario Hospital Association.
58. See, for example, McCarthy, Angela and Coleborne, Catharine. 2012. 1 *Migration, Ethnicity and Mental Health, International Perspectives 1840–2010*, eds 73–90. New York: Routledge.
59. *Handbook of Identity Theory and Research*, edited by Seth J. Schwartz, et al., Springer, 2011. ProQuest Ebook Central, https://ebookcentral.proquest.com/lib/HUD/detail.action?docID=763293.
60. Al-Azzawi Y. 2016. *Safety and autonomy in the Australian mental health services sector: recommendations based on a review of the international literature*, Melbourne: University of Melbourne.
61. Covello, Vincent & Mumpower, Jeryl. 1985. Risk Analysis and Risk Management: An Historical Perspective. *Risk Analysis*. 5. 103–120; Callaly, Tom, Dinesh Arya, and Harry Minas. 2005. 'Quality, Risk Management and Governance in Mental Health: An Overview.' *Australasian Psychiatry* 13 (1): 16–20.
62. Crossley, Nick. 2006. Contesting Psychiatry. Social Movement s in mental Health. London: Routledge.
63. Foucault, Michel and Colin Gordon. 1980. *Power/knowledge: Selected Interviews and Other Writings, 1972–1977*. Brighton, Sussex: Harvester Press.
64. Rhys, Jean and Angela Smith. 1997. *Wide Sargasso Sea*. London: Penguin.
65. The Madness and Literature Network, available at: http://www.madnessandliterature.org/index.php.
66. See for instance Kafka, Franz. 2009. *The Trial*. London: Vintage.
67. Plath, Sylvia. 1977. Johnny Panic and the Bible of Dreams. London: Faber and Faber.
68. Parker, Dorothy. 1944. 'The Lady's Reward'. In The Portable Dorothy Parker. New York: The Viking Press.
69. Dostoyevsky, Fyodor (transl. Magarshack, David). 1951. Harmondsworth: Penguin.
70. Ibid.
71. Camus, Albert. 1942. L'Etranger. Paris: Gallimard.
72. Emma Healey. 2014. Elizabeth is Missing. Harper Collins: New York.

PART I

Shifting Perspectives in the Industry of Madness

CHAPTER 2

Accepted and Rejected: Late Nineteenth-Century Application for Admission to the Scottish National Institution for the Education of Imbecile Children

Iain Hutchison

The Scottish National Institution [SNI] opened near Larbert in central Scotland in 1862. Like Baldovan Asylum, 65 miles away near Dundee, and established in 1855 as Scotland's other institution for mentally impaired children, the SNI aspired to train 'imbecile' children to become self-supporting in adulthood.[1] The SNI accepted children under three financial categories—private fee-paying children who were often accorded special status as 'parlour' boarders; pauper children who were housed in more rudimentary accommodation paid for by parochial boards under the

The research for this chapter was aided by Wellcome Trust Grant 203,443/Z/16/Z, and the Marc Fitch Fund provided additional support.

I. Hutchison (✉)
University of Glasgow, Glasgow, UK
e-mail: iain.hutchison@glasgow.ac.uk

R. Ellis et al. (eds.), *Voices in the History of Madness*, Mental Health in Historical Perspective,
https://doi.org/10.1007/978-3-030-69559-0_2

provisions of the Poor Law (Scotland) Act of 1845; and elected boarders who were poor, but not paupers—selected through an annual competition from lists of applicants placed before the institution's philanthropic subscribers.

Childhood in Scotland offers great scope for ongoing historical research; however, 'othered' children have received attention in a variety of contexts[2] including Junghans' chapter within this volume. Such othered children in Scotland were the focus of often religiously inspired and motivated intervention by the country's respectable classes, flavours of which are found in Olive Checkland's exploration of philanthropy.[3] Callum Brown's studies of Scottish religious belief and practice have concluded that religious conviction for evangelicals was demonstrated by behaviour and action such as 'good works as expressions of faith';[4] therefore bodies such as the SNI were a popular focus for religious piety in action. However, as occupants of an almost unique carceral institution, the children of the SNI are only now being explored because of the very recent archival deposit of its administrative and inmate records that offer opportunity for new historical insights to imbecile children in confinement.[5] William W. Ireland (1832–1909) was the SNI's medical superintendent for the decade commencing in 1869. He wrote about childhood imbecility during his SNI tenure and afterwards, while recent historical work on this category of mental impairment has been contributed by the writers such as Mark Jackson.[6]

This chapter investigates the SNI admission process, making use of application papers and supporting correspondence. Over 3000 applications have survived, dating from the 1860s to the 1940s. Significantly, they include all three financial categories, and rejected as well as successful applications. Resources such as SNI annual reports and admission registers play a contextual role. However, central to this exploration are application papers for individual children. These draw attention to children rejected for a variety of reasons such as age, epilepsy, additional impairment (physical or sensory), and need for additional nursing or support. By employing further sources, such as decennial census returns, the chapter traces the lives of a small sample from the 3014 surviving application folios. This makes it possible to give personality to children, yet also highlights children's lack of voice, and the subdued, reverential nature of parental voices, in a process where medical doctors and clergymen were the authoritative players in deciding children's fates. The SNI therefore presents the challenge for historians to hear the voices of silenced children and of their reverential parents and guardians.

A survey of applications demonstrates high demand for entry to the institution. By the end of the century, the SNI had a licensed capacity of 250, although to the consternation of John Fraser, Commissioner in Lunacy, occupancy often substantially exceeded this.[7] Demand was encouraged by parents' perception of the SNI as providing 'life chances' to mentally impaired offspring, but admission might also represent removal of 'problem' children from homes or from poorhouses unable, or unwilling, to cope. The chapter highlights that admission numbers were not reflective of the full demand for places from parents and guardians, yet children's feelings about such life-changing decisions are hidden, whether accepted for admission, or rejected, and the voices of their parents were mostly stifled by the weight accorded to the views of medical professions and 'social superiors'.

Early Ethos and Evolution

In the founding of both Baldovan and the SNI, Scotland was an early instigator of residential institutions for mentally impaired children, this being highlighted in this section of the volume by Jennie Sehr Junghans in her examination of the innovatory role of Copenhagen University Hospital, with which some comparisons can be made, although that facility in Denmark was not opened until almost a century later. When the SNI at Larbert was being planned, it aimed to accommodate up to thirty children and 'to furnish special means of education for those young persons who, from mental weakness or peculiarity, are unfit for the training of ordinary schools, but who ... may be rendered capable of education to self-guidance and some measure of usefulness'.[8] Opening coincided with the passage of the 1862 Lunacy (Amendment) Act and this caused uncertainty as to whether the SNI should be licensed under the Board of Lunacy, which would mean classification of the institution's pupils as also being children who 'could be benefitted by curative treatment'. While the licensing dilemma rumbled on unresolved through the 1860s, the directors decided early on that 'the Institution will be a HOME, but more especially a SCHOOL, for the imbecile [original emphasis]'.[9] While developing its primary function, SNI directors 'considered that more credit was likely to accrue ... by the treatment of children susceptible of improvement, than by ... [being] an asylum of helpless and unimprovable cases'.[10] There was therefore enduring ambiguity surrounding a role for the SNI in providing physiological and psychiatric intervention, but also education and skills training.

The SNI directors, dependent upon charitable subscriptions, were conscious that empathy towards mentally impaired children was not enough—the institution had to be shown to be making a difference and it was positive outcomes that their rhetoric had to articulate to potential supporters. A selection process evolved through which 'promising' cases took precedence over 'hopeless' cases, seen in the ability-graded classification system adopted. In 1865, the SNI, in placing before subscribers the prospectuses of children presented for election, emphasised that 'the voting papers [indicate] the class in which each child had been placed by the medical man who had visited and reported', and directed voters to 'those cases [that] would have the best chance of success … [and] offered most prospect of improvement'.[11] It was a controversial strategy, the directors observing, in 1867, loss of some subscribers who wished to support 'specific lower-rate cases', action that they attributed to 'misconception of the real position of these pupils'.[12] The process underlines the primacy of clinical voices over those of parents, but also in this instance over financial supporters.

As the SNI expanded, the classification system became increasingly detailed. In the mid-1880s, revisions of its Constitution suggested a tightening of admission criteria for elected cases to those for whom 'there was reasonable ground for expectation of [their] deriving benefit from being treated at the Institution', and from 1885 there were no longer Grade I children on the roll.[13] By the end of the nineteenth century, the five 'grades' used were:

I Can neither speak nor understand speech;
II Understand speech, but do not speak;
III Can speak a few words;
IV Can be taught to read and write;
V Can read books for themselves.

Each grade was further categorised by ability to perform certain tasks. Grade III for example included 'at alphabet, distinguish colour, can sing, can dance, can sew, can knit', and so on, but without any indication of scales of proficiency within these vague markers. The 1899 annual report summarised resident children as follows:

Various acquirements and capacities of the pupils

Grade	*Male*	*Female*	*Total*
I	0	0	0
II	25	10	35
III	54	38	92
IV	62	45	107
V	20	9	29
Total	161	102	263

USASC, SNI 38th Annual Report (1899), p. 17

In 1900, there were 278 pupils, twenty-eight more than the SNI's licensed capacity—and there were twenty-one Grade I pupils present.[14] These were part of a group intended for onward transfer to 'the home for Uneducable Imbeciles, which is being erected at Lenzie by the Glasgow Parish Council', yet by 1909, there remained twenty-four Grade I children at the SNI, out of a total of 304, who could 'neither speak nor understand speech'.[15] Grade I children nonetheless remained a minority group.

To give a flavour of the range of admissions to the SNI, in the year 1889 there were forty-eight new arrivals. Their ages upon admission were:

Six years	1
Seven years	4
Eight years	9
Nine years	3
Ten years	6
Eleven years	6
Twelve years	5
Thirteen years	7
Fourteen years	5
Fifteen years	1
Twenty-eight years	1

Source: USASC, SNI Admission Register 1888–99, RS/1/2/1

The twenty-eight-year-old was Janet, an 'imbecile from birth,' and she remained at the SNI for eighteen months until being removed to Westmains Private Asylum, Kirkintilloch.[16] In April 1890, at the other end of the age spectrum, was the admission of Harold, age two years and four months, and he remained for three years when he was taken home by his family.[17] One reason for the extreme relaxation of the rules for Janet and Harold was financial inducement—the willingness of parents to pay generous private fees, £100 p.a. for Janet, and £80 p.a. for Harold. Of the 1889 admissions, sixteen were paupers paid for by parochial boards, twenty-two were poor elected cases, and ten were private patients for whom fees paid ranged from £30 to £100 p.a.[18]

Using this sample overview year of 1889, with the exception of one designation of 'epilepsy', all have 'imbecility' as the mental disorder, but the physiological status of each child was also noted. There were six broad categories of 'bodily condition', these showing that good physical health in children sought by the SNI was often an aspiration rather than a reality. The forty-eight new admissions were accordingly defined as: Good—18, Fair—10, Spare—9, Reduced—7, Feeble—3, Extremely Feeble—1. Outcomes for these children therefore assume additional poignancy because, in addition to their mental state and any improvement achieved while in the SNI, physiological circumstances could be critical. Physical wellbeing should therefore be considered when surveying discharge arrangements after what typically was a five-year residence, a process in which there is no indication of children being invited to express their feelings and aspirations, or exercise any agency over their lives.

Half of the twenty-two elected cases from 1889 are simply noted as being discharged when 'election period expired', while a twelfth case departed 'vastly improved' but with no specific destination shown—these are presented as time-served departures and as such involved no discussion or negotiation with the children's families. Eleven children, predominantly private cases, are noted returning to their families (but not necessarily to take up permanent residence), and three pauper children were removed by their parochial boards. Four children were placed under the 'boarding out' system employed in Scotland and described in detail by Harriet Sturdy and William Parry-Jones.[19] Six were transferred to other mental institutions: three to district asylums; Alexander to the lunatic wards of Dumbarton Poorhouse; Amelia, an elected case, was accepted by Baldovan Institution when she was seventeen, and Janet, as already mentioned, went to a private asylum (a proprietor-run establishment, a few of which continued to operate after their regulation was enforced by the 1857 Lunacy (Scotland) Act). Twelve children from the 1889 intake died while in the SNI, including the singular 'extremely feeble' child, two of the 'feeble' children, one who was 'reduced', and two who were 'spare' upon admission. But deaths also included three 'fair' cases and three 'good' cases, suggesting that weeding out of potential applicants due to poor physical health was not a foolproof basis of selection.[20]

Selected and Rejected: Outcomes

While many children from all three categories of admission came from central Scotland, some came from further afield including paupers from island parishes such as Malcolm from Coll in 1889, Ewen from North Uist in 1890, and Lachlan from Islay in 1897.[21] Cases presented for election were generally from Scotland, but the origins of private cases were more varied. Indeed, the directors liked to show international recognition, annual reports citing cases from far-flung origins as diverse as China, South Africa, and USA.[22] These were private, fee-paying cases where publicising them might be seen as having a marketing objective to attract additional children from families able to pay. However, this international flavour has to be placed in context because, where it is possible to identify 'foreign' cases, they frequently appear to be offspring of Scottish expatriates—such as five-year-old Grahame, a doctor's son arriving from Aix les Baines, France, and seven-year-old Ronald, his father an engineer in Shanghai—and were therefore a reflection of Scottish continental and imperial commercial activity rather than the SNI engaging in unfettered import of mentally impaired children from across the globe.[23]

In 1880, forty-three cases were presented to subscribers for consideration for the twelve places available by election, the number of votes available to each subscriber being in proportion to their philanthropic largesse and commencing at one vote for an annual subscription of ten shillings. Major benefactors wielded considerable voting power. The results of the 1880 election show that Helen polled the highest number of votes—11,097, while twelfth on the list, William, was elected with 2328 votes. At the bottom of the poll was Alasdair with a disheartening three votes.[24] All children admitted, whether by election, by agreement with parochial boards paying a set pauper fee, or private cases where the fee—and facilities offered—were often the subject of negotiation, went through an application and evaluation process. Some of these applications will now be examined, beginning with Helen, William, and Alasdair.

The application procedure entailed submission of the SNI's prescribed questionnaire by parents or guardians, the SNI's standard medical certificate completed by a doctor, and other supporting documents that applicants might care to add. The application form advised the operation of a four-stage classification system: Class I—very hopeful of responding to treatment proposed; Class II—hopeful; Class III—less hopeful; Class IV—identified children 'subject to fits, severe and frequent'. The form also informed applicants that 'Cases of Insanity, of Confirmed Epilepsy, of the Deaf and Dumb and of the Blind, are ineligible for admission except upon Payment', that is, private cases such as Helen.

Helen's doctor believed her to be a 'Class II—Hopeful' case, but the SNI disagreed and accorded her Class III, so that we see elite voices engaging in debate and negotiation, but with the SNI's power articulating the stronger voice as the final arbiter. Helen's impairment was attributed to a fall when three weeks old. Helen's parents being deceased, her application was submitted by her widowed stepmother, and these tragic family circumstances may have aided the accrual of the massive 11,097 votes that saw her elected as first preference on the ballot.[25] Helen remained at the SNI for ten years, being discharged in 1890 as a 'healthy young woman', aged nineteen, when she was transferred to Dundee Royal Asylum.[26] While her physical state may have been good, in Dundee she was variously described as an 'idiot' or 'imbecile'; the vast majority of the Dundee inmates were designated as 'lunatic', but Melling et al. have highlighted the problematic use and inter-changeability of what were often loose classifications.[27] However, not only was Helen still there twenty years later, suggesting that the confidence of the SNI electors in 1880 had been overly optimistic, but when she died in Stracathro Hospital in 1958 at the grand age of eighty-seven, her residence was recorded as Gowrie House, Liff (this being the former Dundee Royal Asylum).[28] While we do not have first-hand insight to Helen's world, her term at the SNI did not result in adolescent transition to adult independence, her adult life being a wholly institutionalised one.

Twelfth-placed in the 1880 ballot for elected cases, with considerably less votes than Helen, was William of Charlestown, Fife, where he lived with his parents and five siblings. His father, a ploughman, offered £30 annually towards William's upkeep at the SNI and their doctor enthusiastically endorsed him as Class I, adding 'very hopeful case'.[29] Nine years of age upon application, the SNI's wish to avoid receiving children with epilepsy was probably instilled among many of the electors, and the votes cast for William may have been prejudiced by the admission that he had had epileptic seizures until five years old 'when the fits ceased entirely'.[30] In 1885, upon completion of his term, William was optimistically returned to his parents 'considerably improved' while his successful admission via the ballot may have been aided by his father's voice generating more resonance by his offer of a financial contribution towards the care of son.[31]

Thirty-one children were rejected by subscribers in the 1880 ballot, none more emphatically than Alasdair, born 1872, of Carmyllie in the county of Angus. Alasdair's application was completed by his parents' minister, Rev. George Anderson, who described them as 'plain working people', adding that 'the father's wage will never be high'. Anderson described Alasdair's habits positively and his estimate of the benefit that Alasdair would achieve through admission was corroborated by the family's doctor who judged him to be a Class II case. While approved by the SNI to be placed on the ballot, his meagre three votes must have been cause of despair. However, for Alasdair, aged seven, there remained future opportunity and he secured admission three years later.[32] There was not however a positive outcome—four years following his admission in 1883, he died, age fourteen, from enteric fever and was 'buried in Larbert', generally meaning the burial ground of Larbert Old Parish Church and signifying that his family could not afford their own interment arrangements.[33]

Besides Alasdair, another six applicants attracted less than 100 votes. Applications survive for three of these. Charles (11 votes) was a case of suspected hydrocephalus, his application made by Royal Infirmary of Edinburgh physician and surgeon Alexander Bruce.[34] Hugh (20 votes) was the son of an Ayrshire harness weaver and the application was completed for his family by William Wilson (1806–88), Episcopalian Bishop of Glasgow and Galloway.[35] An application for Christine had previously been made in 1876, completed by her mother who was perhaps too forthright and it was rejected by SNI secretary, A. J. Fitch, who judged: 'Case getting worse. Too bad for admittance'.[36] A new application in 1880 was supported by the eminent psychiatrist, John Batty Tuke (1835–1913). Submitted by Christine's father, who was emphatic that he was 'unable to pay', it claimed that she was 'improving'; she was placed on the 1880 ballot, but received only seventy-eight votes.[37] It might be expected that the support of such people as the bishop and Tuke would carry considerable influence, but voters were the people with power and they were apparently of independent minds—theirs were the voices that counted.

The SNI Register of Applications confirms that unsuccessful cases were sometimes recommended to reapply after a time lapse.[38] Charles was admitted in 1881, and Christine in 1882. Hugh, however, remained at home with his parents and four young siblings. He was labelled an 'imbecile' in the 1881 census, but ten years later that tag had disappeared and he was employed as a weaver.[39] Despite rejection from admission to the SNI, Hugh, it seems, flourished for a time, even if that was not to be sustained. Indeed, the resilience of his working life is thrown into some doubt by his admission, in 1897, to Ayr District Asylum (ADA) where his case-notes claimed that 'he had never been able to earn a livelihood, but was willing to do little odd jobs, go messages and the like for his relatives and neighbours'.[40] Yet, five years after his admission to ADA, where he was classified 'lunatic', he was credited as 'keep[ing] himself tidy … does a little work in the garden'.[41] Arguably, Hugh's existence, even within the values of the period, had not been 'worthless' when, in 1903, he died of tuberculosis, aged thirty-six.[42] The high points of Hugh's life suggest that there were times when he had been able to express himself coherently and to advance his life positively.

The children in the 1880 ballot had already been through a vetting process in order to reach that stage, so there were also children who were rejected out of hand for admission and therefore not included in the ballot. In 1875, medical superintendent W. W. Ireland (1832–1909) lamented that not all cases presented could be accepted because SNI funds were limited and that, consequently, 'a preference should be given to those who seem to promise most improvement under training'. Ireland continued:

> I have found it to be a difficult and painful task to visit those for whose benefit applications were made … and to report upon the condition and probable sequence of the malady. These visits have shown to me, in a very vivid manner, the great misery and hardships which the parents and relations of idiots have often to undergo, and how much better off and happier they are when included in a community which is accustomed to their deficiencies, understands their wants, and cultivates their capacities.[43]

Home circumstances, and the voices of desperate parents trying cope with family life and create a harmonious domestic environment while also doing their best for a mentally traumatised child, did, it seems, resonate with Ireland as he tried to balance demand and need for places against the constraints under which he had to work.

Some applications failed for the applicants simply to 'disappear'. Eliza's mother was a tobacconist on the Isle of Cumbrae.[44] Eliza was an example of a child with an international aura—she, and her older brother, John, were born in Shanghai where the family may have enjoyed comfortable lives before their father died. Eliza attended Cumbrae School from

December 1883 until January 1889 when, having reached the school leaving age of thirteen, was recorded in the school register as thereafter being 'at home'.[45] Four months later, her mother applied for Eliza to be admitted to the SNI, but the application was rejected because Eliza was deemed too old, had epilepsy, and was 'unimprovable'.[46] Two years later, the family appear to have left Scotland.

The application for Richard, ten years old when placed before the SNI in March 1868, was also rejected even although his application, endorsed by David Low, master of the burgh school at Burntisland, Fife, was judged by James Carmichael, the local medical officer, to be a Class I case, that is, 'very hopeful'.[47] Like Eliza, there are gaps in the paper trail, but apparently Richard's family and supporters did not give in and acceptance was secured in September 1870.[48] Richard is another case that suggests that voices of support from both parents and 'professionals' could have variable influence, but that there were instances when persistent parents could eventually secure their child's admission. In 1873 and 1874, the SNI medical superintendent's report listed Richard as a Grade III pupil, that is, one who 'Can Speak and Can be Taught to Work', a grading which also included knowledge of the alphabet, and ability to sing, dance, sew and knit. However, Richard was only credited as being able to distinguish colours.[49] In 1874, to extend his stay, a further application was 'completed'—the questions on the form were not addressed, Rev. Edgar Hill of Burntisland, as an 'influential party', simply writing across the document that Richard's 'particulars' were unchanged and adding that he was 'anxious that [Richard] should be retained [in the SNI]'.[50] Richard's stay was continued for a further year until August 1875, by which point, when discharged to the care of his father, he was noted as being able to sing as well as identify colours.[51] There were seven children in the household where Richard's elder brother, John, was also noted as 'imbecile' and who, unlike Richard, had not 'enjoyed' what the SNI frequently alluded to as 'the benefits of the institution'.[52]

Richard remained at home until his death in 1893, aged thirty-four. His mother had predeceased him and his father and grown-up siblings continued to care for brother John for a further year until his death in 1894.[53] While we do not know the dynamics of the household, Richard had both adolescent institutional experience and adult home experience, while John remained at home throughout his life, perhaps contributing to great family misery and hardship as suggested by Ireland—but perhaps not.

Of ten 'declined' applications made between the end of 1877 and end of 1878, the decisions in eight instances were not elaborated upon in the Register of Applications, but for two cases it is revealed that, at five years of age, Dick was deemed 'too young', while seven-year-old Elizabeth was 'declined except as a payment pupil', suggestive that, as previously noted, if the financial arrangements were acceptable, other admission criteria could be flexible.[54] Of the remaining eight rejected cases, application papers survive for six children. These provide information presented to the SNI selectors, but for three, James, Alice, and Caroline, there are also brief, informal annotations indicating the reasons for rejection.

James's father offered to pay the SNI three shillings weekly (£7–16 s p.a.), a substantial amount for an unskilled labourer, but James was rejected 'in consequence of dangerous propensities'—he had a tendency to throw objects when lapsing into 'moody passionate fits'.[55] Here, the SNI placed perceived difficulties in managing James above his father's willingness to contribute towards the boy's maintenance. The application from London for eight-year-old Alice was 'declined in consequence of being an English child and better fitted for an Institution nearer home'. Alice's father was a London commercial traveller, but he was 'at present out of situation' and the SNI would have demurred following his assertion that he was unable to contribute towards her board; and by a perception that minor physical impairment from infantile paralysis might place additional care demands on the institution.[56]

Application as a 'reduced payment' case was made for Caroline, daughter of a deceased clergyman. Caroline's mother pled precarious annual income of £75, yet supporting her son at the prestigious Watson's School in Edinburgh and another daughter undergoing teacher training. At the time of the application, Caroline had a place at Baldovan Institution. The application was refused by the SNI on the basis that the 'board offered [is] quite insufficient'.[57] In a previous application of 1870, endorsed by Thomas Balmer, Commissioner for the Duke of Richmond, Caroline's mother was able to pay £5 annually, plus an additional £5 'by friends', but on that occasion the plea was 'rejected on account of fits'—epileptic seizures then occurring several times daily.[58] The mother's 'poverty' was relative to the superior social position that she perceived as her continuing station in life.

In the three instances where the application files, like the Register of Applications, carry no notes of explanation, we can only make judicious conjecture for their refusal. In the case of six-year-old Mary, the form notes several points that may have been factors—her young age, an earlier history of seizures, inability to stand without support, and uncontrollable bowels.[59] The application of Sandy of Paisley was placed by a relative. The form indicates that Alexander was a nine-year-old 'destitute' orphan and the information volunteered suggests that his abilities, temperament, and medical assessment should have presented no concerns for the SNI. His rejection for admission, or inclusion on the election roll, may therefore have been because it was felt he should be the responsibility of the parochial authorities from which the SNI would have been able to extract a fee.[60] Thirteen-year-old Gilbert was from Kilchoman, Isle of Islay, where his father was 'an occasional labourer at small wages'. Gilbert had five siblings, three of school age. There was no record of seizures, he had received all the required vaccinations, the family had never called upon poor relief, and the certifying doctor endorsed him as 'a proper object for admission'. Without elaboration, the application was disposed of with the single word, 'Rejected'—he may have been considered too old, but at thirteen years was this too harsh?[61]

Following rejection of the five cases resident in Scotland, subsequent life stories, it seems, were tragically short:

Caroline (1863–1881) died from phthisis in Nazareth House, Aberdeen, an orphanage and industrial school run by the Sisters of Nazareth.[62]

Gilbert (1863–1880) remained with his family on Islay until his death from diphtheria, age 17, in 1880.[63]

James (b.1865) was living with his family in 1881, age 16; there is no trace of him after this date.[64]

Sandy (1868–1880) was sent to Smyllum Orphanage, Lanark, by an uncle who paid annual board of £16, but successfully sought poor law support, pleading that the financial burden was 'heavy on him'. Sandy died at Smyllum from scarlet fever, age 11.[65]

Mary (1872–1889) was the illegitimate daughter of a domestic servant in Thornhill, Dumfriesshire, and, along with an elder sister, was boarded with an aunt.[66] Durrisdeer Parish provided out-relief for her support from 1877 when her mother was removed from the Poor Roll 'having gone to service', Mary being entered on the Roll in her own right 'separated from parent'.[67] At the age of 16, Mary died from 'congenital imbecility and bronchitis' in her aunt's home.[68]

Beyond the Gates of the SNI

Longer-term outcomes can be difficult to reconstruct, partly because of the 100-year closure on decennial census enumerators' returns and variable closure periods on hospital and asylum records. This final section nonetheless re-assembles the lives of three girls received by the SNI, two later discharged and one withdrawn by her family.

Agnes was admitted to the SNI as an eight-year-old pauper from the Midlothian parish of Kirkliston in 1898. Agnes's application papers have not survived, but the admission register indicates that she remained at the SNI until aged twenty-four, being transferred to Stirling District Asylum (SDA) in 1915.[69] Her SDA casenotes help fill some of the void in the SNI records as they are descriptive and conformed to the practice of photographing patients introduced in 1890. The historian Katherine Rawling exploits this medium as revealing intriguing diversity in patient/institution interaction in the presence of the camera, in her chapter in this volume (Fig. 2.1).[70]

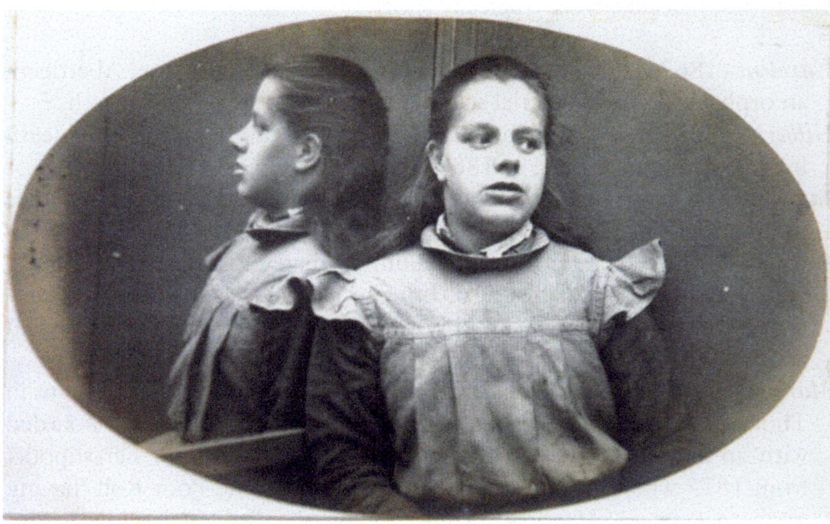

Fig. 2.1 Agnes, upon admission to Stirling District Asylum from the SNI, age 24. (Reproduced with permission of NHS Forth Valley Archive, University of Stirling Archives)

We are therefore visually introduced to Agnes, her portrait poignantly depicting her as a pleasant young woman in pensive mood. Her medical notes re-enforce this photographic impression to a degree, describing how 'she sits for hours at a time with a vacant expression taking no interest in her surroundings', 'sits staring vacantly into space', and 'sits quietly by the fire all day, speaks little and unintelligibly'.[71] This has a certain resonance with Foucault's assessment of madness in the early modern period as the 'experience of nothingness' and 'the head that will become a skull is already empty', and with Rawling's photographic example of Elizabeth D at Holloway Sanatorium in 1903 who 'sits all day in the attitude depicted'.[72] Agnes, it seems, was detached from her surroundings, institutions providing the parameters to her world from 1898 until 1961 when, reclassified as 'infirm', she was discharged from the SDA, now Bellsdyke Hospital.[73] Agnes lived for a further nine years, but her 'liberation' from a life of institutionalisation does not appear to have worked. When she died in Bellsdyke Hospital in 1970, aged seventy-nine, from bronchopneumonia and fracture of the head of her left femur, this former district asylum had again become her normal residence.[74]

Hannah was born in Orkney in 1871 where her father was a newspaper manager in Kirkwall.[75] Her socio-economic circumstances were markedly different to those of Agnes. Applying for a place at the SNI in 1879, by which time Hannah had six siblings, her father wrote that, 'It is not good to have my little girl as a companion for children younger than herself and I earnestly wish to place her where she will receive such a training as I hope will fit her in some measure to be useful'.[76] Apart from a two-month intermission in 1881, when Hannah's return to the SNI following home leave was delayed while her father unsuccessfully endeavoured to board her out in Orkney, she remained until 1885.[77] On 9 June 1887, she was admitted to Earlswood Asylum, Surrey, casenotes revealing that in the intervening period she had been in 'private care away from home'.[78]

In the decade that followed, her Earlswood notes regularly referred to her as spiteful, destructive, vicious, restless and making 'no improvement mentally', although revealing that she had some rudimentary ability in understanding and articulation.[79] She was discharged as 'relieved' on 30 November 1898 when she was transferred to private care in Painswick, Gloucestershire. Correspondence in Hannah's Earlswood casenotes reveal that Washwell Cottages, Painswick, operated as a 'home' and had a warm working relationship with the Surrey asylum.[80] In 1900, Washwell's proprietor, Eliza Steele, informed Earlswood of her retirement, advising that

Hannah had been sent to Scotland, that 'she had grown so refractory that one person could not struggle alone with her' (Hannah weighed only seven stones), 'she was the worst patient I have had to manage', and 'I do not think that her people knew how bad she was'. Steele revealed she had spelled sentences to a helper in Hannah's presence only to find that 'to my utter astonishment [Hannah] coolly told me what I had spelled'.[81]

Hannah arrived at Lanark District Asylum, Hartwood, on 14 April 1900, but as a private rather than pauper inmate and where she was described as 'cannot comprehend simple questions' and 'silly and feckless'.[82] During Hannah's post-SNI years, institutional opinions were voiced that did not concede her ability to understand—and to articulate both verbally and by her actions as, although credited with having 'a kind and an affectionate nature' on admission in 1900, Hannah was considered 'destructive and homicidal' by 1904.[83] Hannah died of acute lobar pneumonia in Lanark District Asylum on 9 October 1908 when she was 36 years old.[84]

Despite her father's wish that admission to the SNI might 'fit her in some measure to be useful', Hannah's adult years were marked by contradictory forms of self-expression, but despite certain benefits of being a private patient, institutionalisation nonetheless remained her lot until her early death. The voices of the SNI's young inmates are exasperatingly silent, but Hannah is perhaps an exception, her behavioural outbursts being expressions of her frustrations and, in contrast to Agnes, displaying awareness of her surroundings and deprivation of agency (Fig. 2.2).

Agnes and Hannah had been admitted to the SNI, both aged eight, Agnes a pauper and Hannah a private patient. While the SNI had received both girls and not rejected their applications, rejection could be a two-way dynamic, as seen when Hannah's family had prevaricated about her return to the SNI in 1881. So parents could reach a point where *they* rejected the continued services of the institution. Susan, admitted in 1892, was such a case.[85] Her parents, joiner William and his wife, Elizabeth, seem to have excelled at fulfilling the Victorian middle-class ideal of rational and responsible behaviour desired of the working classes.[86] When putting Susan forward for election to the SNI, a move that was successful, William offered to pay what he could afford for her upkeep, £10 annually. A year earlier, when Susan was eight, she was attending school and her parents were persevering with her advancement despite her slow mental ability.[87] After four years at Larbert, the directors noted that her parents perceived improvement in Susan's mental health and withdrew her, claiming that

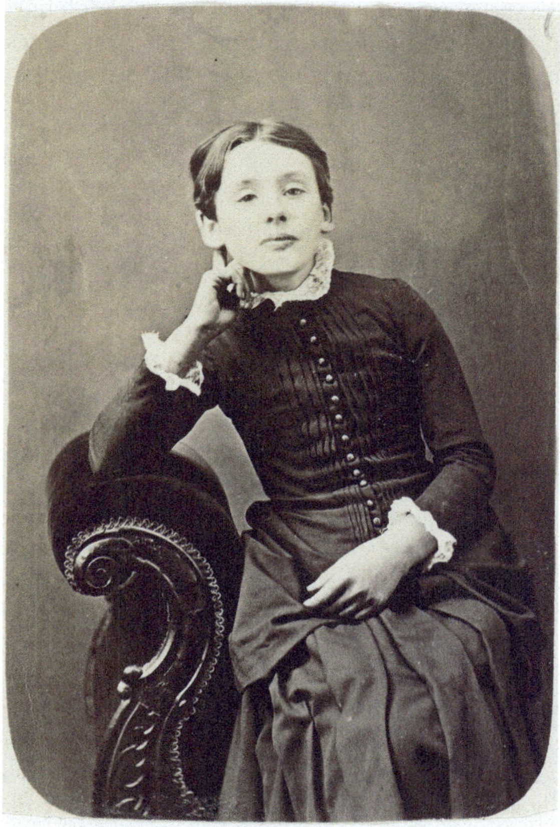

Fig. 2.2 Hannah while she was a private patient of the Royal Earlswood Asylum. (Reproduced with permission of the Surrey History Centre. Copyright of Surrey History Centre)

'we will be able to get on with her nicely at home'.[88] And that is what transpired. In 1901, while recorded as an 'imbecile', she nonetheless played a domestic role as 'mother's help' and, ten years later, although there had been substantial changes to the family structure through deaths, marriages, and births, she was still part of that evolving family network.[89] That appears to have remained the case until Susan died in 1944 at the age of sixty-one, her death registered by one of her nephews.[90] While the quality of Susan's adult life can only be speculated, she might nonetheless be considered a success story in that throughout her adult life she escaped the cycle of institutional confinement experienced by Agnes and Hannah. Indeed, Susan may have been adept at voicing her needs and emotions to her family circle, with her family proactive in those conversations.

Conclusions

An ambiguous identity surrounded the Scottish National Institution from its opening in 1862—was it a school for mentally impaired children or was it an asylum for juvenile 'imbeciles'? The SNI played up its aims of providing education and training to prepare its children for self-sufficient adult lives, although the emphasis gradually moved away from schooling to training in simple crafts and chores. In the SNI's efforts to 'improve' children, it endeavoured to admit only those considered educable. Children who it was felt would not advance under the SNI's regime were to be refused, as were cases of epilepsy, sensory impairment, and chronic ill-health, while it also endeavoured to stipulate age criteria based on physical age rather than developmental progress. While the criteria were frequently circumvented, there was nonetheless a selection process for acceptance and rejection governed by the SNI's regulations, by the fees offered for private cases, and by high demand across the three admission categories.

The SNI's purpose was brought into question at its founding and it consequently came under the scrutiny of the Commissioners of Lunacy who made biannual inspections across Scotland of homes and institutions for mentally impaired people.[91] Archival deposits for Scotland's royal asylums and district asylums might sometimes contain personal casenotes, but these do not survive for the SNI. The large body of application papers partially fills this void by providing insight to children's medical and social circumstances on admission. But, importantly, they also showcase applicants who were refused entry to the SNI.

The SNI directors were conscious of persuasive, wealthy parents aspiring to have children admitted whose care needs were complex because of other impairing circumstances. They were wary of poor boards seeking admission for pauper children who were problematic to them for reasons other than mental impairment. And in trying to aid admission of poor children by election, they were conscious of their duty to distribute a limited number of places by selection of 'eligible' cases for the annual ballot, and then guiding electors about the prospects of each child to be considered. Application papers for all three categories give insight to the diverse array of children for whom admission was sought.

The SNI registers reveal eventual outcomes for successful applicants. These suggest that judgements on prospects for improvement, including medical expertise, were inevitably speculative. Not all successful admissions resulted in even modestly positive outcomes, there being, for example, physical decline or illness resulting in death, or eventual discharge that was followed by lifetime incarceration in adult asylums. It is also apparent that some initially rejected cases eventually secured admission to the SNI, perhaps even with encouragement from SNI officials. Equally, there are instances of rejected children remaining in evolving family settings throughout their lives and, although these cases may have been perceived as failures in the late nineteenth century, twenty-first century perspectives on mental health care might now see these as offering positive life experiences. This chapter not only presents a small sample of children accepted and rejected by the Scottish National Institution in the late nineteenth century, but demonstrates that prognosis and classification of mentally impaired children were an imprecise arts, and that outcomes deemed both positive and negative could result for the 'promising' cases received—and in respect of the 'hopeless' cases rejected. Even though it is almost impossible to hear the children's voices, this chapter argues that it is possible to reconstruct life journeys as a means of giving some voice to those who were otherwise silenced. In considering children directed to the SNI, both families and professionals expressed voices to varying degrees, with mixed levels of success. For example, Devine writes of the huge influence of the Protestant churches in public life, of the clergy being 'among the social and intellectual leaders of Scotland,' and of social policy after 1850 being 'driven by religious vision which equated social improvement with moral improvement'.[92] Yet as seen in the cases of Alasdair and Hugh, even the power of the clergy had its limitations. There was a hierarchy to the weight of verbal input in securing places within the SNI and, at the apex of that hierarchy, the institution's administrators and voting subscribers were all-powerful.

Notes

1. Iain Hutchison, 'Institutionalisation of mentally-impaired children in Scotland, c.1855–1914,' *History of Psychiatry*, 22, no. 4 (2011): 416–433; Guthrie Hutton, *The Royal Scottish National Hospital: 140 years*, (Larbert: Forth Valley Primary Care NHS Trust, 2000).
2. Lynn Abrams, *The Orphan Country: Children of Scotland's Broken Homes from 1845 to the Present Day* (Edinburgh: John Donald, 1998). Marjory Harper, 'Boarding Out at Home and Abroad: Rescuing and Rehabilitating Scotland's Destitute Children from the 1860s to the 1960s', *Northern Scotland* (2007) 27:1, 99–115, and *Adventurers and Exiles: The Great Scottish Exodus* (London: Profile, 2003). Iain Hutchison, 'The disabled child in an industrial metropolis: Glasgow's children's hospital, Scottish convalescent homes 'in the country' and East Park Homes for Infirm Children' in Iain Hutchison, Martin Atherton and Jaipreet Virdi (eds), *Disability and the Victorians: Attitudes, interventions, legacies* (Manchester: Manchester University Press, 2020), pp. 145–63. Helen J. Macdonald, 'Boarding-out and the Scottish Poor Law, 1845–1914', *Scottish Historical Review* (1996), LXXV (2): 200, 197–220.
3. Olive Checkland, *Philanthropy in Victorian Scotland: Social welfare and the voluntary principle* (Edinburgh: John Donald, 1980); Callum G Brown, *Religion and society in Scotland since 1707* (Edinburgh: Edinburgh University Press, 1997).
4. Callum G. Brown, *The Death of Christian Britain, 1800–2000* (London: Routledge, 2001).
5. Iain Hutchison and Dee Hoole, 'Discharge, Disposal, and Death: Outcomes for Child Inmates of the Scottish National Institution, Larbert, and Stanley Hall, Wakefield, to 1913', *Journal of Family History* (2019), 45, no. 2, (2020): 207–227.
6. William W. Ireland, *Idiocy and Imbecility* (London: Churchill, 1877), *The Mental Affections of Children: Idiocy, Imbecility and Insanity* (London: Churchill, 1898). Mark Jackson, *The borderland of imbecility: medicine, society and the fabrication of the feeble mind in later Victorian and Edwardian England* (Manchester: Manchester University Press, 2000).
7. University of Stirling Archives & Special Collections (USASC), Scottish National Institution (SNI), 40th Annual Report (1901), p. 23.
8. USASC, SNI 1st Annual Report (1862), p. 6; 3rd Annual Report (1864), p. 5.
9. USASC, SNI 2nd Annual Report (1863), p. 8; 3rd Annual Report, p. 5; 7th Annual Report (1868), p. 9.
10. USASC, SNI 3rd Annual Report, p. 12.
11. USASC, SNI 4th Annual Report (1865), p. 5.

12. USASC, SNI 6th Annual Report (1867), p. 7.
13. USASC, SNI 25th Annual Report (1886), p. 6; 26th Annual Report (1887), p. 22.
14. No Grade I cases were recorded at the SNI between 1887 and 1899—USASC, SNI Annual Reports, 1862–1901.
15. USASC, SNI 39th Annual Report (1900), pp. 15, 17; 48th Annual Report (1909), p. 22.
16. USASC, SNI Admission Register 1888–99, RS/1/2/1, Case 742.
17. Ibid., Case 781.
18. USASC, SNI Admission Register, RS/1/2/1.
19. Harriet Sturdy and William Parry-Jones. 'Boarding out insane patients: the significance of the Scottish system, 1857–1913,' in *Outside the Walls of the Asylum*, ed. Peter Bartlett and David Wright. (London: Bloomsbury, 1999), 86–114.
20. USASC, SNI Admission Register, RS/1/2/1.
21. Ibid., Cases 733, 77 and 1166.
22. USASC, SNI 35th Annual Report (1896), p. 12; 38th Annual Report (1899), p. 15.
23. USASC, SNI Admission Register, RS/1/2/1, Cases 1016 and 1232; SNI 38th Annual Report, p. 15.
24. USASC, SNI Voting Paper for 5th May 1880, RS/2/19.
25. USASC, SNI Admission Application, RS/1/3/312.
26. USASC, SNI Register of Discharges & Removals, RS/1/4/2.
27. J. Melling, R. Adair and B. Forsythe, "'A Proper Lunatic for two years', pauper lunatic children in Victorian and Edwardian England, child admissions to the Devon County Asylum, 1845–1914,"' *Journal of Social History*, 31, no. 2 (1997): 371–405.
28. Registration of Death, Stracathro, 1958.
29. £30 in 1880 equates to c.£2000 today—http://www.nationalarchives.gov.uk/currency-converter/. Accessed 11 Jul 2019.
30. USASC, SNI Admission Application, RS/1/3/334.
31. USASC, SNI Register of Discharges & Removals, RS/1/4/2.
32. USASC, SNI Admission Application, RS/1/3/452.
33. USASC, SNI Register of Deaths, RS/1/5/1; Registration of Deaths, Parish of Larbert, 1887. I thank Eleanor Thomson of Falkirk Council Bereavement Services for her help in exploring SNI burials.
34. USASC, SNI Admission Application, RS/1/3/358.
35. USASC, SNI Admission Application, RS/1/3/356.
36. USASC, SNI Admission Application, RS/1/3/162.
37. USASC, SNI Admission Application, RS/1/3/365.

38. USASC, SNI Register of Applications, RS/1/1/1—see for example the 1880 entries where two unsuccessful applicants were recommended to reapply after twelve months.
39. Decennial Censuses, Ayr, 1881 and 1891.
40. Ayrshire Archives (AA), Ayr District Asylum (ADA), Casenotes, p. 368, AA17/1/3/41.
41. Decennial Census, Ayr, 1901; AA, ADA, Casenotes, p. 368, AA17/1/3/41.
42. Registration of Death, Ayr, 1903; AA, ADA, Register of Deaths, AA17/1/39—which inaccurately gives his age at death as 37 years.
43. USASC, SNI 14th Annual Report (1875), pp. 11/2.
44. USASC, SNI Register of Applications, RS/1/1/1; Decennial Census, Cumbrae, 1881.
45. AA, Cumbrae School Admission Register, N14/02.
46. USASC, SNI Register of Applications, RS/1/1/1.
47. USASC, SNI Admission Application, RS/1/3/69.
48. USASC, SNI Register of Discharges & Removals, RS/1/4/1.
49. USASC, SNI 12th Annual Report (1873), p. 15; 13th Annual Report (1874), p. 12.
50. USASC, SNI Admission Application, RS/1/3/156.
51. USASC, SNI Register of Discharges & Removals, RS/1/4/1; SNI 14th Annual Report, p. 14.
52. Decennial Census, Kirkcaldy, 1881.
53. Decennial Census, Kirkcaldy, 1891; Registration of Deaths, Kirkcaldy & Abbotsford, 1893 and 1894.
54. USASC, SNI Register of Admissions, RS/1/1/1.
55. USASC, SNI Admission Application, RS/1/3/227.
56. USASC, SNI Admission Application, RS/1/3/268.
57. USASC, SNI Admission Application, RS/1/3/277.
58. USASC, SNI Admission Application, RS/1/3/19.
59. USASC, SNI Admission Application, RS/1/3/285.
60. USASC, SNI Admission Application, RS/1/3/296; Registration of Birth, Paisley, 1868; Decennial Census, Paisley, 1871.
61. USASC, SNI Admission Application, RS/1/3/279.
62. USASC, SNI Admission Application, RS/1/3/277; Registration of Death, Old Machar, Aberdeen, 1881.
63. USASC, SNI Admission Application, RS/1/3/279, Registration of Birth, Kilchoman, 1863; Decennial Census, Kilchoman, 1871; Registration of Death, Kilchoman, 1880.
64. USASC, SNI Admission Application, RS/1/3/227; Decennial Censuses, Paisley, 1871 and 1881.
65. Renfrewshire Heritage Services, General Register of Poor, Paisley, 8:34, ref. 70/78; Children's Register of Poor, ref. 5/78; Statement of Cases,

11–19, ref. 18,000; Paisley Parochial Board Committee Minute Book, 7:30, pp. 272/3, 446/7. Registration of Death, Lanark, 1880. For more on placement of orphans during this period, see Lynn Abrams, *The Orphan Country* (Edinburgh: John Donald, 1998).

66. USASC, SNI Admission Application, RS/1/3/285; Register of Births, Morton, 1872; Decennial Census, Morton, 1881.
67. Dumfries & Galloway Archives, General Register of Poor, Durrisdeer, ED7/12/6; Durrisdeer Parish Minute Book, 1877–95, ED7/12/2.
68. Registration of Death, Morton, 1889.
69. USASC, SNI Admission Register 1888–99, RS/1/2/1, Case 1236.
70. John Sibbald, Commissioner in Lunacy, commended SDA Medical Superintendent, Dr. John Macpherson for his many improvements, including record keeping: 'Each case is prefaced by a compendious schedule of particulars of great value; a photographing of each patient is inserted; and accurate details of examinations made with the best scientific appliances are added.' USASC, Stirling District Lunacy Board 21st Report, 15 May 1891, p. 17. Patient case books compiled prior to 1890 subsequently had sheets of photographs of patients who were resident in advance of the policy, being added as an appendix or occasionally in the notes themselves, e.g. USASC, SDA, Male Case book, commencing 1886, SD/1/4/9. Katherine D B Rawling, "She sits all day in the attitude depicted in the photo': photography and the psychiatric patient in the late nineteenth century', *Medical Humanities*, 43 (2017), 99–110.
71. USASC, Stirling District Asylum (SDA), Female Case Book XIX 1914/15, SD/1/4/54.
72. Gary Cutting, *Michel Foucault's archaeology of scientific reasoning* (Cambridge, Eng: Cambridge University Press, 1989), 70. Rawlings, 105–6.
73. USASC, SDA Admissions Register 1909–1915, SD/1/1/8, Case 8701.
74. Registration of Death, Larbert, 1970.
75. Registration of Birth, Kirkwall, 1871.
76. USASC, SNI Admission Application; father's letter to A J Fitch, 17 Feb 1879, RS/1/3/302.
77. USASC, SNI Institution and Visiting Committee Book 1881–1899, p. 15, RS/2/4/2/3.
78. Surrey Heritage Centre, Earlswood Asylum, Female Case Book 1878–88, 392/11/14/3, p. 892.
79. Ibid., pp. 892–5.
80. Ibid., p. 895.
81. Ibid., letter, Eliza Steele to Earlswood Asylum, 7 May 1900.
82. North Lanarkshire Archives (NLA), Lanark District Asylum (LDA), State on Admission No. 2, LK29/4/53, p. 368; Case Book Female B, p. 535, LK29/5/3.

83. NLA, LDA, Case Book Female B, pp. 535/6, LK29/5/3.
84. Ibid., p. 536; Registration of Death, Shotts,1908.
85. USASC, SNI Admission Application, RS/1/3/815; Admissions Register RS/1/2/1, Case 897.
86. For example, see Hamish W Fraser, 'Necessities in the Nineteenth Century,' in *A History of Everyday Life in Scotland, 1800 to 1900*, ed. Trevor Griffiths and Graeme Morton (Edinburgh: Edinburgh University Press, 2010), 60–1.
87. Decennial Census, Barony Parish, 1891.
88. USASC, SNI 36th Annual Report (1897), p. 19; SNI Superintendent's Letter Book 1895–1900, Alexander Skene to SNI Secretary A J Fitch to RS/3/1/3, p. 240.
89. Decennial Census, Glasgow, 1901; Glasgow, 1911.
90. Registration of Death, District of Springburn, 22 Jan 1944.
91. USASC, SNI 2nd Annual Report (1863), p. 8. The Commissioners in Lunacy first inspected the SNI as 'a statutory visit' on 31 December 1864. They found the governor [Dr Brodie] absent so had to rely on extracting a verbal report from the housekeeper, nonetheless concluding that 'even during a visit paid under disadvantageous circumstances, [we formed an impression] of a very favourable and hopeful character.'—General Board of Commissioners in Lunacy, 7th Annual report (1865), pp. 229–30.
92. T. M. Devine, *The Scottish Nation, 1700–2000* (London: Penguin, 1999), pp. 364–6.

CHAPTER 3

Mental Health in the Vernacular: Print and Counter-Hegemonic Approaches to Madness in Colonial Bengal

Pradipto Roy

The most practical, and therefore most contentious, area of engagement between Hindu and Western science lay in the field of medicine.
—David Arnold *(Science, Technology, and Medicine in Colonial India*, The New Cambridge History of India, III, 5 (New York: Cambridge University Press, 2000), 176*)*

The original version of the chapter was revised: The funding acknowledgement was included in the footnote of the first page of chpater 3. The updated version of this chapter can be found at https://doi.org/10.1007/978-3-030-69559-0_20

This chapter is part of my doctoral research work carried out at the NIMHANS, India, under aegis of the Wellcome Trust *Turning the Pages* project at the institute (Grant Number: WT096493MA).

P. Roy (✉)
Early Career Researcher, Kolkata, India

R. Ellis et al. (eds.), *Voices in the History of Madness*, Mental Health in Historical Perspective,
https://doi.org/10.1007/978-3-030-69559-0_3

Prelude: Epistemic Challenges in the Concept of Psyche in Modern South Asia

Mind has often been defined, either through its assumed opposition to matter, or where it is included within matters, in its illuminative relationship with consciousness, in respective philosophical and epistemological doxographies across the world. Studies ranging from applied philosophy of sciences, applied ethics to advanced genetic and neuro-imaging studies, attempt to unpack different aspects of the amorphous mind-sciences, albeit often with ambiguity.[1] Scholars working in intellectual history and history of emotions in the Western world, locate the ambiguity of the present psych-sciences in their contested origin and development through the early-modern and modern era: 'The modern problem of mind and its relationship to matter cannot be solved alone through logical and epistemological reflection. It is a problem that can only be clarified through historical investigation since it rests upon contingent decisions made in seventeenth-century debates', argues Rhodri Hayward.[2] In the context of Europe, the seventeenth-century debates appear crucial since 'it is in the writings of Descartes that we find the full-blown paradox of the mind-body dichotomy. His method of radical doubt led to a single certainty: *I think, therefore I am* – a theory of knowledge based on subjectivity linked to a theory of ultimate reality based on *thinking substances* as one class of existence. Mind was being put forward as a self-contained sphere of enquiry.'[3] This specialised enquiry of mind occupied a central position in the Enlightenment discourses of the seventeenth- and the eighteenth-century Europe, subsequently influencing all major psychiatrists, thinkers and contributors to the modern fields of Western psych-sciences.[4]

In south Asia, formal Western psych-sciences began to take root via the lunatic asylums established by the British East India Company in and around their settlements from the mid-eighteenth century. Throughout the nineteenth century, with the consolidation of British Rule over the subcontinent, a number of lunatic asylums were built up for the Indians as well. The large-scale systematic custodial care of the insane was a new thing in south Asia, as was the entire repertoire of colonial apparatus of power-discourses, that attempted to survive by 'recognition and disavowal'[5] of cultural and racial differences. Western knowledge attempted to survive by subordinating the local knowledge as backdated, superstitious and inadequate, as well as by claiming the universality and authenticity of Western science.[6] Thus in south Asia, it was the nineteenth century that witnessed significant rupture from the evolving late medieval and early modern indigenous perceptions of health and mind in the subcontinent, and it is against that background that the modern debates on psych-sciences in south Asia need to be contextualised.

Despite acknowledging the long and significant history of contact between the Occident and the Orient, scholars in intellectual history emphasise this rupture in nineteenth-century south Asia, often taking cues from Edward Said: 'the modern period of imperialism and nationalism provides a specific rupture with the past because of the externality of imperial power and the ideological emphasis on the difference of modern society from both its own past and from other so-called backward societies',[7] and 'in this era of rupture with the past, desires of restoration fought with passions of innovation'.[8] Indeed, several such novel strategies of innovation—including but not limited to creation, appropriation, re-appropriation, domestication, braiding, acculturation, and rejection of ideas and practices—are seen to operate in nineteenth-century south Asia, especially in the realms of everyday health and diseases.

In the following sections, I first reflect briefly on the concept of madness in premodern India, and then delve into the world of printing and vernacular publications from colonial Bengal to probe the chequered development of modern notions of madness and mental health against the interactional space of nineteenth-century south Asia.

The Concept of Madness in Premodern South Asia

Sanskrit texts from ancient and medieval south Asia give voice to ancient concepts of madness. They mention the term *unmada* to refer to serious mental illness: 'The condition was recognised as a serious problem for the affected individual, the social network of relatives, friends and day-to-day contacts, and for society at large'.[9] Specific management for the *unmada* was prescribed in ancient medical texts (Ayurveda), such as the application of various medicinal preparations, ritual oblations, medical care-taking, social-familial-peer supports, and at times occasional restraints with 'gentle but firm' ligatures.[10] Yet, while medical priorities of diagnosis and treatment of the *unmada* concerned Ayurvedic texts, other aspects of *unmada* pertaining to liberation, social norms, and expectations were considered in religio-philosophical and politico-legal texts since Vedic and classical times. The politico-legal texts of *Dharmasastra* and *Nitisastra* are concerned with a broad range of social interactions, including, but not limited to, protecting people with *unmada*. Scholars emphasise the reference to a social order respectful of caste and sanctioned behaviour (*dharma*) implicit in all the texts.

Later healing practices (including Ayurveda, Unani, Siddha and various local traditions), and medical as well as socio-religious texts in premodern south Asia are seen to centre on specific social milieu from which those emerge, and different from current bio-medical perceptions of mind and mental health. The term *unmada* thus is rarely used nowadays in current social and clinical settings in south Asia, albeit its meaning is well known: 'Among popular notions of mental illness, apart from professional concepts such as depression or schizophrenia, people more commonly refer to various forms of "tension," which has become a vernacular term in many parts of India. Other terms are also commonly used, such as *pāgalpan* in Hindi, for madness or insanity. It is not a clinical term, but more a way of characterising a seriously disordered condition, or in everyday speech to dismiss bizarre behaviour or ideas, usually derisively but sometimes playfully. Used to describe an individual, referred to as crazy or insane (*pāgal*), the term is stigmatising. In other regional Indian languages related terms are also used, such as *pagalāmi* in Bengali or *pagalvanu* in Gujarati, both denoting madness'.[11]

Much later, during the colonial era, different voices of madness emerged. In Bengal, the world of print, and specifically the vernacular health writings, offer interesting insights into the popular medical space of colonial Bengal, where important transformations regarding the notions of mind, madness and mental health indeed took place. Using the world of print in colonial Bengal as a backdrop, the next section explores the tensions arising from different voices, the traditional and the new, resulting from the impact of the British Raj.

The World of Print in Colonial Bengal

The potential of print media not only to dominate or dictate but also to create culture, and shape everyday perceptions and practices, has long been recognised, by both the colonial actors and recent scholars. 'The Press is a great system of circulation … a very small quantity of printing even in a language not more generally understood than English in India, is enough to furnish materials for a great quantity of manuscript, as well as of declamation, conversation, dissemination of rumours and alarms',[12] noted Mountstuart Elphinstone, one time governor of Bombay

(1819–1827). The first printing press in colonial India was established in Hooghly (near Calcutta) by protestant English missionaries in 1778, and in the same year, Bengali typography was created by Charles Wilkins with the help of Panchanan Karmakar, a Bengali blacksmith. That very year, Halhed's *A Grammar of the Bengali Language* was printed from that press in Hooghly.

William Carey, the missionary and later teacher of Bengali at the Fort William College, supported this vernacular printing world, through his association with the Serampore Press from 1800. Besides biblical literature, the Mission started printing vernacular textbooks for both the elementary schools and Fort William College. With increasing cost of importing papers, the Mission erected its own paper mill in 1811, and it was boosted up with a twelve-horsepower steam engine in 1820. Financial constraints led to the closure of the press by 1837, yet within the short span of three decades (1800–1832), more than two lakh (212,000) copies of books were issued from it in forty different languages.[13]

Indigenous enterprise in printing began from the very first decade of the nineteenth century and soon paralleled the European publications. *Friends of India*, the missionary newspaper noted in 1821 that 'within last ten years native works were being printed by the natives themselves'.[14] More than thirty thousand such native works were in circulation by around 1825.[15] Few places in the Empire had similar exposure to print technology, especially of vernacular script, at such an early date. A vast corpus of materials, previously confined to painstakingly handwritten manuscripts, started appearing in a stable and affordable form, thereby causing significant increase in the circulation and readership of the vernacular texts.

A number of Bengali entrepreneurs, mostly from the middle and lower-middle classes, joined the printing industry, and by the middle of the nineteenth century, at least fourteen hundred Bengali books and pamphlets were in circulation. Some of these had a print order of over thirty thousand.[16] The diverse texts included mythological fables, popular oral narratives, religious instruction manuals, literary pieces (mostly farces and parodies), as well as educational books on history, geography, arithmetic, medicine, grammar, and so on. They were mostly written in simple Bengali on cheap or affordable papers.[17] The century-long traditions of '*kathakata*' prevalent in local societies of Bengal seem to have modelled the ways in which print culture was initially adapted in local life: the printed Bengali texts were often read out to the unlettered fellows by the literates or semi-literates.[18]

The milieu print culture set in nineteenth-century Bengal was not unique. Similar developments were observed in other contexts such as the printing industries of Europe from sixteenth to the late nineteenth century, which served semi-literate populations, along with the gentry, with specific regional variations.[19]

The growth of production technologies marked 'a complete transformation of the printing trade'[20] by the second half of the nineteenth century: 'With the development of the rotary press, introduction of cheap paper in place of expensive linen rag material, and the implementation of faster modes of transport such as trains and steam boats, the potential for production, marketing and distribution of print media increased dramatically'.[21] Besides small quantities of reformist high literature, the dominant and voluminous corpus of cheap print culture that flourished in Bengal, popularly known as *bot-tala* books (referring to the locality in the black town, the older part of the city with Indian conglomeration, where most of such Indian printing presses were located), share many similarities in their production and consumption patterns with the popular eighteenth- and nineteenth-century English and Continental chap-books.[22] Scholars have tracked the common circumstances and interests that produced the publishers and consumers of these chap-books in Europe and Bengal, and their reach to the remotest parts of the country have been affirmed beyond doubt.[23]

Medical Books in the Vernacular

As mentioned earlier, one of the major categories of the printed texts in Bengali belonged to pedagogical medical texts. Their popularity and usage continue even today as one takes a walk down the alleys throughout the subcontinent.[24] A mid-twentieth-century scholar observed the lives of majority of Bengali people to be heavily influenced still by those popular chap-books and manuals. He noted that thousands of doctors, compounders, Ayurvedic practitioners in the villages actually learn to feel the pulse from *Narhi-gyan Shiksha (Learn how to measure pulse)* and in 1950s Calcutta many doctors were practising by reading *Patent Oushadshiksha*[25] *(Learning Patent Pharmaceuticals)*.

The first medical text in Bengali appeared around 1818, and most of the medical texts written in vernacular before mid-nineteenth century were books. Similar to other categories of printed texts, medical publishing in Bengali flourished enormously post mid-nineteenth century: Ten such books were published within the first six years of the 1850s, compared with fourteen medical books published between 1818 and 1850,[26] while James Long's 1857 report on the Bengali press notes four thousand popular medicinal texts in circulation. It was however not until the 1880s that Western medical terms like 'malaria' or 'nerves' started appearing uniformly in the vernacular medical texts and during that time, specific health periodicals started to emerge in the vernacular. The following sections engage with the entries pertaining to mental health in those health periodicals of late-nineteenth and early-twentieth-century Bengal.

Mental Health in Vernacular Health Periodicals

The selection of health periodicals selected for study here has been limited by their availability in the archives. *Svasthya (Health), Svasthya Samacara (Health Bulletin), Chikitsa-sammilani (Healing-compendia/ Compendia of Healing Traditions), Chikitsaka o Samalocaka (Treatments and Criticisms), Chikitsaka (Healing), Anubikshan (Microscope), Bhisaka-darpana (Doctors' Mirror)* are the surviving health periodicals that this chapter has been able to look into, along with occasional relevant entries from other general periodicals and newspapers. There are entries ranging from *Nisi-paon* (Somnambulism), *ahifen*(opium)-cocaine-ganja(cannabis) addiction, jealousy, violence, selfishness, narrow-mindedness, insomnia, hysteria (*bhute-paoa/ bhablaga*) to nocturnal emission (*swapno-dosh*).

In most of the cases the doctors were called into patients' homes to examine them, applied a hybrid set of therapies, and interestingly, the doctors would almost always relate those cases to the then prevalent popular-modernist discourses of rationalism and utilitarianism. These popular discourses were mostly distinct from the then occasional alternative, non-medical attitude towards colonial systems, which often took the 'problems of mind as a critique of the colonial experience'.[27]

All these Bengali health periodicals came in late nineteenth century, almost a century after the first lunatic asylum was erected in Calcutta. By the second half of nineteenth century the number of lunatic asylums increased significantly. Yet, there is little mention of lunatic asylum practices in these popular medical spaces. Even the government-sponsored Bengali health periodical *Bhisaka-darpana (Doctors' Mirror)*, which contained translations of English articles appearing in *British Medical Journal* and *Journal of Mental Science* (the present *British Journal of Psychiatry*), mentions little about lunatic asylum practices. Regarding mental health, *Bhisak-darpana* included only translations of those articles which dealt with management of patients at their home or in clinics. This was perhaps suited to the need of the targeted audience of the journals, viz., the Indian general practitioners who were treating patients outside the institutions, mostly by paying home visits. The rest of the vernacular health periodicals were run by the Indians, and the targeted audience included other practising physicians, quacks, trainee doctors, and also patients. The absence of mention of lunatic asylum practices in these vernacular health periodicals could be explained by taking a look in the mental health-related entries in these periodicals, which I turn to shortly.

The first psychology book discussing 'rules for the advancement of mind' (*Chittokarsa Bidhan*) appeared in Bengali in two volumes around mid-nineteenth century (1849). *Manastatva Sar Samgraha* (Collection of the Essence of Psychology) in three volumes by Radhaballabh Das appeared later in the same year. *Manobijnan* (Psychology) by Gopalchandra Ghosh was published in 1874 and *Mesmerism Ba Sakticalan Vidya* (manual on applying hypnotism) by Kunjabehari Bhattacharya appeared in 1887. Discussions on mind sciences, mental health and hygiene, appeared in general non-specialist or literary periodicals mainly concerned with rationalism, utilitarianism and positivism, rather than psychology or psychiatry per se. While there is a sense of an implicit drive to situate the local understanding at par with superiorly posited Western knowledge, at places there are explicit, strong anticolonial stances as well within these up-to-date and scientific socio-health discourses, as may be evident in their bleak sarcasm against the asylum doctors (vide, infra), or in their criticism of contradictory colonial policy on opium and hemp.

Scholars working with these periodicals have noted criticisms of the received knowledge in these journals. But as I show in the following section, there were few criticisms of Western scientism, rather there was a claim for at par and at times superior Indian knowledges, armed with empiricism and scientificity. I find the dissent, not in the received knowledge, which was appropriated, re-appropriated and braided with the Indian traditions and experiences, but in the direct or indirect criticism of colonial policy, together with occasional mockery of Western institutions (such as the lunatic asylum), where the discourses in these periodicals became polemic. Here it reminds me of the nature of religious dissent in nineteenth-century wider imperial space, where the radical anticolonial anticlerical universalism (against the then prevalent Christian and racial notions of British superiority) and anti-Christian polemics centred around notions of *Religionswissenschaft* (the science of religion).

I argue that this was the same as the case with mental health. An article in 1875 titled *Manasik Rog* (mental illness),[28] hesitantly noted the relative unavailability of categorisation and in-depth study of mental illness in indigenous medical systems, yet then pointed out that remedies for specific mental illnesses were yet to be discovered, thus implying a deficit in Western medicine. Taking the view that disorders of mind were caused by an excess or absence of natural thoughts, the author urged fellow medical men to engage with efforts to find remedies, as otherwise enmity between races and men would never end. Just as the ethical spirituality and universalism of the rational religion of modern Hinduism—loaded with intellectual systems and critical epistemologies—debunked Christianity of its hedonist materialism, idiosyncrasies and inconsistencies, the call for fellow countrymen and medical men to take up the challenge of solving the riddles of mind sciences that even the West was unable to achieve, appears to subvert the Western subjection of the native mind so implicit in the then prevalent imperial medico-scientific discourses.

As the radical anticolonial and anticlerical universalism of Theosophy challenged notions of Christian (read Protestant) and racial superiority in Britain (and later in India), the popular health rhetoric about mental health in nineteenth-century India privileged non-asylum discourses. This would be further evident as we probe briefly the career of James Esadaile and mesmerism in nineteenth-century Bengal.

James Esdaile (1808–1859), the Scottish surgeon and mesmerist with the British East India Company in Calcutta, had 'manoeuvred himself on to the margins of his professional group'[29] by believing and practising the healing approach of animal magnetism (aka mesmerism), which most of his contemporaries condemned. Despite much controversy, Esdaile's methods gained considerable popularity among the Indians (and some Europeans as well), many of whom not only consulted him with their problems, but were actually part of his healing team in conceptualising and delivering mesmeric services. Operations were carried out under mesmeric trances and by around 1847, Esdaile 'claimed to have successfully treated both European and Indian patients who suffered from insanity and epilepsy'.[30] Despite the great popularity of Esdaile's hospital of magic (or *jadoo hospital*, as it was known popularly) among the lower classes, it received fierce criticism from majority of his professional colleagues, who assigned that popularity to the general superstitious nature of the Indians. Esdaile himself recognised and acknowledged the similarity of his treatment methods with those of indigenous healing systems, and yet to achieve strong footing amidst the approved Western medicine, he 'tried to locate his approach squarely within contemporary Newtonian scientific thinking'.[31]

It could be Esdaile's non-reliance on the psychological concept of hypnotism, or his conviction regarding the material existence of an animal fluid on which magnetism should work, that led to his non-acceptance among Western professional circles, as Waltraud Ernst suggests. But the racial overtone implicit in colonial administrator-doctors' discourses (e.g.lunatic asylum superintendents, Inspector Generals or Assistant surgeons) was absent in Esdaile—rather, his ideas emphasised the subaltern character of popular medicine and advocated for the scientific status of the same. In so doing, Esdaile's *jadoo hospital* might have conveyed a sense of subterranean anticolonial antihegemonic subaltern undercurrent, which could have been the reason why so many Indian and European lower classes flocked there. In his criticism of E. P. Thompson's emphasis on the exclusive plebeian nature of radical mysticism, Peter van der Veer notes, 'class background does not determine people's interest in one crucial area that is engaged by radical mysticism, namely the area of healing and medicine. It is in this field that animal magnetism or mesmerism, herbalism, crystal-ball gazing, and astrology enjoyed great popularity among all classes'.[32]

The popular medical space in colonial Bengal enjoyed great popularity as well, and almost every approach claimed to be scientifically superior, more relevant and legitimate than the other. Parallel to the rise of institutional psychiatry and medicine, interest in popular medical space was escalating throughout the nineteenth century. Thus long after Esdaile's departure from the scene, we find books and articles describing methods of hypnotism through practice of mesmerism, appearing in Bengali in the late nineteenth century.

Indeed the print media in vernacular became a great booster to the popular medical space as the Indian physicians (of plural lineages and hybrid practices), writing in those periodicals used to narrate some of their patients' stories in simple lexicon, citing those at times as their patients' own voices, albeit mostly interspersed with medical terms. Indirectly, this might have given some primacy to patients' concerns for the emerging disciplines of health in south Asia. However, those were not actual patients' voices by any means, just as such patients' voices could not be found in lunatic asylum annual reports or mental hospital clinical records or case descriptions, after all, all these were being written by doctors of some kind or the other. Yet, unlike the custodial care of the lunatic asylums, it could be argued that at times, such patients' stories might had helped patients and their caregivers to assume some agency in the popular medical space over their own mind and body, as and when they went through such health manuals, written in simple languages, aiming to promote individual practices (and repute), and to aid in practices of less qualified medical men. Unlike the institutional care at other places, where 'evidence does not suggest that they (i.e., patients) were consulted'[33] while designing therapeutic options, the very nature of home- and clinic-based mental health care provided by the Indian doctors in the community ensured that patients' concerns needed to be prioritised to ensure their popularity. And this popular practitioners and rhetoric of value-laden mental health care continued to push mental health as an emerging and viable discipline in early twentieth-century south Asia, though distinct from modern psychiatry, psychology or neurology, as was being practised in contemporary West.

The near absence of sarcastic references to lunatic asylums in this popular medical space indeed tells a tale of contested development of mental health practice in the subcontinent, where popular enthusiasm centred on the plural healing world, and bureaucratic institutional care was perceived, at best, to serve refuge and custodial functions. The Bengali journal *Anubiksan (Microscope)* noted sarcastically in 1875, "Readers may remember that when Prince of Wales stepped in this city, on the grace of such occasion, an insane hospital, i.e. a treatment centre for mad persons, was constructed at the northern fringe of the city. A few rich persons from this country have donated more than lakhs of rupees for it. With a lot of curiosity, we went to visit the treatment centre. First, we had to cough up Rs. 25 as 'entry fee' and felt that money will be of a waste! ... While thinking this, as we advanced a few steps ... There were plenty of visitors like me. I also saw a few doctors for the insane. Some of them appeared like men of knowledge but some appeared like insane! At least in the first glance I took a person to be an insane but after introduction I found him to be a doctor!"[34]

The bleak sarcasm towards colonial administration and their farcical medical establishment, did not remain hidden here. Not only was the mockery directed against the government for his vain attempt to show off before the visiting Prince of Wales, but by sarcastically confusing the sanity of the doctors and the patients, it reduced the entire enterprise of nineteenth-century colonial (institutional) psychiatry to a redundant non-medical bureaucratic entity. The passage also testifies the prevalent custom of visiting lunatic asylum patients, which continued in the Indian mental hospitals at least till the end of the twentieth century. The asylum practice of earning, not only from patients' labour, but by having them displayed as objects of curiosity as well, led to bullying of the confined mad within the asylums and mental hospitals, an issue that has only changed recently.[35]

The ill running of the overcrowded lunatic asylums in colonial south Asia did not leave enough room for the Indians to consider such asylum provisions as the mainstay of therapeutic options for the mentally ill. Indeed, by probing into the productive language of the colonial archives, Jim Mills holds lunatic asylum doctors responsible for the construction of notions of abnormality and insanity. For the Indian people those categories were merely linguistic and thus little relevant. They used the asylum provisions on their own, as and when they needed such a place either for refuge of themselves or for custodial care of nonconforming family members.[36] The government's rule of payment for every patient (sometimes at quite high rates) received public criticism as well. The lowest rate of maintenance being fixed at Rs. 12 per month sometime in late nineteenth century, appears logistically impossible even for the middle class of that time. While welcoming the decision of the colonial government to pick up the wandering lunatics from the street, a Bengali daily insisted on the necessity of detaining not only the 'non-violent' and 'poor' lunatics from the street, but those 'unruly' in their home as well. It objected to the high rates proposed by the government, which made it impracticable for the Indians to seek admission in the lunatic asylums.[37] Despite several new asylums being built from 1860 to 1880s in British India, the problem of overcrowding worsened, attracting criticism both from the government and the Indians. An editorial in the Indian Medical Gazette in 1877 severely criticised the government for rampantly admitting the destitute, as it held that 'Parish relief' should not be the duty of the medical community. The article titled 'Poor House or Hospitals?' expressed annoyance towards the government for being unable to recognise feigned illnesses by 'professional beggars'.[38] Indeed, like France (and many other places), as Jane Freebody shows in her excellent chapter in this volume, occupational therapy in colonial south Asia, despite being premised theoretically towards therapeutic goals, in practice, was being directed by the economic priorities of running the overcrowded and underfunded mental health institutions, which grossly limited the medical benefits of such work in the Indian asylums as well.[39] Further, many asylum superintendents in colonial India further managed to economise food provisions for the patients and Indian patients were always treated differently, subject to harsh experimental treatments and compulsory hard labour.[40] It is obvious that the Indians could not relate to the colonial asylum system with mutual trust and reliance. This may provide some explanation for the near absence of mention of lunatic asylum practices in popular medical space.

The Bengali health periodicals flourished mostly from 1875 to 1930s–40s. There was little stability or specificity in the contents and forms of these varied and protean literature. Various such journals, mostly born out of small entrepreneurial ventures (often of the doctor-editors themselves), used to appear and disappear with great regularity. Instead of focussing only on specific specialised issues, each of the journals, as their names suggest, tried to incorporate as many divergent topics as possible (ranging from surgery to hygiene and public health) and accommodate different conceptual and therapeutic approaches regarding each topic. Of the numerous Bengali medical periodicals that emerged in the second half of nineteenth century, only a few survived for longer periods, viz., *Bhisaka-darpana* (continued for at least 23 years since 1890), *Chikitsa-sammilani* (at least 12 years since 1887) and *Svasthya* (at least 7 years since 1897). Most of the other periodicals did not survive beyond the first two years. Of the periodicals appearing in early twentieth century, *Svasthya Samacara* survived for a significant period of at least 16 years (1912–1928). Entries related to mental health are fewer than medico-surgical topics in these periodicals.

The periodicals were in no sense strictly medical, as almost all have entries pertaining to ethics, moral values, man–woman relationships and related social-familial issues; thus the term health periodicals seems more appropriate than medical periodicals. In the popular space of nineteenth- and early twentieth-century Bengal, health is thus observed to be perceived and practised as part of a more general social-familial entity, and not as part of a strict biomedical entity championed by the medico-bureaucratic institutions of the colonial state, over which the colonial subjects had little direct control. Institutional (and later biomedical) notions of health were appropriated, re-appropriated, braided into Indian knowledges and circulated in the popular medical space, but were almost always wrapped in social–ethical messages. This may explain how institutional psychiatry and later psychology–psychoanalytical approach lost direct relevance in popular medical spaces: both were perceived as extra-social categories, the former as a hegemonic colonial enterprise and the latter as refined conceptual categories of the sophisticated urban educated. The popular medical space mediated the naturalisation and popularisation of the mental health ideas and practices of different horizons, albeit in a socio-familial-health perspective, thereby promoting emergence and consolidation of the modern categories of 'tension' rather than *unmada* or insanity. My final section explores this with the example of '*dhatu-dourbalya*', a condition that illustrates contrasting medical philosophies.

Bhisaka-darpana, the demi-official government publication mostly published translations of English articles published elsewhere. The major contributions here included the disciplines of obstetrics, gynaecology and surgery. Largely, the Indian Medical Service (IMS) doctors and the sub-Assistant surgeons used to contribute to this journal, though at times references to other medical systems such as Ayurveda could be noted. One Dr. Lalitmohan Chattopadhyay contributed on 'dhatu-dourbalya/ sexual disability' in successive issues. The discussion on *dhatu-dourbalya* covered almost every medico-social periodical of late nineteenth- and early twentieth-century south Asia, and thus predates the current psychiatric diagnosis of *dhat-syndrome*, a similar yet much more consolidated and unitary disease entity usually attributed to certain cultures.

The late nineteenth-century Bengali physicians, as it appears from the writings of Dr. Chattopadhyay and others, did not merely equate *dhatu* loss with loss of semen, since they conceptualised *dhatu* with all necessary and major body parts, and *dhat* with constitutions or nature of a person. *Dhatu-dourbalya* thus referred to a wider dissonance between mechanical and functional aspects between the connected body parts, incorporating into it a number of related disease entities, from Western medicine—such as 'entic dyspepsia', 'sexual debility', 'impotency', 'spermatorrhoea'—and also from non-specific entities of the popular medical space such as 'sadharan dourbalya' (general weakness), 'snayubik pirha' (nervous disease), 'swapna-bikar' (dream disorders), 'constipations', 'nervous phimosis' and so on. Popular medical texts in the vernacular such as Radhagobinda Kar's *Bhisak Suhrid*, notes monomania, dementia, epilepsy, nervous asthma, strabismus, paralysis and impotence as the main symptoms of *dhatu-dourbalya*, among many others. Often other authors are seen to attribute additional symptoms to these, such as Dr. Pulinchandra Sanyal and Kaviraj Avinashchandra Kaviratna, joint editors of the periodical *Svyastha Samacara*, held burning sensation during micturition as symptomatic of *dhatu-dourbalya*.

Often, the symptoms alone are seen to emerge as disease entities in these vernacular texts. While many of these varied and protean symptoms were taken up from the pre-existing plural healing market of south Asia, where they might have catered to the sale of specific pharmaceuticals, the linking of such symptoms with nerves or mental illness is observed to be a phenomenon happening in south Asia for the first time in the nineteenth century. Telegraph, electricity, dissection of the cadaver at the medical colleges with revelations of the nerves, tales of cure by electrotherapy—all these might have contributed to the popular understanding of the nervous categories of mental illness in late nineteenth- and early twentieth-century Bengal. The way epilepsy, monomania or dementia were conceptualised as the symptoms of ***dhatu-dourbalya*** in the same way as impotence or nervous asthma, actually led to the de-pathologisation of serious categories of mental afflictions such as monomania, epilepsy or dementia, almost turning them to an extension of general nervousness. This, I argue, led to the consequent de-stigmatisation of serious categories of fatal or morbid mental illnesses requiring occasional institutional admission and/or prolonged care.

There was a quite active group of Indian physicians with training (and degrees, at times from the United Kingdom) in Western medicine and knowledge of indigenous healing traditions, albeit without having the privilege of joining the hierarchical Indian Medical Service, where only Europeans were allowed to move to the higher ranks, until the second decade of the twentieth century. Instead, they joined the popular medical space spread across the subcontinent. Numerous indigenous practitioners, pharmacists and quacks were already active there. Together, this larger group of practitioners might have paved the way for a certain kind of popular professionalism of mental health in the subcontinent in nineteenth and early twentieth century, a kind of professionalism distinct from the disciplinary professionalism that psychology, psychiatry and neurology attained in modern West during the same time. Readings of the vernacular health periodicals suggest popularisation of socio-spiritual-ethical-health paradigms for mental health and sanity. Being largely aloof to the lunatic asylum practices and manuals, albeit appropriating and braiding notions and categories across the disciplines, the nineteenth- and early twentieth-century popular medical space in south Asia de-stigmatised notions of both the mad-bad-sad lunatic and the ***unmada***, turning both the categories into preventable conditions by adoption of a balanced, stress-free, socio-ethical living, or at worst, as symptom clusters mostly amenable to a few medications; here I find the transformation from the premodern concept of ***unmada*** to the modern vernacularisation of the "tension" complexes relevant.

Closing Remarks

The argument for popularisation of mental health and naturalisation of madness gains stronger support as we delve deeper into the vernacular medical texts. The majority of earlier discussions in these periodicals centred more on reports or translations narrating advancements of Western medicine. Later discussions criticised such direct narration of developments in Europe, and more authors were sending descriptions of their own patients and/or analysis of their own theories. Many of the Indian doctors came from traditional physician families and underwent training at the medical college in Calcutta, possessing knowledge of both traditional as well as Western medicine. Further, newer developments in therapeutic options across the globe were available in Calcutta.

In practice, these doctors used to employ a set of hybrid therapies. On many occasions, their treatment modalities were even more efficacious than the IMS doctors, and they often stimulated novel approaches in both treatment and research. In the early twentieth century, as an extension of extra-institutional care for the mentally ill, the editor-cum-publisher of the Bengali health periodical *Svasthya samacara*, Dr. Kartickchandra Bose, a quite popular and busy practitioner, even arranged to send extracts of a popular Indian medicine, *sarpagandha* roots (reserpine) for trial at the then Indian Mental Hospital in Ranchi.[41]

By historicising the voices of the Indian doctors in the popular medical space, this chapter argues the need to look at the widest domain of mental health ideas that permeated the popular space in late nineteenth- and early twentieth-century south Asia, and impacted the Indian attitudes towards madness and mental health. The Indian doctors in independent practice never accepted the Western medical discourses in their original form, rather, ideas were significantly appropriated and re-appropriated and were braided carefully into relevant local contexts and notions. For example, although insomnia and sleep disorders were an oft-repeated topic in these Bengali health periodicals, as was hysteria and *dhatu-dourbalya*, none of these ever came without being wrapped in familiar social-ethical messages. 'The Bromide Sleep: A New Departure in the Treatment of Acute Mania', an important article in history of use of bromides in psychiatry, that appeared in the *Journal of Mental Science* in January 1900, got immediately translated and published in April of the same year in the Bengali periodical *Bhisaka-darpana*. An article in the June 1900 issue of the same periodical notes nervous debility as one form of *dhatu-dourbalya*. The same article relates madness to the uncontrolled or extravagant lifestyle of the younger generations.

Increasing numbers of English words and Latin medical terms were cited in these Bengali texts, probably to claim authenticity. I would like to argue here that gradually all these might have led to the consequent naturalisation and popularisation of specialised biomedical disease concepts, many of which lost their strict medicalised essence in the process of becoming part of everyday colloquial lexicon. Hysteria cases were described in almost all issues of each of the periodicals. Gendered localisation of such disease category is quite explicitly visible there, yet not even the most cynical of the authors took the hysteric women neither as completely pathologised nor as entirely manipulative. Instead the physician-authors and editors appear more keen to establish even quite serious mental afflictions as manageable realities of everyday life, which may happen at times, mostly due to loss of balance in socio-economic-familial world. Indeed, it was each of their treatment options and suggestions they each felt proud of, and subsequently posited such claims before the public through their writings in the health periodicals.

It was Quentin Skinner, who once urged us to think of historical knowledge by bracketing our own, better knowledge: 'No agent eventually be said to have meant or done something which he could never be brought to accept as a correct description of what he had meant or done. … Otherwise the resulting account, however compelling, cannot be an account of his statement or action'.[42] Interpretations of both the Whiggish medical historians as well as the staunch post-colonial scholars of medical history, regarding history of mental health in south Asia, thus appear to me too far from these contexts of nineteenth- and early twentieth-century popular medical spaces that this chapter has tried to contextualise. Comparative discussions between hysteria, hypochondria, psychosomatic medications all ranged these periodicals, yet emphasis was never on the diagnostic categories, rather emphatic participation with the patients and moral encouragement were always solicited to relax the patients in almost all the cases. Later institutional developments in twentieth-century south Asia witness lack of consolidation of psychiatric professionalism, which is often seen to sway between biochemical, genetic, neurological or psychological paradigms. Whether and to what extent nineteenth- and early twentieth-century naturalisation of madness and popularisation of mental health have any legacy in that later and present context, is difficult to gauge, and beyond the scope of this chapter, but it is a fascinating tale that this author takes up elsewhere.

Notes

1. See for e.g., Richard Rorty, *Philosophy and the Mirror of Nature*, 1. paperback print (Princeton, NJ: Princeton University Press, 1980); H.P. Rickman, 'The Philosophic Basis of Psychiatry: Jaspers and Dilthey,' *Philosophy of the Social Sciences* 17, no. 2 (June 1987): 173–96: G.E. Berrios, 'Phenomenology and Psychopathology: Was There Ever a Relationship?,' *Comprehensive Psychiatry* 34, no. 4 (July 1993): 213–20; G. Bryan Young and Susan E. Pigott, 'Neurobiological Basis of Consciousness,' *Archives of Neurology* 56, no. 2 (February 1, 1999): 153–57: William R. Uttal, *The New Phrenology: The Limits of Localizing Cognitive Processes in the Brain*, Life and Mind: Philosophical Issues in Biology and Psychology (Cambridge, Mass: MIT Press, 2001); Ed Diener, 'Neuroimaging: Voodoo, New Phrenology, or Scientific Breakthrough? Introduction to Special Section on FMRI,' *Perspectives on Psychological Science* 5, no. 6 (November 2010): 714–15; Russell A. Poldrack, 'Mapping Mental Function to Brain Structure: How Can Cognitive Neuroimaging Succeed?,' *Perspectives on Psychological Science* 5, no. 6 (November 2010): 753–61; Eric Kandel, 'The New Science of Mind and the Future of Knowledge,' *Neuron* 80, no. 3 (October 2013): 546–60.
2. Rhodri Hayward, 'Medicine and the Mind', in Mark Jackson, ed., *The Oxford Handbook of the History of Medicine*, The Oxford Handbooks (Oxford, United Kingdom: Oxford University Press, 2013), 524.
3. R. M. Young, 'The Mind-Body Problem', in R C. Olby et al., eds., *Companion to the History of Modern Science* (London; New York: Routledge, 1990), 703.
4. 'All the great philosophical ideas of the past century—the philosophies of Marx and Nietzsche, phenomenology, German existentialism, and psychoanalysis—had their beginnings in Hegel', noted Maurice Merleau-Ponty (1908–1961), the French scholar on phenomenology, in Maurice Merleau-Ponty (trans. Herbert L. and Patricia Allen Dreyfus), *Sense and Nonsense*, Northwestern University Press, 1964, p. 63.
5. Homi K. Bhabha, 'The Other Question…,' *Screen* 24, no. 6 (November 1, 1983): 26.
6. Ibid; For specific discussion on areas relating to mental health and mind sciences see, China Mills, *Decolonizing Global Mental Health: The*

Psychiatrization of the Majority World, Concepts for Critical Psychology (London ; New York: Routledge, Taylor & Francis Group, 2014).
7. Peter van der Veer, 'Nation, Politics, Religion,' *Journal of Religious and Political Practice* 1, no. 1 (January 2015): 8.
8. Ibid., 13.
9. Mitcell G. Weiss, 'Madness (Unmāda)', in *Brill's Encyclopedia of Hinduism*, Vol. II (Leiden: Brill, 2010), 798.
10. Ibid., 801.
11. Ibid., 804.
12. Quoted in Edward Colebrooke, 'Memoir of the Honourable Mountstuart Elphinstone,' *Journal of the Royal Asiatic Society of Great Britain and Ireland* 18 (1861): 298.
13. Nikhil Sarkar, 'Printing and the Spirit of Calcutta', in Sukanta Chaudhuri, ed., *Calcutta, the Living City*, vol. 1 (Calcutta; New York: Oxford University Press, 1990), 130. Also see, Sri Pantha [Nikhil Sarkar], *Jakhan Chapakhana elo*, Kolkata: Paschimbanga Bangla Academy, 1996 [1977].
14. 'On the Effcet of the Native Press in India', *Friend of India*, Quarterly Series, 1 (1821), p. 133.
15. 'On the Progress and the Present State of the Native Press in India', *Friend of India*, Quarterly Series, 4 (1825), pp. 149–50.
16. James. Long, *A Descriptive Catalogue of Bengali Works* (Calcutta: Sanders, Cones & Co, 1855).
17. Ibid.
18. For e.g., the Hindoo Patriot dated the 3rd May, 1855, notes 'very few even among the unlettered peasantry are willing to forgo the pleasure of having popular books read to them by some fortunate neighbour who understands better than they the mystic symbols of the alphabet'.
19. R.A. Houston, *Literacy in Early Modern Europe: Culture and Education, 1500–1800* (London: Longman, 1988).
20. David. Reed, *The Rise of the Popular Magazine in Britain and the United States, 1880–1960* (Toronto, 1997).
21. David. Finkelstein & Douglas M. Peers, "A Great System of Circulation': Introducing India into the Nineteenth-Century Media'., in David Finkelstein & Douglas M. Peers, ed. *Negotiating India in the Nineteenth-Century Media*., Macmillan Press Ltd. UK, 2000.
22. In Europe, in the heyday of cheap book trade on topics of popular interest (sixteenth till the end of nineteenth century), each country had their own variety, but catering to the common interest of semi-literate people. In UK, such books were known as chap-books after the name Chapman that was used to denote the peddlers of these books. Like early-modern and modern Europe, in nineteenth-century Bengal, the cheap books, manuals, periodicals and pamphlets printed were distributed through a network of

peddlers to the neo-literate readers and their numerous unlettered listeners in remote areas. For more details please see, Nikhil Sarkar, 'Calcutta Woodcuts: Aspects of a Popular Art', in Ashit Paul (ed.), Woodcut Prints of Nineteenth-Century Calcutta (Calcutta: Seagull Books, 1983); & Sri Pantha, Battala (Calcutta: Ananda Publishers, 1997).

23. Please see, Sumanta Banerjee, 'Calcutta's Battala Books in Nineteenth-Century Bengali Popular Culture', in Preben Kaarsholm, ed., *The Popular and the Public: Cultural Debates and Struggles over Public Spaces in Modern India, Africa and Europe* (London: Seagull, 2009), 159–82; Also, Anindita Ghosh, *Power in Print: Popular Publishing and the Politics of Language and Culture in a Colonial Society, 1778–1905* (New Delhi: Oxford University Press, 2006).
24. Interesting ethnosociological works are under way to assess the impact of such popular pedagogical manuals on various aspects of life; but a critical appraisal of such treatises on mental health is yet to be taken into account.
25. Benoy. Ghose, *Kolkata Culture (*Calcutta: Bihar Sahitya Bahvan, 1956).
26. James. Long, *A Descriptive Catalogue of Bengali Works (*Calcutta: Sanders, Cones & Co, 1855).
27. Amit Ranjan Basu, 'Emergence of a Marginal Science in a Colonial City: Reading Psychiatry in Bengali Periodicals,' *The Indian Economic & Social History Review* 41, no. 2 (April 2004): 104.
28. Anonymous, 'Manasik Rog', *Anubiksan*, Aswin 1282 BS/ 1875 AD, 88.
29. Waltraud Ernst, "'Under the Influence' in British India: James Esdaile's Mesmeric Hospital in Calcutta, and Its Critics', *Psychological Medicine* 25, no. 6 (November 1995): 1113.
30. Ibid., 1117.
31. Ibid., 1120.
32. Peter van der Veer, *Imperial Encounters: Religion and Modernity in India and Britain* (Princeton, NJ: Princeton University Press, 2001), 61.
33. Jane Freebody, '"The root of all evil is inactivity": The response of French psychiatrists to new approaches to patient work and occupation, 1918–1939', in. Rob Ellis, Sarah Kendal, and Steven J Taylor, eds., *Voices in the History of Madness: Personal and Professional Perspectives on Mental Health and Illness*, Mental Health in Historical Perspective (UK: Palgrave Macmillan, 2021).
34. Anonymous, 'Insane Hospital', *Anubiksan*, Agrahayana-Caitra, 1282 BS/ 1875 AD, 165–72, cited in Amit Ranjan Basu, 'Emergence of a Marginal Science in a Colonial City: Reading Psychiatry in Bengali Periodicals', *The Indian Economic & Social History Review* 41, no. 2 (April 2004): 103–4.
35. Several newspapers till late 1990s report the same, and also recounted by numerous public, patients and psychiatrists in India. For an indirect ref., see, Tapan Sinha, *Adalat O Ekti Meye (The Law and a Lady)*, Feature

(D. K. Films, 1981), secs. 1:14:53–1:15:44, http://www.imdb.com/title/tt0155473/
36. James Mills, *Madness, Cannabis and Colonialism: The 'native Only' Lunatic Asylums of British India, 1857–1900* (Basingstoke: Macmillan, 2000).
37. Dainik o Samarchar Chandrika, 3 April 1894.
38. Indian Medical Gazette, 12 (1877), 76.
39. Jane Freebody, '"The root of all evil is inactivity": The response of French psychiatrists to new approaches to patient work and occupation, 1918–1939', in. Rob Ellis, Sarah Kendal, and Steven J Taylor, eds., *Voices in the History of Madness: Personal and Professional Perspectives on Mental Health and Illness*, Mental Health in Historical Perspective (UK: Palgrave Macmillan, 2021).
40. Waltraud Ernst, '"Useful both to the patients as well as to the State": Patient work in colonial mental hospitals in South Asia, c. 1818–1948', in. *Work, psychiatry and society, c. 1750–2015*, ed. Waltraud Ernst (Manchester: Manchester University Press, 2016).
41. For a critical appraisal of the account see, Pradipto Roy, 'Global Pharma and Local Science: The Untold Tale of Reserpine', *Indian Journal of Psychiatry* 60, no. Suppl 2 (February 2018): S277–83.
42. Quentin Skinner, 'Meaning and Understanding in the History of Ideas', *History and Theory* 8, no. 1 (1969): 28–29.

CHAPTER 4

"The Root of All Evil is Inactivity": The Response of French Psychiatrists to New Approaches to Patient Work and Occupation, 1918–1939

Jane Freebody

Introduction

This chapter focuses on the varied responses of French psychiatrists to new theories of patient occupation emerging after World War I (1914–18). The voices that come across in this chapter are those of psychiatrists; the psychiatrists who criticised the way work and occupation were organised and who advocated the adoption of the new ideas in French asylums, and those who chose to ignore them. It is argued that the voices of the psychiatrists in favour of the new methods were "drowned out" by competing pressures, such as the desire of French psychiatrists to be

This research was funded by the Wellcome Trust (Grant No. 108615/Z/15/Z).

J. Freebody (✉)
Oxford Brookes University, Oxford, UK
e-mail: jfreebody@brookes.ac.uk

R. Ellis et al. (eds.), *Voices in the History of Madness*, Mental Health in Historical Perspective,
https://doi.org/10.1007/978-3-030-69559-0_4

regarded as "scientific", financial expediency and staff resources. The voices of the patients are not heard in this study. Without access to patients' medical records, to which letters, poems, journals and other personal accounts were sometimes appended, it is difficult to gauge what the patients themselves felt about the activities in which they were expected to participate. There is an assumption that patients preferred to be occupied, rather than left with nothing to do, but the evidence does not suggest that they were consulted. The asylum records studied (the annual reports made by the psychiatrists in charge of patient care within the asylums to the local Prefecture) give us an idea of the daily routines, the living conditions, food and the variety of treatments, including work, that comprised the patient experience, but the patients' opinions on these matters are not recorded. In fact, one of the striking impressions of one French psychiatrist, on witnessing the new methods of occupation in practice, was the silence observed whilst patients were working, suggesting that patients' voices were not meant to be heard.

Patients had been given work to do since the advent of asylums in the early nineteenth century. The work comprised helping in the kitchens, laundry and workshops, labouring on the farm or in the grounds and performing household chores such as cleaning and polishing. This work was originally perceived as therapeutic by the early nineteenth-century moral therapists, but as the century wore on, the benefits of patient work to the institution began to take priority over its benefits to patients. The new theories regarding the occupation of patients emerging in the early twentieth century re-emphasised the therapeutic properties of work and recreational activities and required intensive input from asylum staff. While these new ideas were greeted very positively by some, most French psychiatrists did not put them into practice. Patient work failed to evolve significantly during the interwar period in France, remaining similar in character to the decade before 1914. The chapter examines the ideological, organisational, social and economic factors that contributed to a lack of support for the new theories by psychiatrists working in asylums, specifically the Asile Clinique in Paris, the most prestigious of the Seine department's six asylums, and the Asile de la Sarthe in Le Mans, a town 185 kilometres south-east of Paris, in the rural department of La Sarthe.

One of the most significant contributory factors was ideological and related to the way French psychiatrists interpreted the causation of mental disorder. Since the late eighteenth century, psychiatry has been characterised by competing explanatory theories regarding the origin of mental disorder, one emphasising psychosocial factors that portrayed insanity as an illness of the mind or spirit brought on by external factors such as personal circumstances, emotional issues or family matters, and the other indicating an organic, or physiological cause that located the origin of mental symptoms in the brain or central nervous system.[1] In the early twentieth century, most French psychiatrists were "organicists", that is, they interpreted mental disorder physiologically, or as "matter", as Pradipto Roy argues in Chap. 3. This perspective discouraged the use of psychological treatments, such as occupational therapy. Other factors contributing to a failure to adopt the new methods included the internal management structure of French asylums; economic pressures following World War I and the need to keep asylum running costs down; the poor quality and inadequate quantity of French mental nurses and other support staff; and overcrowding (which made the delivery of any treatments difficult). These impediments meant that new methods of occupational therapy were only introduced to French psychiatric hospitals (as asylums were renamed in 1937) after World War II.

Historiography

Patient work is often described in studies focusing on individual asylums or on moral treatment, but has rarely been assessed in its own right, despite its centrality to the daily asylum regime. There are notable exceptions, including an edited volume by Waltraud Ernst (2016), and studies by Véronique Fau-Vincenti (2014), J-P. Arveiller and Clément Bonnet (1991); Jennifer Laws (2011); Vicky Long (2013, 2006); Geoffrey Reaume (2006); and Jean-Pierre Goubert and Rémi Remondière (2004).[2] Ernst's edited volume constitutes the first attempt to analyse patient work in a range of psychiatric institutions, but to date, little has been written on patient work in interwar France.

Patient Work before 1918

Work formed an essential aspect of moral therapy, which emerged in the context of the humanitarian ideology of the Enlightenment during the late eighteenth century. Moral therapy was a psychological method of treatment aimed at developing a patient's ability to control his/her symptoms. Philippe Pinel (1745–1826), the French pioneer of moral therapy, advocated a balanced regime of work, recreation and rest for patients in his *Traité* of 1800. The next generation of French psychiatrists, including

Jean-Étienne Dominique Esquirol (1772–1840), Maximien Parchappe (1800–1866) and Jean-Pierre Falret (1794–1870), continued to advocate moral therapy and extol the virtues of therapeutic work. French psychiatrists' commitment to patient work was indicated by the fact that France was the only country in Europe where legislation (introduced in 1838 and amended by the Ministerial Circular No. 7, dated 20/3/1857) ensured its provision for patients. The 1857 circular emphasised the therapeutic importance of patient work and the role of the doctor in prescribing it. Article 150 stated that "Work is instituted in the establishment as a means of treatment and distraction for patients", while Article 154 declared that "The chief medical officer (*le médecin en chef*) alone decides which patients should work and the type of work they are able to do".[3]

Support for moral therapy waned by the mid-nineteenth century, as an organicist interpretation of mental disorder, based on the theory of hereditary degeneration proposed by Bénédict-Augustin Morel (1809–73) in 1857 gained popularity. Morel's theory, that a neuropathic (i.e. physiological) predisposition to mental disorder was transmitted through heredity, soon dominated interpretations of mental illness by psychiatrists in France and elsewhere on the Continent.[4] Degeneration theory remained influential in Denmark, for example, until the 1940s, as Jennie Sehr Junghans observes in Chap. 5. Morel's theory of hereditary degeneration provided psychiatry with a "convincing biological explanation"—in the absence of any other—about how mental disease was acquired.[5] It also helped explain the accumulation of incurable cases that were causing overcrowding in most French asylums, rendering impossible the delivery of effective moral therapy. The therapeutic pessimism surrounding degeneration theory, which contradicted the views of the moral therapists, led to a concept of the asylum as a custodial institution, where patients were routinely managed rather than cured. Patient work continued to be part of the daily regime for patients, independent of its original context. By the early twentieth century, when most public asylums were overcrowded and underfunded, particularly those in Paris, patient work became increasingly geared towards institutional profit. "Idleness" was not tolerated amongst the pauper class of patients who were expected to contribute to the costs of their care, according to the legislation of 1857. This insistence on "usefulness" is echoed in Iain Hutchison's chapter on the Scottish Institution for the Education of Imbecile Children where the more capable inmates were expected to do some form of work.

The Aftermath of World War I

The French economy was shattered by World War I. France had lost 7.2% of its human capital, 25% of its domestic assets and 49% of its overseas assets as a result of the conflict; 31% of its GDP was spent on the war effort.[6] The destruction caused by the war was evaluated at 34 billion Francs by the Reparation Committee.[7] Government finances were therefore extremely stretched. Meanwhile, the asylum system was in disarray following the disruption caused by the war. Two particularly vociferous psychiatrists from the French Asylums' Medical Society (*la Société Médicale des Asiles*), namely Édouard Toulouse and Henri Colin of the Villejuif Asylum, described the post-war state of the Seine asylums as "deplorable". They were unhygienic and overcrowded; they lacked outdoor space and adequate laboratories. Distractions (including occupation), considered so important for patients whose conditions were beginning to improve, were practically non-existent.[8] Treatment for curable patients was compromised by mixing curable and incurable patients in the same quarters, while the ratio of 400 patients per doctor prevented the application of any effective treatment for more than a few patients.[9] Most asylums lacked the equipment necessary for delivering modern treatments, such as hydrotherapy, UV-ray treatment, electrotherapy and radiography. Many patients, who, in more favourable conditions, might be cured or improved, remained in asylums far longer than was necessary. Toulouse and Colin maintained that services for the mentally ill were "a long way from the peak of psychiatric science" and that the paucity of equipment and facilities was an embarrassment when doctors visited from abroad.[10] Various reforms were put forward, at the heart of which was the provision of separate facilities for the care of incurable and curable cases. It was understood that the reforms would be costly; it was therefore suggested that the economic value of patient work be enhanced.[11]

Criticisms of Patient Work

A focus on the financial benefits of patient work led to criticism from certain psychiatrists who believed that patient work was not being used to its full *therapeutic* potential. Julien Raynier (1888–1936)[12] and Henri Beaudouin (1885–1968),[13] whose publication *L'Aliéné et les Asiles d'Aliénés au point de vue administrative et juridique* (1924, 1930) became known as the "bible" for asylum doctors, maintained that patient work was neglected or poorly organised in many asylums.[14] Work, the authors reminded doctors, had been accepted as beneficial to a patient's mental and physical well-being since the early nineteenth century. Among the benefits, a patient gained "social dignity" through productive work, even if minimal results were achievable.[15] Work accelerated convalescence from acute psychosis and provided an excellent treatment for chronic patients. Farm work (which also provided the asylum with nutritious, fresh food) was considered particularly effective. However, the purpose of the work was therapy, and patients should not be expected to be as productive as "normal" individuals. It was essential that the personnel directing patient work understood this and treated patients appropriately.[16]

Psychiatrists Charles Ladame[17] and Georges Demay[18] tried to advance contemporary thinking on patient work in their work, *La thérapeutique des maladies mentales par le travail* published in 1926.[19] They highlighted that in the past, patient work had been indicated for convalescent and calm, chronic patients, but not for patients at the acute stage of their illness, nor for those suffering from severe mania or melancholia. They suggested that medical thinking on this matter had evolved and that work could be appropriate for acute patients, although not at the very beginning of their illness, when bed-rest was indicated. They believed, for example, that it was not considered necessary to wait until the agitation of delirious patients had completely disappeared. Work could fix their attention, channel their energy and facilitate a change in habits.[20] The benefit of work as a distraction was illustrated by the case of a patient suffering from delusions of persecution who remained perfectly calm when working in the fields for six days out of seven, but on Sundays (when patients did not work) his delirium returned, resulting in noisy monologues and gesticulations.[21] Work was considered beneficial for melancholic patients, either as a means of encouragement to engage with their surroundings, or as a refuge and a distraction. In Ladame and Demay's opinion, some patients suffering from dementia[22] were also capable of work, including those suffering from dementia praecox.[23] They noted that Bénédict-Augustin Morel found work helped to retard the deterioration of dementia praecox patients, while Eugen Bleuler (1857–1939) claimed that work was one of the most effective means of treating schizophrenia.[24]

Patients at the acute phase of their illness were required by chief medical officers to remain under medical surveillance. If acute-stage patients were to be given work, workshops had to be situated within the interior of the patient quarters. This was most unusual in French asylums; an enquiry had revealed that only two out of the 25 French asylums surveyed had interior workshops.[25] Most of the work available for patients took place in the asylum workshops situated in the maintenance areas away from the wards, or in the kitchens, laundry or grounds for cultivation. Establishing interior workshops was recommended by Ladame and Demay since they could provide work (such as basketry, mat-making, brush-making, book-binding, knitting or sewing) for a large group of patients who would otherwise be left unoccupied. The authors suggested the introduction of local industries, such as lace-making, glove-making or weaving, with which patients may have been familiar. They cited the example of the Third Section of the Villejuif Asylum in Paris, where even the most "difficult" patients worked in small workshops in the interior of their quarters.[26]

The Villejuif Asylum's Third Section for criminal and dangerous patients, established by Henri Colin in 1910, was one of the few French asylums where interior workshops existed, and could provide a model for other establishments. Whilst the primary purpose of work for these criminal patients was to ensure that they contributed to the costs of their care, as they would have been expected to do in prison, it was clear that the work also had a beneficial effect on their behaviour.[27] Colin, who had outlined the work of the Third Section in the journal *Annales Médico-psychologique* in 1912 and 1913, claimed that although doctors had not sent agitated or violent patients to the workshops in the past because they required continual surveillance, many of these patients were excellent workers.[28] By situating the workshops (including shoe-repair, machine-knitting, tailoring, furniture repair and carpentry workshops) within the patient quarters, productive work could be achieved, supervised by nurses experienced in manual labour.[29] An economic benefit for the institution could therefore be derived from patients whose labour had not previously been "exploited" at the same time as improving behaviour.

As Dr Calmels highlighted in a paper presented to the congress of French alienists and neurologists in Geneva in 1926, in which he outlined the work regime of the Villejuif's Third Section, interior workshops would enable the employment, not only of the criminally insane or of potentially dangerous patients, but of many other hitherto unoccupied patients. Patients suffering from chronic delirium,[30] dementia praecox or general paralysis of the insane (chronic mental disorder associated with late-stage syphilis), for example, who were forced to remain in their quarters with nothing to do, despite being capable of simple work, could be employed.[31] The atmosphere of boredom and sadness, so often evident in quarters where patients were idle, could be replaced by one of activity and purpose. Furthermore, claimed Calmels, chronic patients could fulfil a useful, social role.[32] Calmels was advocating the provision of work for these patients on the grounds of both humanity and economy; on the one hand relieving the boredom of patients unable to leave the ward, and on the other hand, enabling the institution to benefit from another source of labour.

Ladame, Demay and Calmels were clearly advocating that work should be provided for a wider cohort of patients, with a more diverse range of conditions, than had previously been considered beneficial from a medical perspective. The average percentage of patients given work in French asylums was not given in Ladame and Demay's 1926 report, but Dr Lautier quoted a figure of 50–55% in 1929.[33] Demay maintained in an article in *L'Hygiène Mentale* in 1929 that the figures regarding patient workers in Swiss and Dutch asylums were "unknown in France".[34] In the Swiss asylum at Wil, under Dr Schiller, 83% of male and 75% of female patients were working, while at the Santpoort asylum in Holland, 90% of patients worked.[35] Demay suggested that French doctors were being "too timid" in their allocation of work to patients. The peaceful, chronic patients and the inoffensive, intellectually impaired, together with the convalescents, were sent to work, but most of the other patients were consigned to overcrowded quarters and remained unoccupied all day, apart from a small number cleaning the wards. Demay said that it was time to get the agitated, the impulsive, the perverse, the violent and the escapees to work, by making the appropriate arrangements, such as introducing interior workshops and ensuring that adequate security measures were in place.[36] He believed that it was possible to occupy most patients in some sort of work. "The acute phase of psychosis should not present an obstacle" to work and the only contra-indications were "senility, physical weakness or illness" according to Demay.[37]

"More Active Therapy"—A New Theory Regarding Patient Occupation

Demay's ambitions to occupy more patients were encapsulated by the new method of "more active therapy" (MAT), developed in Germany by Dr Hermann Simon (1867–1947), director of the Gutersloh Asylum in Westphalia. Simon, writing in 1929, maintained that "idleness" was not only the "root of all evil ... but also of impending idiocy".[38] He claimed that "powers that are not used diminish" and that "inactive loafing around breeds bad moods, moroseness, irritability" and brought patients into conflict with one another.[39] His new approach, which he described as a method of "psychotherapy", involved the re-education of the patient through the establishment of a regular routine of occupation, rest and recreation. Although the therapeutic value of occupation was paramount, patient work had to serve a useful purpose as this was an important aspect of the re-education process. Patients needed to feel that their work was real and serious, only then would they take an interest in it. Simon insisted that a patient be pushed to "the upper limits of their abilities" as this was the only way to make progress. Identifying tasks of the appropriate level of complexity for each patient was "one of the most important as well as most difficult tasks for the psychiatrist".[40] The first review of Simon's work appeared in France in *L'Hygiène Mentale* in 1929.[41]

French support for the German model might initially seem surprising since the French had been traditionally hostile to everything German since the defeat of France by Germany in the Franco-Prussian War of 1870–71.[42] This defeat intensified the French sense of inferiority with regard to Germany, initiated by the loss of French scientific and medical supremacy to Germany earlier in the century.[43] The university chair established in Germany in 1863 demonstrated German psychiatry's scholarly and scientific legitimacy, while the ground-breaking work of Emil Kraepelin (1856–1926), whose influential *Textbook of Psychiatry* was published in eight editions between 1883 and 1915, sealed their victory over French psychiatry.[44] Postgraduate students flocked to Kraepelin's clinic in Munich, rather than Paris, to study psychiatry under the "new master".[45] French psychiatrists were anxious to re-establish their reputation by emulating, or surpassing, German achievements. Recommendation of MAT may have been part of a conscious or unconscious attempt to ensure that French asylums kept pace with developments in Germany.

Simon's ideas were enthusiastically communicated to a French audience by psychiatrists Paul Courbon and A. Porot, following a visit to the Dutch asylum at Santpoort where his methods had been put into practice in 1926. Courbon and Porot shared their observations in the French journals *Annales Médico-psychologique* (1928) and *L'Hygiène Mentale* (1929). What so impressed Paul Courbon when he visited Santpoort in 1928 was the silence. Patients worked from 0900 to 1200 and from 1400 to 1700 and were not allowed to speak whilst working.[46] The moment patients became agitated they were removed from the work room for half an hour to rest and then brought back again. If they re-offended, they were removed for a longer period; if this proved insufficient, the patients were given a sedative. Courbon found the results of this method were "extraordinary", while for Porot they were "revolutionary".[47] The application of MAT totally transformed the atmosphere of asylums; everywhere there was silence, concentration and an impressive discipline.[48] Porot believed that the methods he had witnessed at Santpoort and other Dutch asylums were not simply a way of filling the time and occupying idle hands, but an effective means of therapy that countered agitation and other symptoms. It was, as Courbon claimed, "*une véritable rééducation*".[49] This enforced silence was reminiscent of moral therapy and its attempts to induce self-control (or *la police intérieure* as Pinel called it) amongst patients and to encourage them to behave like people who were regarded as sane.

Simon elaborated his views in an article in the French journal *L'Hygiène Mentale* in 1933, explaining that "all psychotherapy is above all an education ... it acts on the will of patients with the goal of improving their ability to adapt to their environment".[50] Patients lacked judgement and understanding, so doctors and nurses assumed the role of "spiritual guide", rather like that of a mother using her authority to guide a child in the appropriate direction.[51] Simon maintained that authority was the basis of all successful psychotherapy; not force or strict rules, but the "spiritual superiority" of the therapist. This, he insisted, had been recognised by the great psychiatrists of the past such as Pinel, Reil, Griesinger and Conolly.[52] It was important not to treat patients as "mad" but as sane individuals capable of "normal" behaviour. Patients were to be respectful of others, and to remain calm and orderly. They were not to use foul language or shout, to shred their clothes or march up and down. These objectives were best achieved by encouraging patients in an occupation, teaching them good working habits, and developing their sense of responsibility.[53] Patients who behaved well and showed a willingness to work were rewarded with certain privileges such as greater freedom or attendance at special events (parties, concerts, theatrical performances). In contrast, those who engaged in antisocial behaviour were deprived of certain benefits.[54] As a patient improved, s/he would be given work involving greater responsibility. It was important to keep raising the patient's expectations of him/herself to maintain progress.[55] Outside working hours, the patient's mind should still be kept occupied with lectures, conversation and physical exercise. Patients should not be allowed to discuss or dwell upon their troubles; work and activities should distract them.[56]

Patients were thus expected to maintain certain standards of "normal" behaviour, based on contemporary perceptions of what that comprised. They were effectively being silenced by the asylum staff whose duty it was to enforce the "no talking" rule and to act as mentors to the patients, setting an example of hard work and self-discipline. Compliance was encouraged through a system of rewards and non-compliance resulted in expulsion from the working environment and periods of sedation. Although there was no evidence of restraint or punishment, signs of agitation or attempts by patients to discuss their concerns were clearly met with disapproval. Everyone was expected to perform some sort of work. Simon maintained that although work could not cure physiological conditions, such as brain disease, it could nonetheless strengthen a patient's physical and mental faculties.[57] He believed that every patient, even those at the acute stage of their illness, should be set to work on admission to hospital as this was one of the best means of combatting agitation, impulsivity and a tendency to violence.[58]

The Effect of the New Theory on Practice in Asylums

The accounts written by French psychiatrists appearing in the professional journals between 1928 and 1936 regarding Simon's new approach to patient work indicate a considerable level of interest in developing the practice of therapeutic occupation for French asylum patients. However, the evidence does not indicate that the organisation of patient work changed significantly during this period. The percentages of patients who worked in the Asile Clinique and the Asile de la Sarthe did not increase. At the Asile Clinique, the percentage of patient workers fell from 28% to 20% between 1921 and 1926, although it increased to an average of 30% between 1927 and 1939 as a result of the drafting in of additional chronic patients.[59] At the Asile de la Sarthe, the annual reports indicate that the percentage of patient workers fell slightly. In 1923, 59% of male and 58% of female pauper patients worked, and by 1937, these figures had fallen to 49% and 51% respectively.[60] These figures are clearly well below those achieved at the asylums at Gutersloh and Santpoort (*c.* 90%), and there is no indication that the chief medical officers adapted their daily regimes or their allocation of work to patients to accommodate those who were confined to their quarters. This might seem surprising given the absence of any other effective cures, at least at the start of the interwar period.[61] Furthermore, the pressure on asylums to deliver "cured" patients back to the workforce, to aid the post-war reconstruction effort and to repopulate the factories which had lost so many young male workers during World War I, was intense, as General Councillor Louis Dausset reported in 1918.[62] The new method was not only believed to be curative, but also fulfilled a rehabilitative function and was therefore allegedly helpful in returning recovered patients to work outside the asylum. There are a number of reasons, however, for an adherence to the *status quo* with regard to the prescription of patient work by French psychiatrists. These were related to the professionalisation of French psychiatry and mental nursing, and to the political and economic instability of the interwar years.

Impediments to the Adoption of More Active Therapy

Professional Orientation of Asylum Psychiatrists

As Porot highlighted in his 1929 article, the organicist stance of many French psychiatrists, who regarded mental disorder as a physiological, rather than a psychological, condition, presented a barrier to the replication of MAT in French asylums.[63] Adherence to this organicist model of mental disorder allowed psychiatrists to demonstrate their scientific credibility and, as Jean-Christophe Coffin put it, "to be part of the flow of new knowledge stemming from biology and general pathology".[64] This credibility was further enhanced by attempts to forge an alliance between psychiatry and the most prestigious of the medical disciplines in *fin-de-siècle* France, neurology. Neurologists, who specialised in diseases of the brain and the central nervous system, also took a physiological view of mental disorder and preferred biological over psychological methods of treatment. In a sense, psychiatrists were prevented from developing an independent voice by forging this alliance with neurology. The French, as Harry Paul observes, were especially proud of their scientific heritage, as the foundation of various scientific institutes (such as the Pasteur Institute, founded in 1888) during the nineteenth century, and state investment in scientific research during the early twentieth century attest.[65] This pride helps to explain the emphasis within French medicine on scientific method and the keenness of French psychiatrists to be regarded as scientific.

Patient work and occupation were not sufficiently scientific to enhance psychiatry's under-developed professional reputation.

A neurological approach to psychiatry was pursued at the Asile Clinique. It would be inaccurate to conclude that a neurological orientation precluded the prescription of work for patients as this was still deemed a useful means of distraction for chronically ill and incurable patients. However, neurologically oriented psychiatrists, with a preference for biological over psychological treatments, were less likely to be interested in the adoption of occupational therapy as a means of treating acute cases, since occupational therapy did nothing to enhance the scientific credentials of the psychiatrists. This is indicated by the small proportion of patients engaged in work at the Asile Clinique. This was also the case at the Asile de la Sarthe. The organicism and neurological approach of Dr Christy (chief medical officer 1935–39) was made explicit in his first annual report of 1935, in which he sought to impress upon the prefecture the "scientific trends" that guided his treatment methodology.[66] He divided patients into two categories, the intellectually impaired, who were incurable, and the mentally ill, who responded to treatment. The two categories, he maintained, required different therapeutic techniques. The intellectually impaired required treatment for any physical ailments; support; comfort; and the moral discipline provided by work. The mentally ill, on the other hand, required "aggressive biological treatment".[67] The two types of treatment required different medical skill sets. When treating the intellectually impaired, the doctor had to be a psychologist, while the skills of a neuro-psychiatrist were required to treat the mentally ill. This distinction had important implications for patient work. Christy made it clear in 1936 that he was more interested in neuro-psychiatry than psychological medicine.[68] He wanted to focus on acute, curable patients, whom he would treat biologically.[69] Christy's distinction between work for chronic patients and biological treatment for curable patients, and between the different skill sets required of doctors for each type of treatment (the first, psychological and the second, neuro-psychiatric) highlight the alignment between French psychiatry and neurology and suggest that Christy did not support the principle of treating acute patients with occupational therapy. It was not until the replacement of such a rigid physiological interpretation with a more environmental or social approach to mental disorder that occupation became recognised as an effective *treatment*. This was also the case in Denmark, as Junghans highlights.

Management Issues

Had the chief medical officers of the Asile Clinique or the Asile de la Sarthe believed that the new methods of occupational therapy comprised an essential aspect of treatment (as many of their British colleagues did), they would have needed the authority to introduce them. As Simon emphasised, the successful introduction of MAT into asylums depended on control of the institution by a medical director, someone with the authority to ensure that all staff shared the same therapeutic ethos. Medical control of the work regime was essential to ensure that the work was oriented towards a therapeutic goal, rather than an economic one, a point emphasised by Seine asylum physician Jacques Vié in 1934.[70] The psychiatrist was the only person qualified to decide on the type of work to be allocated to each patient. At Simon's asylum in Gutersloh, Germany, the psychiatrists and senior nurses began each day dividing the work between patients and work teams, based on their knowledge of the patients, their conditions and their aptitudes. Each work team had a particular therapeutic goal which could be achieved by a certain type of work. Simon emphasised that these therapeutic goals might not always be in harmony with the interests of economic exploitation. Those responsible for asylum administration, claimed Vié, must be united in serving the best interests of patients, since any discord between the medical and economic teams could lead to severe difficulties and compromise the potential benefits of patient work.[71] In France, although the legislation stated that work should be prescribed by the chief medical officer, overall responsibility for decisions regarding asylum management did not rest in the hands of a single medical director.

Unlike elsewhere on the continent, in France, responsibility for management of the asylum was shared between the chief medical officer and the asylum director, who controlled administrative and financial matters. The chief medical officers had autonomy in most medical matters, but patient work, which impacted on the financial management of the asylum, as well as being a means of therapy, was a contested area and a potential source of friction between the medical and administrative teams. As doctors Legrain and Demay wrote in their 1934 report (published in *L'Aliéniste français* in 1936), "it is clear that patient work is regarded differently by the economic and technical services and by the medical services".[72] They observed that for the Administration, patient workers were divided into two groups, good workers and the rest, while for the medical team, productivity was not the main aim of the work.[73] Compared with their Dutch colleagues, as Courbon and Porot observed, French doctors lacked the authority to insist upon a therapeutic objective for patient work.[74] The voice of the French chief medical officer was effectively weakened by the management structure of French asylums. A medical director, as Demay maintained, invested with both medical and administrative authority, could balance the interests of patients and asylum management.[75] Under the French asylum system, any proposed changes to the existing organisation of patient work that might compromise its contribution to the budget were likely to be rejected by the asylum director.

Financial Issues

The contribution made by patient work to asylum finances was particularly important following the economic devastation caused by World War I. By 1925, the social care budget of the Seine department was overstretched. In the light of the escalating costs of maintaining the Seine's mentally ill population,[76] the General Council was seeking ways of reducing the paid asylum workforce of the Seine, so the work provided by patients was crucial.[77] The General Council emphasised that using patient labour in the asylum workshops served to "lighten the maintenance costs which weighed so heavily on the collective purse".[78] Concerns regarding the potential loss of the financial contribution made by patient work delayed the decision to transform the Asile Clinique from a general asylum serving a mix of curable and chronic patients, to one specialising in acute, curable patients. Work was not considered suitable for patients at the acute stage of their illness, according to the traditional view of patient work. By specialising in acute cases, the Asile Clinique risked losing its workforce of calm, chronic patients, who would be transferred to other asylums. A solution to the problem was eventually found in 1923 (although the project was not implemented until 1927/8), involving the drafting in of 170 chronic patients (120 males and 50 females), accommodated in separate "workers' pavilions", to perform the duties required by the establishment workshops.[79] These chronic patients brought the total number of patient workers to an average of 334 between 1929 and 1938, or *c.* 30% of all patients.

Had the Asile Clinique employed the MAT method of occupation, a much higher percentage of patients would have been employed, since Simon maintained that patients at the acute stage of their illness could be given work. However, while the numbers of employed patients would have increased, much of the work performed would not have been productive. Furthermore, the acute patients would have required careful supervision, taking staff away from other duties. Paradoxically therefore, it was financially more expedient to remain with the existing system of allocating work to fewer patients (the chronic and convalescent patients) who were capable of *productive* work.

Productivity was carefully monitored at both the Asile Clinique and at the Asile de la Sarthe. At the Asile Clinique, the work carried out in each of the workshops, which collectively employed 25–40% of the patient workforce, was monitored carefully, and the number of days worked by patients in each was recorded. The value of the work provided by the patients was evaluated and appeared in the asylum accounts as the *produit du travail des aliénés*, while the value of produce harvested from the market gardens and farm (cultivated using patient labour) was recorded as the *produits recoltés*. Interestingly, it was the asylum director who reported on patient work in the asylum annual reports, emphasising its administrative function, rather than its therapeutic value. At the Asile de la Sarthe, for example, frequent references were made to the 'profits' generated by the asylum bakery and by agricultural exploitation in the asylum director's annual reports, which were separate from those produced by the chief medical officer.[80] In 1920, the asylum director commented that the farm had given good results that year, saving the asylum 38,718F. The products, including bacon, eggs, chicken, fruit and vegetables, were all consumed on the premises, thereby benefiting the establishment, as well as the patients involved in their production.[81]

Staffing

The adoption of MAT required the co-operation of all members of the asylum staff; in French asylums this was rendered problematic by the dual management structure indicated above. Staff training and numbers also presented impediments to the introduction of MAT. Although workshop managers were responsible for supervising the patient workers assigned to their workshops, they lacked training in how to manage and respond to mentally ill patients. Demay observed in 1929 that workshop managers appeared unaware of the nature of mental illness and many showed neither kindness nor patience towards the patients working in their workshops.[82] Reporting to the asylum director, they were overly concerned with productivity and failed to prioritise the therapeutic, re-educative purpose of patient work. Patients were sometimes excluded from workshops for being disruptive, or too placid, or for showing a "lack of respect" for an employee. Demay recommended that each workshop manager should undergo a period of training in medical services.[83] The existing relationship between workshop managers and the medical team was an impediment to the institution of MAT.

Highly trained nursing staff were also required for the successful introduction of MAT, since, as Legrain and Demay highlighted in their 1934 report, the application of therapeutic work rested with the nurses.[84] Nurses needed to have the skills to motivate patients, to direct the activity of distracted or confused patients, to intervene if a patient became agitated and to modify the work according to how a patient was coping. They needed to be familiar with their patients' conditions, interests and capabilities, and able to handle them with patience and tact.[85] However, formal training in mental nursing was rare in France in the immediate aftermath of World War I. It was provided in some departments, including the Seine, where a mental nursing school had been established at Ste Anne's in 1882, but many departments, including La Sarthe, lacked a school.[86] As a result, the skills of French mental nurses compared unfavourably with those of their Dutch colleagues. After visiting the Dutch asylum Santpoort in 1928, French psychiatrist Paul Courbon observed that Dutch nurses regarded the profession as a vocation, rather than just a job, and they were recruited from a more highly educated and cultivated class than in France.[87] Nurses tended to be recruited from peasant or labouring stock and lacked a vocational calling to their profession.[88] In 1935, it was estimated that only 5% of the Seine's mental nurses held a certificate of primary education, and some were illiterate.[89] These comments did not augur well for the ability of Asile Clinique nurses to take on the additional responsibilities associated with MAT.

At the Asile de la Sarthe, the quantity of nurses was just as much an issue as their quality. In 1920 the Asile de la Sarthe director reported that they had barely enough staff to give nurses a rest day every week.[90] In 1933, the new chief medical officer, Dr Schutzenberger, highlighted that although "on paper" there might be an appropriate ratio of patients to nurses, in reality, the actual number of nurses was insufficient.[91] Nurses were often required to be somewhere other than the patients' quarters (such as delivering patients to the workshops), and days off and holidays had to be taken into consideration.[92] Despite a salary rise in 1920, few applicants were able to satisfy the asylum's requirements for nursing experience gained at other local hospitals or asylums. The introduction of the 40-hour week in 1937, requiring an increase in the number of male nurses from 46 to 125, compelled the Asile de la Sarthe to recruit individuals with no experience of nursing.[93] As a result, the chief medical officer Dr Christy, reported that he had been obliged to organise courses for all male nurses, including elementary instruction in anatomy, physiology and hygiene, since he could achieve little if his staff lacked any understanding of and had scant interest in their work.[94] These nurses were unlikely to have the time, knowledge or inclination to adapt to new, more intensive methods of patient occupation.

The Asile de la Sarthe also experienced difficulty recruiting junior medical staff. Until the mid-1930s, the chief medical officer had been the only medically qualified member of staff. Dr Schutzenberger highlighted that it was impossible for a single doctor to treat *c.* 850 patients without either a medical assistant or interns.[95] Le Mans was a small town without a university (at that time), which made the recruitment of interns difficult. Christy concluded that without interns, he could not offer his preferred modern treatments, particularly as he was also running courses for the male nursing staff.[96] Given the level of involvement expected of medical staff in the application of MAT, the prospect of its introduction at the Asile de la Sarthe was remote.

Conclusion

This chapter has argued that the voice of the French psychiatrists who advocated a new approach to patient occupation during the interwar period failed to be heard by the chief medical officers of asylums. This was in part to do with an adherence to an organicist interpretation of mental disorder by doctors who were anxious to augment their professional credentials by moving more closely towards mainstream medicine, specifically neurology. This approach, which favoured biological means of treating acute cases, was at odds with the psychotherapeutic method of MAT. Patient work continued to be considered beneficial for convalescent, incurable and chronic patients, as it had been since the nineteenth century, but biological treatments were prioritised for acute patients. Furthermore, any change to the status quo in terms of the supply of patient labour could have compromised its economic contribution to institutional running costs. This would have generated problems for asylum directors who were tasked with managing asylum budgets, which were particularly tight during the challenging financial climate in the aftermath of World War I and the Great Depression of the early 1930s. Chief medical officers were not in a position of sufficient authority to insist upon a wholly therapeutic rationale for patient work. Even if they had had this authority, issues related to staff quality and quantity, together with overcrowding and poor facilities, would have posed difficulties for the introduction of MAT. Inadequate training and low levels of educational attainment, coupled with a lack of commitment to caring for the mentally ill, meant that French mental nurses were ill-equipped to deliver MAT. Doctors were too few in number to devote sufficient time to the method. Workshop managers in the asylum service departments were too focused on productivity and a lack of space, due to overcrowding, precluded the installation of interior workshops. Together, these factors served to quash the voices of psychiatrists seeking to reform the organisation of patient work in French asylums. The patients' views about how they were occupied failed to come across. Reform of the asylum system begun tentatively just before the outbreak of World War II, and gathering pace after Liberation in 1945, eventually led to the introduction of occupational therapy in the 1950s.

Notes

1. Mark S. Micale, "The Psychiatric Body", in *Companion to Medicine in the Twentieth Century*, ed. Roger Cooter and John Pickstone (London: Routledge, 2000), 323–346, 323.
2. Waltraud Ernst, ed., *Work, Psychiatry and Society, c.1750–2015* (Manchester: Manchester University Press, 2016); Véronique Fau-Vincente, "Valeur du Travail au Troisième Section de l'Hôpital de Villejuif: Entre thérapie et instrument de discipline", *Savoirs, Politiques et Pratiques de l'exécution des peines en France au XXe siècle* (2014). http://criminocorpus.revues.org/2788. Accessed 15 April 2016; J.P. Arveiller and Clément Bonnet, *Au Travail, les activités productives dans le traitement et la vie du malade mental* (Toulouse: ERES, 1991); Jennifer Laws, "Crackpots and Basket-cases: A History of Therapeutic Work and Occupation", *History of the Human Sciences* no. 24 (2011): 65–81; Geoffrey Reaume, "Patients at Work: Insane Asylum Inmates' Labour in Ontario, 1841–1900", in *Mental Health in Canadian Society: Historical Perspectives*, eds James Moran and David Wright (Montreal: McGill Queen's University Press, 2006), 69–116; Jean-Pierre Goubert and Rémi Remondière, "Les Origines Historiques de l'Ergothérapie en France", *Revue Sociologique Santé* no. 20 (2004): 247–68.

3. Ministère de l'Intérieur, Bulletin Officiel sur le règlement intérieur des asiles d'aliénés, Circulaire No. 7, 20/03/1857, 57. www.gallica.bnf.fr. Accessed 13 March 2019.
4. Ian Dowbiggin, "Degeneration and Hereditarianism in French Mental Medicine 1840–90: Psychiatric Theory as Ideological Adaptation", in *The Anatomy of Madness: Essays in the History of Psychiatry*, ed. W.F. Bynum, Roy Porter and Michael Shepherd (London and New York: Tavistock Publications, 1985), 188–232, 210.
5. Ernst Abel, "Bénédict-Augustin Morel (1809–73)", in *American Journal of Psychiatry* 161, no. 12 (2004): 2185.
6. Jari Eloranta and Mark Harrison, "War and Disintegration, 1914–1950", in *The Cambridge Economic History of Modern Europe*, eds Stephen Broadberry and Kevin O'Rourke (Cambridge: Cambridge University Press, 2010), 133–55, 149.
7. Pierre-Cyril Hautcoeur, "Was the Great War a Watershed? The Economics of World War I in France", in *The Economics of World War I*, eds Stephen Broadberry and Mark Harrison (Cambridge: Cambridge University Press, 2005), 169–205, 199.
8. Archives de Paris (hereafter ADP) D.10K3/27/20, Louis Dausset, *Rapport Général au nom de la 3e Commission sur les propositions budgétaires pour le Service des Aliénés* (Paris: Conseil Général de la Seine, 1918), 27.
9. Ibid.
10. Ibid., 28.
11. Ibid., 43.
12. After serving on several professional commissions of the Superior Council of Public Hygiene, Raynier was appointed inspector general of administrative services for the Ministry of the Interior in 1935.
13. Beaudouin, a respected clinician, was Chief Medical Officer of the Maison Blanche asylum, 1926–55.
14. The importance of the work in the Raynier and Beaudouin volume has been highlighted by Michel Bénézech. See: Michel Bénézech, 2013. "Une Bible Oubliée de la pratique psychiatrie asilaire: Le Traité des docteurs Raynier et Beaudouin", in *Annales Médico-psychologiques* 171 no. 1 (2013): 51–3.
15. J. Raynier and H. Beaudouin, *L'Aliéné et les Asiles d'Aliénés au point de vue administratif et juridique, assistance et législation* (Paris: Librairie Le François, 1924), 313.
16. Ibid., 314.
17. Director of the Bel-Air Asylum in Geneva.
18. Chief Medical Officer of the Clermont Asylum in Clermont Ferrand, Oise.
19. C. Ladame and G. Demay, *La thérapeutique des maladies mentales par le travail* (Paris: Masson, 1926).

20. Ibid., 22.
21. Ibid.
22. Defined as a temporary or permanent loss of brain function causing incoherence that could affect people of all ages. See: Edward Shorter, *A Historical Dictionary of Psychiatry* (Oxford: Oxford University Press, 2005), 71–6.
23. Dementia praecox (*démence précose*) was first identified in 1860 by Morel as a form of hereditary dementia affecting teenagers; its classification was further developed by Emil Kraepelin in 1893. In 1908 it was then reclassified by Eugen Bleuler as schizophrenia, to include milder and broader categories. See: Shorter, *Historical Dictionary of Psychiatry*, 267–75.
24. Ladame and Demay, *La thérapeutique*, 24.
25. Ibid., 7.
26. Ibid.
27. The disciplinary and therapeutic aims of work for patients in the Third Section are the subject of research by Véronique Fau-Vincenti. See footnote (2) above.
28. Henri Colin, "Le Quartier de Sureté de Villejuif (Aliénés criminels, vicieux, difficiles, habitués des asiles)", *Annales Médico-psycholoique* (novembre 1912): 370–91, (décembre 1912): 540–8; (janvier 1913): 36–65, (février 1913): 170–7.
29. Colin, "Le Quartier de Sureté", *Annales Médico-psychologique* (février 1913): 171–2.
30. Delirium is defined as acute brain failure resulting in reduced awareness of the environment such as loss of orientation, confusion, hallucinations and irrational fears; chronic delirium refers to the condition when it has become entrenched. See: Shorter, *Historical Dictionary of Psychiatry*, 70–1.
31. M. Calmels, "Le Travail par petits ateliers à la troisième section de l'Asile de Villejuif", *Annales Médico-psychologique* (janvier 1927): 283.
32. Ibid., 283.
33. Dr Lautier, "Les Exagérations de la Thérapie par le Travail", *L'Hygiène Mentale* no. 2 (1929): 191.
34. G. Demay, "Les conditions de la thérapeutique par le travail dans les asiles", *L'Hygiène Mentale* no. 2 (1929): 33.
35. Ibid.
36. Ibid., 34.
37. Ibid.
38. Hermann Simon, "Active Therapy in the Lunatic Facility (1929)", in *From Madness to Mental Health: Psychiatric Disorder and Its Treatment in Western Civilisation*, ed. Greg Eghigian (New Brunswick: Rutgers University Press, 2010), 271–5, 272.
39. Ibid., 273.

40. Ibid.
41. P. Schiff, "Le movement d'hygiène mentale an Allemagne", *L'Hygiène Mentale* no. 8 (1929): 232–3.
42. Jacques Postel and Claude Quetel, *Nouvelle Histoire de la Psychiatrie* (Paris: Dunod, 2012), 350.
43. George Weisz, "Reform and Conflict in French Medical Education, 1870–1914", in *The Organisation of Science and Technology in France 1808–1914*, eds Robert Fox and George Weisz (Cambridge: Cambridge University Press, 1980), 61–94, 64–5.
44. Jan Goldstein, *Console and Classify: The French Psychiatric Profession in the Nineteenth Century* (Chicago and London: University of Chicago Press, 2001), 350; Paul Lerner, *Hysterical Men: War, Psychiatry and the Politics of Trauma in Germany, 1890–1930* (Ithaca, NY: Cornell University Press, 2003), 16.
45. Ibid.
46. Paul Courbon, "Un Voyage d'études dans les asiles en Hollande", *Annales Médico-psychologique* (février 1928): 289–306 and 385–405, 396.
47. Ibid., 397; A. Porot, "L'Assistance par le travail dans les asiles Hollandais", *L'Hygiène Mentale* no. 2 (1929) 41–54, 52.
48. Porot, "L'Assistance par le travail", 52.
49. Ibid.
50. Hermann Simon, "La Psychothérapie à l'Asile", *L'Hygiène Mentale* no. 1 (1933): 16–28, 21.
51. Ibid., 22.
52. Ibid.
53. Ibid., 23–5.
54. Ibid., 26.
55. Ibid.
56. Ibid., 27.
57. Ibid., 20.
58. Simon, "Active Therapy in the Lunatic Facility (1929)", 273.
59. These figures were gleaned from the Asile Clinique asylum directors' reports to the Paris prefecture 1921–39.
60. These figures were gleaned from the Asile de la Sarthe directors' reports to the Le Mans prefecture 1919–39.
61. Malaria therapy was introduced into French asylums between 1924 and 1932, but this was only for patients suffering from general paralysis of the insane (GPI), a condition associated with tertiary syphilis.
62. ADP/D.10K3/27/20, Dausset, *Rapport Général*, 1918, 26.
63. Porot, "L'assistance par le travail", 52.
64. Jean-Christophe Coffin, ""Misery and Revolution": The Organisation of French Psychiatry, 1900–1980", in *Psychiatric Cultures Compared:*

Psychiatry and Mental Health Care in the Twentieth Century, Comparisons and Approaches, eds M. Gijswijt-Hofstra, H. Oosterhuis and J. Vijselaar (Amsterdam: Amsterdam University Press, 2005), 225–48, 227.

65. Harry W. Paul, *From Knowledge to Power: The Rise of the Science Empire in France 1860–1939* (Cambridge: Cambridge University Press, 1985), 2, 340.
66. Archives De La Sarthe (hereafter ADS) 1X964/5, Rapport du Médecin en Chef de l'Asile de la Sarthe (Le Mans: Préfecture de la Sarthe, 1935), 7.
67. Ibid.
68. ADS 1X964/5, Rapport du Médecin en Chef, 1937, 12.
69. Ibid.
70. J. Vié, "Le traitement des malades mentaux par le travail", *L'Aliéniste français* (janvier 1934): 589–98, 597.
71. Ibid., 596.
72. D.-M. Legrain et G. Demay, "Le Travail des Aliénés Convalescents", *L'Aliéniste français* (décembre 1936), 281–97, 283.
73. Ibid.
74. Courbon, "Un voyage d'études", 403; Porot, "L'Assistance par le travail", 50–1.
75. G. Demay, "Les conditions de la thérapeutique par le travail dans les asiles", *L'Hygiène Mentale* no. 2 (1929): 40.
76. Between 1924 and 1925 the maintenance costs rose by 11 million Francs and were set to rise by another 6.3 million in 1926.
77. ADP/D.10K3/38/83, Chausse, *Rapport Général*, 1925, 7.
78. ADP/D.10K3/38/75, François Latour, *Rapport au nom de la 6e Commission sur les comptes du directeur de l'Asile Clinique en 1924* (Paris: Conseil Général de la Seine, 1925), 20–1.
79. ADP/D1X3-44/6, Procès Verbal de la Visite de la Commission, 21–4 Avril 1923 (Paris: Commission de Surveillance des Asiles Publiques d'Aliénés de la Seine, 1923), 122.
80. By profits is meant the value of the produce (evaluated according to local market rates) minus the associated costs, including the wages of employees, such as the head gardener or bakery manager, the nominal amount paid to the working patients, raw materials such as seeds or flour, and other costs such as equipment, fertiliser, fencing etc.
81. ADS-1X964/5, Rapport du Directeur de l'Asile de la Sarthe (Le Mans: Préfecture de la Sarthe, 1920), [no page numbers].
82. Demay, "Les conditions", 37.
83. Ibid.
84. Legrain and Demay, "Le travail des aliénés convalescents", 283.
85. Ibid.
86. E. Jean-Louis and A. Valentine, "Un institut au coeur de l'histoire de la profession infirmière", in *L'Hôpital Sainte-Anne, Pionnier de la Psychiatrie*

et des neurosciences au coeur de Paris, eds S. Henry, C. Lavielle and F. Patenotte (Paris: Somogy Éditions d'Art, 2016), 170–1.
87. Courbon, "Un Voyage d'étude", 399.
88. Ibid.
89. Patrice Krzyzaniak, "Georges Daumézon (1912–1979): Un Camisard Psychiatre Et Pédagogue: Une Contribution Singuliere Aux Sciences De L'éducation" (Paris: Université Charles de Gaulles, 2018), 89.
90. ADS-1X964/5, Rapport du Directeur, 1920, 16.
91. ADS-1X261, Rapport du Médecin en Chef, 1933 [no page numbers].
92. Ibid.
93. ADS-1X964/5, Rapport du Médecin en Chef, 1937, 13.
94. Ibid.
95. ADS-1X261, Rapport du Médecin en Chef, 1933 [no page numbers].
96. ADS-1X964/5, Rapport du Médecin en Chef, 1937, 22.

CHAPTER 5

Distant Voices: Treatment of Mentally Ill Children at the Copenhagen University Hospital in Denmark, c. 1935–1976

Jennie Sejr Junghans

Introduction

While it is still possible to see the buildings of either desolate, repurposed or renovated psychiatric hospitals in many European locations, the materiality of the people who once lived, worked and died within these institutions is much more elusive. How can historians of today catch and convey the voices and experiences of those once residing there? And which voices, whose experiences is it even possible to access? Although medical records allow us to get a glimpse of what life at a mental institution of the past might have been like, the medical records present us with a number of methodological pitfalls. Medical records usually only contain material produced by employees of the institution and even when the record contains material produced by the patient itself—for example letters or

J. S. Junghans (✉)
European University Institute, Fiesole, Italy
e-mail: Jennie.Junghans@eui.eu

R. Ellis et al. (eds.), *Voices in the History of Madness*, Mental Health in Historical Perspective,
https://doi.org/10.1007/978-3-030-69559-0_5

drawings—it is often difficult to know under which circumstances it was obtained and why it was deemed important enough to be stored with the other documents of the record. However muffled or manipulated, the patient voices as they appear, seemingly at random, in medical records are the most direct way of accessing the experiences of psychiatric patients of the past, despite these concerns. Approached and interpreted with caution, these voices from below allow us to nuance our traditional understanding of mental institutions.

At the dawn of the twentieth century, mentally ill children and adolescents in Denmark were kept and treated at home, unless their illness was deemed severe in the sense that they posed a threat to themselves or the members of their household. These severe cases would be admitted to an ordinary mental hospital for adults, where treatment efforts were rarely adjusted in any specific way to the age of the child. Medical textbooks and articles dealing with the subject of mentally ill children were few and focused mainly on hereditary factors.[1] By the 1930s, this was slowly beginning to change and one of the most important signifiers of this change was the establishment of a small outpatient clinic for mentally ill children at the University Hospital in Copenhagen in 1935. The clinic was the very first of its kind in Denmark and would be the only one until 1946.[2] In 1944, the clinic was expanded with a bed-ward so that staff was able to conduct more thorough examinations and observations of the most severe cases.

While the history of psychiatry provides a rich and diverse historiography on general psychiatry, much less has been written on the development of child psychiatry.[3] In other related fields, for example childhood studies, history of psychoanalysis and institutional history, the story of mentally ill children and child psychiatry is also fragmented and sparse. Noteworthy examples of recent interest in the early history of mentally ill children and child psychiatry include Steven Taylor's excellent study of child insanity in England, 1845–1907, and the special issue of the French historical journal "*Revue d'histoire l'enfance "irrégulière"*" from 2016, edited by historians Samuel Boussion and Jean-Christophe Coffin, on the construction of child psychiatry as a medical specialty in the first half of the twentieth century.[4] Examining the medical records of over 700 children admitted to county asylums, Taylor focuses on how mentally ill children were identified and dealt with in and by the community, whereas the point of interest in Boussion & Coffins issue is the agendas and professional backgrounds of the participants of the first international child psychiatric conference in 1937. These studies highlight the fact that restrictive regulations concerning access to historical clinical material make it difficult—and in many countries—impossible to conduct studies of psychiatric practices after the start of the twentieth century. Therefore, existing research focuses either on earlier clinical practices or solely on theoretical developments. This is where the clinic at the Copenhagen University Hospital can address a gap in our understanding of the early history of child psychiatry. The archives from the clinic have not been previously examined, despite the fact that they are remarkably well-preserved and provide exceptional insight into the early practices and development of child psychiatry in Denmark. Because the clinic was located in Copenhagen, it is reasonable to assume that practices might have been somewhat similar to child psychiatric clinics in other European capitals at the time (for example, the child psychiatric clinic at the Maudsley Hospital in London (1923) or the child psychiatric clinic at the Oslo University Hospital (1950).)

The current chapter is based on the preliminary studies of over 200 medical records from the clinic, produced in the period from 1935 to 1976. Even though the amount of information in each medical record varies significantly, the medical records as a whole contain an abundance of unique information: case-notes describing the child's milieu, the behaviour of the child leading to the consultation at the clinic and the psychiatric staff's assessment and proposed treatment of the child, along with results of various physical examinations and cognitive tests, photographs, drawings, personal letters and administrative documents of different sorts. To protect and respect the identities of the patients and their relatives, names and other identifying details have been changed in present chapter. The medical records have been selected by birth date and selected to provide a random sample of admittances; therefore, only children with birthdays on the 1st–5th of April and 1st–5th of October were chosen.

Even though the medical records from the clinic at the Copenhagen University Hospital do contain written material produced by the admitted children themselves, the documents do not grant any unmediated access to the voices and experiences of the admitted children. Handwritten letters, drawings and photographs tend to present themselves as neutral, direct ways to access the personal voices of the portrayed individuals, but especially in the case of children under psychiatric scrutiny, we should approach our subjects and their voices with sound scepticism. The voices of child psychiatric patients are muffled at best, because children are more vulnerable than adult patients to various forms of manipulation or coercion and because children are less rhetorically skilled. Thus, in the present chapter, the voices and experiences of the children entering the clinic at the Copenhagen University Hospital will be interpreted bearing this in mind.

At its opening in 1935, the child psychiatric clinic was placed as an extension of the newly built psychiatric ward for adults. According to the written memoirs of Kai Tolstrup, who became the first Danish professor of child psychiatry, the ward had been nicknamed "Iceland" ("Island") by 1944, signalling how employees at the Copenhagen University Hospital thought of it as something strange and distant.[5] The vision of the clinic's first leading physician, August Wimmer, had however been to establish the mental health of children and adolescents as an important medical field in its own right and a field in urgent need of professional attention and resources. Drawing mainly on German and French medical literature, Wimmer had made this point clear in the first Danish child psychiatric textbook, "Degenerated Children" ("Degenererede Børn") in 1909. In the book he had argued that in most cases, the deviant and difficult behaviours of children and adolescents were not caused by bad morals but by a medically sick and malfunctioning nervous system. While Wimmer's understanding of the causes of mental disturbances in children was heavily influenced by explicit and complicated notions on heredity (prevalent not only in Danish, but in most Western psychiatry at the time), his reframing of children's behavioural problems as physical problems included both medical and pedagogical treatment. Thus, even though Wimmer repeatedly noted that heredity was the most determining factor in children's mental health, he did admit that the relationship between heredity and environment was complicated and unclear.[6] By the late 1930s, discussions on the determinant role of heredity in relation to mental illness (and various forms of deviant behaviour) were heated and some psychiatrists even suggested that the very popular diagnosis of 'psychopathy' was without adequate scientific grounding and had been used too uncritically, especially with children and adolescents.[7] Thus, when the child psychiatric clinic opened at the Copenhagen University Hospital in 1935, the scientific basis for child psychiatry as a medical discipline was uncertain and controversial.

Admission

When studying the medical records, it is unclear how strict access to assessment at the clinic was. The vast majority of the admitted children lived at home with their parents and the parents would consult a physician when concerned with their child's behaviour, who would then make a referral to the clinic. However, in a substantial number of cases, a teacher at the child's school or a neighbour expressed concern over the child's behaviour and encouraged the child's parents to seek professional help. When a child had been referred to the child psychiatric clinic at the University Hospital, a letter would be sent to the child's parents stating the date and the time of the first consultation. Parents were requested to confirm the appointment via telephone or mail.

Although the majority of the patients had been referred through a GP, it seems it was—at least in the clinic's first couple of years—possible for parents to contact the clinic directly. The medical records contain a few small so-called consultation-cards stating that the clinic offered "guidance on nervous children" on Tuesdays between 8.30 and 9.30 am, which suggests that the clinic had an hourly open-consultation time where a prior appointment was not necessary. In the case of 11-year old Bjarne, his 13-year old sister brought him to the clinic in 1946 and even though they did not have an appointment, an examination was conducted. Bjarne and his sister brought a letter to the psychiatrist, where their mother asked the psychiatrist to examine Bjarne for dyslexia and regretted that she could not bring Bjarne herself. In the letter, Bjarne's mother also asked to be excused, because she was a single mother to five children and had not been able to take time off from her work as a launderer ("*strygerske*").[8] The fact that the clinic had a weekly hourly open-consultation time could suggest that demand was easily met; however, this does not seem plausible given the fact that the clinic was expanded with a bed-ward in 1944 and because long waiting times were mentioned in the records. Furthermore, the fact that a second child psychiatric clinic was established nearby at the Bispebjerg Hospital in 1958 points to an increased demand for child psychiatric expertise. Therefore, it seems more likely that the weekly hourly open-consultation time was an attempt at reaching parents with children who did not yet attend school.

Unlike Bjarne, most children were taken by one or both of their parents to the first consultation and this was the point where the staff would make their first impression of the child's mental difficulties. Inspired by

Austrian-American psychiatrist Leo Kanners textbook from 1935, the psychiatrist would ask the parent about the behaviour that had led the parents to seek professional help. (Leo Kanner was trained in pediatrics and psychiatry, and his textbook "Child Psychiatry", published for the first time in 1935, became the first internationally renowned textbook on the topic.) The complaints could be anything from bedwetting, hyperactivity or stealing to jealousy, temper tantrums or poor reading skills. Depending on the severity of the symptoms, the clinical examination of the child and the number of other patients at the ward, the staff would offer one of two options: if the symptoms were deemed acute and very serious, the child would be admitted to the bed-ward. Maybe not the same day, but as soon as a bed was available. This was only an option from 1944, when the bed-ward was established. (Prior to 1944, children and adolescents could not officially be admitted to any Danish mental hospital as these were not allowed to take in children, even though they did so anyway in a few rare, serious cases.) If the symptoms were deemed milder, the child and parent(s) were offered psychiatric consultations at regular intervals either at the clinic or over telephone. Due to the limited number of beds, most children were given the last option.

The medical case-notes reveal a fairly simple and consistent procedure whenever a child was brought to the clinic for the first consultation. First, parents would be questioned about the family medical history with regard to mental illness and deviant behaviour of any sort (alcoholism, criminality, sexuality, and more)—usually only siblings, parents and grandparents would be mentioned, but in more complicated cases, other family members could be mentioned as well. Second, parents would be asked to provide information on the child's previous medical history and temperament. In younger children, this would often focus on children's diseases and other physical influences (for example accidents where the child suffered a blow to the head or descriptions of the mother's pregnancy or the subsequent nursing period). Third, the child would be physically examined and be subject to a short conversation and a few tests focusing on cognitive abilities. Thus, the three elements central to the psychiatrist's assessment of the child's mental state and behaviour centred on family history, the child's medical history and an examination of the child's current physical and mental health in the consultation room.

This procedure did of course vary somewhat from case to case and would also become more detailed as the decades went on. Especially descriptions of the child's milieu became more important from the 1940s and onwards, where the case-notes show that assessing the mental capabilities, emotional life and socio-economic status of the parents became just as important as assessing the behaviour and mental state of the child. While this was not so pronounced in the 1930s and early 1940s, where ideas on heredity still lingered on in general psychiatry, it became more important in the post-war decades with the increasing influence of developmental psychology and a new emphasis on environmental factors. Thus, in the 1930s and early 1940s, the case-notes would still place most emphasis on the medical history of the child's family (as this could reveal possible hereditary taint conceptualized as "degeneration") whereas later case-notes focus more narrowly on the child itself and its everyday environment. Generally, it seems as if the psychiatric staff managed to make the consultation room feel like a safe and confidential space where parents could—and would—often readily tell about their own personal lives. However, it is also clear from the case-notes that the staff often made some quite harsh assessments of the parents and a few parents are described as being aware of this and feeling uneasy or "nervous" in their contact with the psychiatric staff. This could be interpreted as reflecting the shift in emphasis from heredity to environment: whereas the notion that children carried their parents' hereditary taint did not leave much room for parental intervention, the notion that children could become mentally ill simply from being in an unhealthy environment implied significant responsibility.

Conflicts

In cases where the social and economic resources were limited, the amount of information that the psychiatrist and the other staff members were able to obtain from the parents was usually also limited. Thus, the psychiatrist often had less background information on which to draw his or her conclusions when assessing the child in these cases. However, with the majority of the children admitted to the psychiatric clinic, it was possible to obtain information from other authorities (for example, school-teachers, kindergarten teachers, local practitioners or physicians involved in previous hospital admittances) and the case-notes reveal that they were often contacted. It seems fair to assume that the staff at the clinic did so to get a more unbiased and diverse impression of the child's behaviour and milieu—not only because parents were unreliable witnesses at times, but also because a child could exhibit concerning behaviour at home, and act more or less normal at school, or vice versa. In cases where parents could only provide little information on their child's upbringing and home environment, these testimonies from external actors usually served as confirmation for the suspicion that the child's home was in some way compromised and to blame for the child's difficulties. Thus, in these cases, the voices of other authorities were given more weight and credibility than those of the parents.

Generally, the medical records only reveal few cases where psychiatrists at the clinic disagreed strongly with other official authorities in the child's environment. The various cognitive and mental tests performed at the assessment might show that the child's behaviour was caused by factors other than those identified by the school or the local practitioner, but this did not appear to lead to any controversies. It seems as if the psychiatrists at the clinic were perceived and respected as specialists and therefore that their assessments were accepted without much opposition from other authorities. This is also reflected in the fact that some children were referred to the clinic by school personnel and the like. Internal conflicts between professional groups at the clinic are plausible but not clearly visible in the medical records; various memoirs from individuals who worked as child psychiatrists at the time have asserted that teamwork was integral and this suggests that differing opinions were respected.

The cases that do show strong disagreement between the psychiatric staff at the clinic and other authorities in the child's environment occur in the medical records of the 1960s and 1970s. This can be explained with reference to two developments: one is that child psychiatry as a scientific specialty had undergone significant changes especially in the post-war decades. Whereas the idea of child psychiatry had seemed somewhat strange and obscure to the Danish medical community in the 1920s and 1930s, child psychiatry in the post-war era was understood as one of the key elements in producing mentally healthy and peaceful citizens in a democratic society.[9] Secondly, the larger number of conflicts between the psychiatric staff and other authorities can also be explained by the more sceptical attitudes towards psychiatry in general in the late 1960s and 1970s (the anti-psychiatric movement). Although its influence is subtler in the medical records, it can be traced more explicitly in the Danish child psychiatric textbooks and articles of the 1970s.[10]

While conflicts between the psychiatric staff and other authorities were few, there are more examples of conflicts and disagreements between the psychiatric staff and the child's parents. In the case of 9-year old Asta, admitted to the child psychiatric bed-ward in 1962, Asta's parents decided to take her home again after only two weeks. They believed Asta was feeling better already and they had not expected that she would have to be hospitalized for more than one month at maximum. Chief physician at the time, previously mentioned Tolstrup, attempted to explain to Asta's parents that she would have to stay for at least 2 months for the staff to complete their observations and tests, but Asta's parents refused. Consequently, Asta was discharged with no assessment of her mental state and no provisions for the future.[11] Why Asta's parents did not follow the advice from the psychiatric staff remains a mystery, as one would assume that Asta's parents had been informed about the duration and purpose of the admission beforehand. Unfortunately, the medical records do not reveal what information parents were given when consulting the clinic.

Despite the fact that there were relatively few direct conflicts between psychiatric staff and parents or other authorities, the child psychiatric consultation should be understood as a place of conflict: generally, in the sense that almost every child brought to the clinic was in some sort of conflict with his/her surroundings and had been deemed to need psychiatric assessment—and more specifically in the sense that the psychiatric staff sometimes had to act in the role of professional mediators. In the case of 4-year old Birte, first seen at the clinic in 1955, the conflict centred on the relationship between her parents who had gone through a messy divorce. The staff at the clinic had to function as a neutral authority advising the judge in the Copenhagen city court on which parent to grant parental custody over Birte. Therefore, Birte's medical record contains only little information on Birte herself, but mostly information on her parents' unhappy marriage and their new romantic relationships following the divorce. According to Birte's mother, domestic violence and infidelity caused the marriage to end—she left the home and moved in with a new man. According to Birte's father, the mother had always been hysteric and ill-tempered, and had not shown any interest in Birte in the last few weeks before she left the home. Birte had since lived alone with her father and when she was brought to a consultation at the clinic, the staff noticed that she was a "*tanned and healthy-looking girl, nicely and appropriately dressed, smiling, but cautious—though not shy.*" They also noted that Birte and her father seemed to have a "*very sweet, warm and natural relationship*". In the official letter to the judge, chief physician at the time, Jens Egsgaard, observed that both Birte's mother and father seemed nice and appealing, but recommended that custody was granted to Birte's father, because Birte seemed to have the closest relationship with him.[12]

Diagnostic Tools and Treatment

The clinic at the Copenhagen University Hospital never functioned as a treatment facility during the examined decades—despite the fact that the bed-ward was established in 1944. A child was seen or admitted in order to be observed, tested and diagnosed by psychiatric staff, not meant to stay for any actual treatment. Children who were seen in the clinic would rarely return and children admitted to the bed-ward were only meant to stay there for a limited period of time, usually no more than a few months. Children admitted to the bed-ward could not bring a parent with them, but parents were allowed weekly visits and allowed to take the child out for a few hours or home for the weekend or holidays (if they were able to do so). Depending on the child's diagnosis, the provisions after the first consultation or after the discharge could be anything from permanent transferral to an institution to a few regular visits to a psychologist. Even though treatment was not officially offered at the clinic, a few of the children did receive different kinds of medical treatment. In the case of 8-year old Ella, who was admitted to the ward because of epilepsy-like seizures in 1937, different kinds of epilepsy medication were part of her treatment during her stay and also after the discharge.[13] The 2-year old Erik admitted to the bed-ward in 1945 was treated with sleeping pills because he was extremely irritable, screaming, crying and so defiant that the staff had difficulties establishing any form of contact with him.[14] The 7-year old Martin, admitted to the bed-ward in 1959, was treated with the antipsychotic drugs, Chlorpromazine and Chlorprothixene, because he suffered from tantrums and extreme compulsive behavior, while seemingly not able to relate to or establish real contact with anyone around him.[15] Other children like Ella and Erik received similar kinds of sedative medication, but there are only few examples in the medical records from the child psychiatric clinic at the Copenhagen University Hospital of children receiving any of the new mood-altering medications appearing from the early 1950s and onwards (such as lithium, chlorpromazine, etc.) like Martin. While various forms of physical restraint were necessary at adult psychiatric wards, there is no mention of it being used at the child psychiatric ward. It seems fair to assume that when children were violent or very restless, they were expected to be easier for the adult staff to physically control and therefore the same array of physical restraints available at adult wards was not needed. Social and creative activities were also a part of the everyday life at the ward and to some extent also a part of the treatment. These included different kinds of crafting, drawing, playing theatre, playing with toys, social interaction with the other admitted children and staff, playing outside, supervised excursions outside the hospital, and more. The purpose of these was of course to keep the children occupied, but also to monitor progress and assess their social and cognitive abilities in various ways.

The kind of diagnoses that admitted children were likely to receive after their psychiatric assessment fluctuated heavily from the 1930s to the 1970s, which is not just because child psychiatry underwent great changes during the period but also because general psychiatry changed significantly. The most conspicuous change occurred in the 1940s, where the diagnoses of "degeneration" and "psychopathy", which had been very popular for children and adolescents in the previous decades,[16] were replaced by the much less controversial, but equally vague, diagnosis of "environmental influence" or "environmental flaws". Previously mentioned Danish child psychiatrist, Tolstrup, who started his medical career at the child psychiatric clinic at the Copenhagen University Hospital in the summer of 1944, compared this shift to a swinging pendulum in his memoirs from 2003. During his long career (he retired in 1990), Tolstrup claimed to have seen the pendulum swing back and forth a few times—from focus on heredity to focus on environment, and back again.[17] Although this imagery seems to be correct when examining Danish psychiatric records and medical textbooks, it does not explain why or how this shift should occur. If we look at the controversies haunting modern child psychiatric diagnoses like autism and ADHD,[18] it is clear that the pendulum keeps swinging back and forth, no doubt because it is still a very difficult task to determine the intricate relationship between nature and nurture.

Extracting any statistical information on the given diagnoses from the clinic is in theory possible, but time-consuming and also connected with a series of methodological pitfalls. On the front cover of the medical records, there is a section where the psychiatrist could state the suspected diagnosis and often did so. The problem is that sometimes several diagnoses would be stated and sometimes one or more would be followed by a question mark. Although this illustrates that an admitted child's condition and diagnosis were subject to ongoing review, it presents the historian with the methodological problem of knowing which of the stated diagnoses were seen to be the most important or the 'correct' one. A few of the medical records contain copies of discharge-papers where lengthier admittances are summarized and finished with the diagnosis given at the end of the stay; these also show that the diagnosis or diagnoses suspected at the first consultation were not always the diagnoses given at the discharge. Furthermore, as diagnoses and ideas on the causes of mental illness in children changed substantially in the period from the 1930s to the 1970s, not only titles but also content and meanings of the diagnoses changed. Thus, when examining the medical records from the Copenhagen University Hospital, statistics alone do not offer an accurate insight into how the diagnoses were constructed or used in the psychiatric practice. However, the records do reflect more subtle yet significant changes in discourse about psychiatry.

During the over forty years the clinic was in function, the number and kind of different methods and diagnostic tools available to the psychiatrists (and the other staff) changed drastically. The medical records demonstrate that a large array of technologies and methods were used over the years, that is, psychotherapy, photographs, drawings, play-therapy, various brain scans, and more. The diversity of these illustrate how the mind of the child was unknown territory that needed to be mapped and that the psychiatrists were open to new approaches. This resonates neatly with the few written memoirs of some of the first Danish child psychiatrists; for example, the memoirs of child psychiatrist Niels Hansen, who described the child psychiatric ward at Aarhus in Denmark as an "anarchistic place" where the staff was passionate, but also very occupied with their own specific theories and ideas so that heated discussions were rife at the staff meetings.[19] Whereas the medical records from the 1930s and 1940s contain less information and generally fewer tests and other documents, the records become more and more detailed from the late 1940s and onwards. This is of course linked to the increasing number of available tools and technologies, but also linked to the establishment of the bed-ward in 1944, as the medical case-notes on children who were observed for months at the bed-ward (instead of just being seen at one or a few consultations in the clinic), are very extensive. The most important purpose of the various tests was to help the psychiatric staff decide whether or not the child had any intelligence deficiency, which is why the Binet-Simon-test is the most common test in the medical records.[20] Other smaller tests focusing on language comprehension, morality, creativity and various other cognitive and emotional skills became increasingly common from the late 1940s and onwards, signalling that the psychiatrists sought to examine other mental skills than just those tied to intelligence. The purpose of brain scans was to clarify if there was any detectable physical cause for the abnormal behaviour of the child. Only rarely did these scans reveal something abnormal, and they were mainly used in cases where the child had had an accident of some sort or the symptoms indicated a neurological defect.

The purpose of the photographs in the medical records is a bit more puzzling. Only a small number of the medical records in the sample contain photographs and they are usually attached to the outside cover of the record. The photographs are not described or even mentioned at all in the medical case-notes, so it does not seem likely that they were given much diagnostic significance (which had been more common in the late nineteenth century). Therefore, the most plausible explanation for the photographs seems to be identification because it was only children who were admitted to the bed-ward who had their picture taken.

The use of psychotherapy, play-therapy and drawings is intimately linked to the increasing influence of psychoanalysis and developmental psychology from the 1950s and onwards. Whereas psychoanalysis only received little interest and support from Danish psychiatrists working on mentally ill adults before the Second World War,[21] the medical records from the child psychiatric clinic show that child psychiatrists were more willing to experiment and adopt new ideas. Along with a more informal and family-like atmosphere, physical facilities designed for children and an interdisciplinary group of staff, all these new methods and tools helped constitute child psychiatry as scientific discipline inherently different from that of adult psychiatry.

Distant Voices?

Even though the voices of psychiatric staff, various official authorities, parents and other relatives are the most dominant, the voices and experiences of the children themselves can be located in the medical records from the clinic at the Copenhagen University Hospital, from time to time, but only in small glimpses. The medical record of 14-year old Anne, who was admitted to the child psychiatric bed-ward in 1956 after a long and complicated period of disease, contains a few postcards and a short essay written by Anne. The postcards were written after Anne had been discharged from the clinic in 1957 and were addressed to a female member of staff, Mrs. Jensen, at her private address.[22] In the postcards, Anne thanked Mrs. Jensen for the attention in relation to her recent Christian confirmation, asked Mrs. Jensen to pass on her regards to the other patients at the ward, apologized for not having been able to attend some meetings at the clinic, and informed Mrs. Jensen that she was feeling well and was happy to be home again. Anne's essay was written while she was still hospitalized, probably in early 1957, but is undated. The essay is titled "My stay at the University Hospital" and like the medical case-notes, Anne describes that, during her stay at the hospital, she was moved back and forth from the adult psychiatric ward to the child psychiatric ward a few times. In the case-notes, the staff describe this as being necessary because Anne at times was too restless and violent in her behaviour to be kept in the children's ward.[23] (In the examined medical records there are no descriptions of children or adolescents being physically restrained, and the fact that Anne was kept in the adult ward implies that there were no means of physically restraining children at the child psychiatric ward.) In her essay, Anne herself explains that she was placed at the adult ward at her initial admittance to the hospital because she needed rest, but she describes being tied to the bed at night as frightful. Anne also describes receiving medication (pills) during her stay, but she does not mention this as being unpleasant. Anne also explains that she does not remember much from the periods where she was very ill and staying at the adult ward, so this could be related to the medication she received. On a more positive note, Anne describes that when she was feeling well enough, she was allowed to stay at the children's ward in the daytime, where activities included various kinds of crafting (woodwork and jewellery-making), trips to the city centre with the nurses and even trips to the cinema every now and then. It should also be mentioned that Anne clearly was one of the more privileged children at the children's ward because her parents had the resources to visit her twice a week; she also describes various presents from her parents and excursions to the cinema and pastry shops. When writing the essay, Anne had stayed at the Copenhagen University Hospital for 4–5 months and she hoped to be able to go home for the Easter holidays.[24]

In the case of 11-year old Eigil, admitted to the bed-ward in 1947, a few letters from Eigil to the staff has been preserved in his medical record. The letters were addressed to J. Koch, who were one of the physicians at the clinic. In one letter, Eigil writes that he misses Koch and that he is doing well at his boarding school. He finishes the letter by mentioning the names of no less than 15 staff members that he wants Koch to give his regards to. Eigil also wishes for Koch and the other mentioned staff to write to him, which indicates that Eigil had had a good relationship with the staff during his stay.[25]

That letters like Anne's and Eigil's are uncommon in the medical records does probably not mean that the admitted children and adolescents had a generally poor relationship with the staff during their stay at the ward but is more likely linked to the socio-economic resources at home and the child's age. Both Anne and Eigil were old enough to write, they were of normal intelligence and school-related problems had not been part of their illness, and they returned to resourceful environments after their stay at the Copenhagen University Hospital. Thus, even though the preserved written testimonies from children are few, they do give the impression of a warm and close relationship between the staff and the admitted children. Apart from written testimonies like those of Anne and Eigil, the drawings (made with crayons, pencils or pens) in many of the medical records is of course also a form of testimony or a concrete expression of the child's inner life, but contrary to written texts they are harder to interpret and the circumstances under which they were produced is unclear (i.e. to what extent were the children encouraged to draw?, Who decided which drawing to store in the medical record? and so on).

Of course, both written testimonies and drawings are dependent on the child having acquired and being able to exert very specific cognitive skills and fine motor skills. In the case of previously mentioned Martin, the staff noted that he usually repeated different fragments of sentences he had heard, but only rarely constructed and uttered his own sentences, which made it difficult for the staff (and Martin's parents) to know what was going on inside him.[26] The medical records contain other examples of children who because of young age, illness or mental difficulties of different kinds were not able to communicate properly, neither in writing nor in speech. In these cases, the voices of the children themselves are truly lost, and the voices of the psychiatric staff, the child's parents, and various authorities is all that is left.

Only very rarely do the medical records from the clinic at the Copenhagen University Hospital contain information on how life evolved for the children after their discharge. In those few cases, where a letter or a short note do reveal a little of the child's later life, it is usually because the staff at the clinic had been contacted by another psychiatric or medical institution and asked to provide information on the child's medical history. Other public authorities could also request information on former child psychiatric patients; in the case of 13-year old Jens, admitted to the clinic in 1957, a prison psychologist requested information on his stay, only a few years after his discharge from the child psychiatric ward.[27] Whether Jens was eventually released from prison or transferred to another kind of institution remains unknown, but the fact that the child psychiatric ward was contacted, suggests that his admittance did play a role in assessing to which extent he could be held accountable for his criminal actions as a young adult. Finally, in a few rare cases, pure chance also played a role: the last note of the case-notes of previously mentioned 14-year old Anne, states that a member of staff met Anne on her bicycle on a street near the Copenhagen University Hospital in the fall of 1961. The staff member noted that Anne looked "healthy and happy" and that Anne was training to become a medical secretary. Thus, had the medical record not contained a follow-up study from 1963, Anne's story would have ended on a positive note. When the clinic at the Copenhagen University Hospital started making follow-up-studies of their patients or how these were performed does not appear from the document in Anne's medical record. However, the follow-up on Anne's case revealed that her life after the discharge from the clinic in 1957 had been difficult because of several readmittances to various mental hospitals and because of her continuing struggle with the administered medication.

Concluding Remarks

Because much current research and literature on the history of psychiatry has focused on abuse, controversial scientific progress and lack of medical ethics, one almost expects to be shocked or saddened when approaching the early history of child psychiatry. In this sense, the medical records from the child psychiatric clinic at the Copenhagen University Hospital provide a surprisingly positive and more nuanced story. It is clear that Wimmer, his successors and the other staff members were moving into unknown and very contested territory when they began observing and diagnosing mentally disturbed children at the clinic in 1935, but also clear that they were very enthusiastic and radical in their approach. While state mental hospitals and other psychiatric institutions in Denmark at the time were quite conservative institutions, the child psychiatric clinic was a place of experimentation and a testing ground for new ideas. Although child psychiatry would not become an official medical specialty in Denmark before 1953, the establishment of the child psychiatric clinic at the Copenhagen University Hospital in 1935 marks the first important step towards the professionalization of child psychiatry. Even though the number of available medical records from the child psychiatric clinic at the Copenhagen University Hospital does not extend to later than 1976, there is no reason to believe that the clinic closed at that point. Because the Danish state's mental hospitals and clinics were reorganized in 1976, the clinic became part of a larger network of child psychiatric clinics in the county of Copenhagen and in the rest of Denmark. Thus, in 1976, child psychiatry was no longer an odd and controversial niche-topic but a psychiatric subfield seen as crucial in producing the mentally healthy and stable citizens of the future. This development of child psychiatry was of course part of a much larger orientation towards children's role in society as individuals and as scientific objects which had gained momentum in the early twentieth century. In searching for a faint echo of the voices of the child patients, this chapter has provided a closer look at Danish child psychiatric practices around the middle of the twentieth century, but hopefully it will be supplemented by many more studies in the near future as archival material become accessible.

Notes

1. Jennie Sejr Junghans, "*Mellem arv og miljø – Dansk børnepsykiatri 1891-1940*" (Unpublished MA-thesis, The University of Copenhagen, 2012).
2. In 1946, the Danish parliament decided that a second national child psychiatric facility should be built in relation to Risskov Psychiatric Hospital in Århus. Mentally ill children were treated as outpatients from the same year, but the new child psychiatric ward was not opened before 1958.
3. Neither the renowned late British historian of medicine, Roy Porter, mentioned children at all in his comprehensive body of work; nor so the American historian Edward Shorter in his acclaimed "*The History of Psychiatry: From the Era of the Asylum to the Age of Prozac*" from 1997.
4. Steven J. Taylor, *Child insanity in England 1845–1907*. (London: Palgrave Macmillan 2017). Samuel Boussion & Jean-Christophe Coffin (eds.), "Le psychiatrie, l'enfant et L'État – Enjeux d'une spécialité en construction, 1900–1950" in *Revue d'histoire l'enfance "irrégulière*, 18:2016.
5. Per Hove Thomsen (ed.), *Børne- og ungdomspsykiatrien i Danmark gennem 50 år. Et jubilæumsskrift*, Børne- og Ungdomspsykiatrisk Selskab i Dannmark, 2003. (Anniversary publication.)

6. August Wimmer, *Degenererede Børn*, København: Gyldendalske Boghandel Nordisk Forlag 1909.
7. Jennie Sejr Junghans, "*Mellem arv og miljø – Dansk børnepsykiatri 1891–1940*" (Unpublished MA-thesis, The University of Copenhagen, 2012).
8. Box 4. P. 01.04.1935. Rigshospitalet, Børnepsykiatrisk Afdeling OB 1935–1976. (Case-material available at the Danish National Archives).
9. The importance of child psychiatry as a tool to prevent another world war and to create stable, peaceful citizens was emphasized at the second International Conference on Child Psychiatry held in London in 1947. See: Flugel, J.C. (ed.), *Proceedings of the international conference on Child Psychiatry 11th–14th August*. (London: H. K. Lewis & Co. Ltd. 1948). (My Ph.D. dissertation deals with this conference in more detail, but due to COVID-19-related circumstances, the completion was delayed, and therefore it was not possible to make more exact referencing at the time of finishing present chapter.)
10. See for example: Kai Tolstrup. *Sjæleligt syge børn*. (København: Munksgaard, 1972).
11. Box 4. V. 01.04.1952. Rigshospitalet, Børnepsykiatrisk Afdeling OB 1935–1976. (Case-material available at the Danish National Archives.)
12. Box 4. A. 01.04.1951. Rigshospitalet, Børnepsykiatrisk Afdeling OB 1935–1976. (Case-material available at the Danish National Archives.)
13. Box 16. I. 02.04.1928. Rigshospitalet, Børnepsykiatrisk Afdeling OB 1935–1976. (Case-material available at the Danish National Archives.)
14. Box 4. P. 01.04.1943. Rigshospitalet, Børnepsykiatrisk Afdeling OB 1935–1976. (Case-material available at the Danish National Archives.)
15. Box 36. B. 03.04.1952. (Rigshospitalet, Børnepsykiatrisk Afdeling OB 1935–1976. (Case-material available at the Danish National Archives.)
16. Jennie Sejr Junghans, "*Mellem arv og miljø – Dansk børnepsykiatri 1891–1940*" (Unpublished MA-thesis, The University of Copenhagen, 2012.)
17. Kai Tolstrup, "Børnepsykiatrien i Danmark i de første år – med nogle personlige erindringer" In *Børne- og ungdomspsykiatrien i Danmark gennem 50 år. Et jubilæumsskrift*, ed. Per Hove Thomsen, 4–7. Børne- og Ungdomspsykiatrisk Selskab i Danmark 2003. (Anniversary publication.)
18. See for example: Bonnie Evans. *The metamorphosis of autism – A history of child development in Britain*. (Manchester: Manchester University Press, 2017). Susan C. Hawthorne, *Accidental Intolerance: How we stigmatize ADHD and How We Can Stop*. (Oxford: Oxford University Press 2014). Matthew Smith, *Hyperactive – the Controversial History of ADHD*. (London: Reaktion Books, 2012).

19. Sven Hagen Madsen (ed.), *Børnepsykiatrien i Risskov gennem 50 år (1958–2008).* (Børne- og Ungdomspsykiatrisk Center, Risskov, 2008).
20. The Binet-Simon-test was invented by the French psychologist Alfred Binet and psychiatrist Théodore Simon in 1905. It was translated into Danish in 1930. Hansen, Carsten Rosenberg. 2010. 'Alfred Binet' in *Den Store Danske*, Gyldendal. Accessed the 6th of May 2018: http://denstoredanske.dk/index.php?sideId=47223.
21. Jette Møllerhøj. *På gyngende grund – Psykiatriens praksisser og institutionalisering i Danmark 1850–1920.* (Unpublished Ph.D.thesis, Institut for Folkesundhedsvidenskab, Københavns Universitet 2006). Ole Sylvester Jørgensen, "Børnepsykiatri" in *Den Store Danske*, Gyldendal 2009. Accessed the 6th of May 2018: http://denstoredanske.dk/index.php?sideId=53156.
22. Because Anne wrote to the staff member's private address, her name has been changed to ensure her privacy in this particular case.
23. Box 76. B. 05.10.1942. (Rigshospitalet, Børnepsykiatrisk Afdeling OB 1935–1976. (Case-material available at the Danish National Archives.)
24. Box 76. B. 05.10.1942. (Rigshospitalet, Børnepsykiatrisk Afdeling OB 1935–1976. (Case-material available at the Danish National Archives.)
25. Box 76. J. 05.10.1935. (Rigshospitalet, Børnepsykiatrisk Afdeling OB 1935–1976. (Case-material available at the Danish National Archives.)
26. Box 36. B. 03.04.1952. (Rigshospitalet, Børnepsykiatrisk Afdeling OB 1935–1976. (Case-material available at the Danish National Archives.)
27. Box 25. H. 02.10.1943. (Rigshospitalet, Børnepsykiatrisk Afdeling OB 1935–1976. (Case-material available at the Danish National Archives.)

PART II

Reconstructing Patient Perspectives

CHAPTER 6

Experiences of the Madhouse in England, 1650–1810

Leonard Smith

The profound influence exerted by Roy Porter in his call for greater focus on the patient's voice has been widely acknowledged by historians,[1] and has been cited by several contributors to this volume. One of Porter's other main historical missions was to underline the key significance of the 'long' eighteenth century in the history of psychiatry.[2] He powerfully highlighted the practices and practitioners that characterised a uniquely creative and productive era. One important aspect was his emphasis on the role and significance of the developing network of private madhouses. Building on the pioneering work of Richard Hunter and Ida Macalpine and of William Parry-Jones,[3] Porter showed that the 'trade in lunacy' produced a good deal more than the pursuit of profit based on unscrupulous exploitation of the miseries of madness. Whilst some madhouses did indeed fit such negative images, Porter illustrated the enlightened

L. Smith (✉)
Social Studies in Medicine, Institute of Applied Health Research, College of Medical and Dental Sciences, University of Birmingham, Birmingham, UK
e-mail: l.d.smith@bham.ac.uk

R. Ellis et al. (eds.), *Voices in the History of Madness*, Mental Health in Historical Perspective,
https://doi.org/10.1007/978-3-030-69559-0_6

approaches and crucial therapeutic contributions of several madhouse proprietors, particularly in the provinces.[4]

Since the publication of Porter's seminal *Mind Forg'd Manacles*, studies by Charlotte Mackenzie, Jonathan Andrews and Andrew Scull, Chris Philo, Akihito Suzuki and others have further expanded on our knowledge of eighteenth-century madhouse provision and of some key practitioners. These authors have largely reinforced Porter's nuanced representations of conditions and practices in private madhouses.[5] It is now clear that private madhouses were becoming an established part of the material and cultural landscape by the late seventeenth century, particularly in the Moorfields, Clerkenwell and Hoxton districts of London, but also in some provincial places.[6] The sector expanded steadily during the course of the eighteenth century. London's position as the main centre for private provision was consolidated, as the numbers of its madhouses multiplied and their geographical locations spread. The Chelsea area concentrated on custom from the higher social ranks, whilst some madhouses in Islington, Clapton, Bethnal Green and Hoxton also competed for a wealthy clientele.[7] Increasingly, however, a significant portion of the large north and east London establishments' business was focussed on providing basic care and containment for numerous pauper lunatics placed by parish overseers.[8] In the provinces, new madhouses opened in several places, with particular concentrations in the western and midland counties. Their clientele derived mainly from the middling classes, although paupers were a growing presence by the early nineteenth century.[9]

The other chapters in this section relate to more recent historical periods and draw upon diverse sources to ascertain patients' perspectives. Rory du Plessis makes use of casebooks and patient letters in his South African asylum study, whilst Tomas Vaiseta employs letters of complaint submitted to state authorities in Lithuania. In their exploration of the closure of an Indiana state hospital facility, Emily Beckman and her associates analyse the contents of a patient newsletter as well as oral evidence from former staff. Similarly, Verusca Calabria and colleagues utilise interviews with former patients and staff of hospitals around Nottingham to identify losses experienced in the shift to 'community care'. Such rich resources are clearly not available for a study covering a much earlier period, where explorations of individuals' perceptions are constrained by scant written source material. Nevertheless, Roy Porter deployed patient testimonies as far as possible, and literary historians like Allan Ingram have followed suit.[10] This chapter specifically considers the voices of individuals who experienced periods in private madhouses, deploying lesser-known sources alongside more familiar ones. These include biographies and autobiographies, polemical pamphlets, newspapers, legal papers and letters. Naturally, most of the authors emanated from the educated, literate middle classes, though their perspectives are no less valuable for that. It tended to be resentful or disgruntled people who produced narratives, normally critical of the madhouse, its proprietor, and those perceived as responsible for their confinement. However, that is not universally the case, and even within the writings of unwilling patients some more subtle attitudes can be discerned.

To the Madhouse

Surviving accounts of the processes of conveyance and admission almost inevitably emanate from people who harboured strong resentments about what had happened to them. Their experiences coloured initial impressions of the madhouse itself. For someone in a state of mental turmoil, the surrounding events could indeed be bewildering. An opaque decision-making process might be followed by a journey undertaken either under duress or by the use of subterfuge. One of the earliest known accounts is that of the Exeter nonconformist minister Reverend George Trosse, whose graphic moralistic recollections of his youthful excesses, descent into florid madness and sojourns in a madhouse in the 1650s were published in 1714, and have since been considered by several historians, including Ingram and Katharine Hodgkin.[11] Trosse's family, alarmed by his frightening delusions, hallucinations and 'miserable, distracted condition', sent for 'a Person dwelling in *Glastonbury*, who was esteem'd very skilful and successful in such Cases.' He 'engag'd to undertake the Cure, upon Condition that they would safely convey me to his House'. This required stern measures, which Trosse actively resisted:

> By their concurrent Strength they at length prevail'd against me … .They procured a *very stout strong Man* to ride before me; and when *he* was on Horseback, they by Force put me up behind *him*, bound me by a strong Linnen-Cloth to *him*; and, because I struggled, and did all I could to throw my self off the Horse, they tied my Legs under the Belly of it.

Thinking that he was 'making a Progress into the *Depths of HELL*', he struggled continually until they reached 'the *Physician's* House' in Glastonbury.[12]

The theologian Alexander Cruden's writings have also attracted interest from historians of mental health.[13] Cruden strongly deprecated the means by which he was twice taken to madhouses. On the first occasion, in 1738, he claimed that he was 'decoy'd' into a hackney coach on the pretext of a ride to country lodgings in Bow, but was instead taken against his will to Matthew Wright's Bethnal Green madhouse. On arrival, he was immediately locked up in a room and was 'at first much dejected'.[14] Some force was used against Cruden when he was again committed in 1753. He related how, following his involvement in an altercation, he was tied up for a prolonged period, after which the Chelsea madhouse proprietor Peter Inskip and a keeper Joseph Woodland 'came at five o'clock in the morning, and violently seized the *Corrector* in his bed, and clothed him in a *Strait-Wastecoat*, to which he made no resistance'. Cruden insisted on saying his prayers before departing, 'and afterwards went with them without any reluctance or disturbance'. A coach was waiting nearby and Cruden was once more advised that he was going to 'country lodgings', though this time he was fully aware of the likely destination.[15]

Complaints of having been 'decoyed' recurred regularly, particularly in cases involving alleged wrongful confinement. In 1745, the family of Edward Goldney, a Bristol haberdasher, questioned his sanity after an incautious one hundred guineas wager on a horse race from Chippenham to London. According to him, a man was sent 'to Decoy and Invite Mr Goldney from London to Bristol under Pretence that some Merchandise was then lately arrived which Mr Goldney had an Opportunity of Purchasing upon very advantageous Terms.' As they neared Bristol, the man persuaded Goldney to take a small detour in order to collect some money from a house, and 'by this means betrayed him' into Joseph Mason's madhouse at Stapleton.[16] Conspiracy and subterfuge were also alleged by Samuel Bruckshaw, a deranged Lincolnshire woolstapler, whose protest narratives have received some historical attention.[17] In 1770, his erratic, flamboyant behaviours were causing great concern both to business associates and his family in Cheshire. Following a confusing train of events in Stamford, Bruckshaw related how he was taken forcibly from the town hall, placed in a garret above the local jailer's house and held there for several days.[18] Eventually John Wilson and his son, the proprietors of a madhouse at Scout Mill near Ashton-Under-Lyne, arrived. With the assistance of several local men, they 'seized me, threw me upon the bed, *clapped irons on my hands and legs*, and dragged me into a chaise'.[19] The journey to Scout Mill took two days, involving several changes of chaise and overnight stops in Newark and Sheffield. Much of that time, according to Bruckshaw, he was kept in leg irons and handcuffs, or chained to a bed-post.[20]

Richard Meux junior, a very troubled member of a prominent London brewing family, endured several admissions between 1806 and 1809. On the first occasion he was taken from the Fleet debtors' prison and 'forced in a strait-waistcoat by two persons in the employ of Mr Warburton of Whitmore House' in Hoxton, then placed in lodgings under Warburton's supervision, from whence a Commission of Lunacy was taken out against him. Nevertheless, Meux subsequently managed to get home and resisted an attempt by Warburton's men to effect his return. This only achieved temporary respite, for '(a) few days after I was stopt by them in the Street; drag'd into a Coffee House I used to frequent in Holborn; the straight waistcoat forced on me … and I was again taken back to Kingsland Road'. He was then allowed home for a period but finally, in April 1807, 'I was forced from my own House in a straight waistcoat by the servants of Mr Warburton and taken to his Madhouse'. Meux's delusional insanity had complicated a family dispute regarding control of the brewery. For his part, he believed himself perfectly sane and that his troubles arose from his wife having prostituted herself to his brothers and other named people, including the portrait painter Sir William Beechey, and that his father and brothers had conspired to have him confined.[21]

Richard Meux was one of many madhouse inmates to express a strong sense of injustice regarding the circumstances leading to their confinement. The publican William Rogers spent fourteen months in three different madhouses in 1714–1715, including that of James Newton in Clerkenwell. He maintained that his committal was the consequence of a conspiracy between his adulterous wife, Newton and several others, and it happened even though 'he was in his right Senses, and all for being in a Passion with a Person, whom (like *Sampson*) he thought Plow'd with his Heifer'.[22] Samuel Bruckshaw described, at considerable length, the various conspiracies, collusions and quarrels that preceded his committal and insisted that, when 'imprisoned' at Scout Mill in 1770–1771, he was 'during the whole time perfectly sane'.[23]

Another who disputed imputations of insanity was the well-connected Warwickshire landowner and gentleman-architect Sanderson Miller, who designed County Hall in Warwick and Lord Lyttelton's Hagley Hall.[24] In 1759, he was sent to a madhouse in Hoxton under the care of Dr Meyer Schomberg, after he was 'seized with the Frenzy' and created a public spectacle in Warwick town centre. Miller nevertheless adamantly maintained that he 'never has been out of his Senses'.[25] He asserted that his confinement was the consequence of a conspiracy involving certain relatives and a Methodist servant, 'whose business was to set every Action of mine in a Mad and ridiculous light'. The 'scandalous behaviour of Dr Schomberg', abetted by 'the Methodists', had then kept him in the 'Inquisition' for several months.[26] Despite such protestations and his undoubted professional achievements, Miller was admitted several more times to madhouses, including those of Dr Francis Willis at Dunston and Michael Duffield in Chelsea, where he died in 1780.[27]

The millenarian self-proclaimed prophet Richard Brothers was extremely aggrieved about his committal to a madhouse. In the feverish political atmosphere of London in 1795, his well-attended public meetings, widely read pamphlets, and predictions of apocalyptic events led to his arrest for treasonable practices. Brothers' sanity was soon called into question and, following examination by two eminent physician mad-doctors, Thomas Monro and Samuel Foart Simmons, he was transferred to Simmons's Islington madhouse, Fisher House. Brothers maintained, among other things, that he was God's messenger and successor to King David, with a mission to lead the exiled Jews back to Israel.[28] He protested bitterly to the Prime Minister, William Pitt:

> all the insults I have received, all the industry that has been used to affix the imputation of lunacy on me, and to render void the revealed word of God … so far from thinking him a prophet, or even a man under any divine influence, that he was arrested as a traitor, and in three weeks after, without admitting the necessary evidence in his favour, surreptitiously condemned as a lunatic.

Brothers warned that government attempts to impede his mission, and 'a continuation of imprisonment and insult', would result in an earthquake causing the destruction of London, the death of thousands, and the fall of the British Empire.[29] Notwithstanding, or perhaps because of, his doom-laden threats and predictions, Brothers remained in Fisher House for eleven years.

In the Madhouse

Once inside the madhouse, patients' perceptions of the surroundings and physical conditions, the people among whom they were placed, and the manner of their treatment tended to be unfavourable, compounding any pre-existing resentments. The naval clerk and poet James Carkesse, confined in Dr Thomas Allen's Finsbury madhouse in the 1670s, described it as 'Where *Dungeon, Chains* and *Physick* me did wait, My Mad-suppos'd *Ambition* to abate'. He also had to put up with rats and mice in his cell.[30] William Rogers protested that, after being taken to James Newton's Clerkenwell madhouse in 1714, he was 'there kept in a sort of a Dungeon, stript of what he had, and iron'd and Chain'd down like a Malefactor'. He was then 'detain'd for several Months in a very miserable, starving and deplorable Condition'.[31] Samuel Bruckshaw related how, on arrival at Scout Mill in 1770, he was placed in a 'dark and dirty garret' known as the 'breaking-in garret', stripped of his clothes and chained to the bed. The windows were kept darkened in the day time, and there was no fire to provide warmth. He remained here for several months before being moved to a more comfortable room.[32]

In a widely publicised court case regarding alleged wrongful confinement and maltreatment at Robert Cope's madhouse in Bethnal Green in 1772,[33] one of the victims, Mrs Mills, graphically related her experiences. She was lured into a coach by a keeper named Gunston, on the pretext that her husband had been arrested and was being held at a public house in Shoreditch. However, she was taken direct to the madhouse. On protesting that she had been 'decoyed', Gunston 'threw her down and dragged her up the stone steps to the door by her legs'. Once inside, she was handcuffed and her hands fastened behind her back with a chain. When Mrs Mills asked Mrs Cope, the proprietor's wife, what sort of place it was, she responded that 'it is a place for mad bitches such as you' and 'declared she should soon have her hair cut off, and her head shaved and blistered'. Mrs Mills was later 'conducted up stairs into a little apartment', where the 'stench' was 'such as made her almost retch', and she was given 'rotten beef' to eat. She was released a few days later, after the outraged magistrates upheld charges against Mr Mills and the Copes.[34] The case, with the testimonies of Mrs Mills and another patient Mrs Ewbank, contributed to a growing public outcry against conditions and practices associated with private madhouses.

Alexander Cruden regarded most aspects of his madhouse sojourns with distaste, including the company. Three days after admission to the Bethnal Green madhouse, in 1739, he was 'much disturbed by the blasphemous cursing and swearing of a Patient in the publick Parlour, which made the place a resemblance of Hell'. Two days later, Cruden was 'the first time brought out of his room into the publick parlour among some of the Patients', but he strongly objected to being placed 'with such disagreeable company'.[35] He subsequently found some more congenial companions in the house, including a French army officer whom he nicknamed 'the Cornet'. Together with this man, Cruden sympathetically observed the people in the neighbouring madhouse, also belonging to Matthew Wright:

> The Cornet and the Prisoner walked up and down, and beheld with Grief the many miserable Objects in the *White-house*, a Sight exceeding disagreeable to any man of a compassionate disposition, there being about forty or fifty Patients, some of them at four or five shillings a week.[36]

The writer Mary Lamb, who was admitted on numerous occasions to madhouses in Islington and Hoxton from 1796 onwards, generally remained silent about her experiences. However, in offering advice to a close friend whose mother was mentally unwell, in 1805, she recalled sympathetically some of her own fellow patients, 'the many poor souls in the kind of desponding way she is in whom I have seen, came afresh into my mind, & all the mismanagement with which I have seen them treated'.[37]

Reverend Robert Hall, a highly intelligent but periodically deranged Baptist minister from Cambridge, who was confined in Thomas Arnold's Leicester madhouse for several weeks in 1804, felt himself adversely affected by the nature and behaviours of some of his fellow inmates. As he told his friend and biographer John Greene:

> Sir, they took away my watch, and confined me in a place which overlooked the ward in which were a number of pauper lunatics, practising all manner of ludicrous anticks. Sir, this night was enough to make me ten times worse; they were as mad as March hares. I was at times quite insensible.

His unhappiness was compounded by a 'lazy keeper' who fastened him down hand and foot in bed from five in the evening until eight the next morning. Hall acknowledged the severity of his own illness, but poignantly recounted his lucid intervals, alone and unable to move—'You cannot conceive of the horror of my situation, when I found myself perfectly sensible'.[38]

The mechanical restraint endured by Hall was an integral part of the treatment regime in many private madhouses and public lunatic hospitals during the seventeenth and eighteenth centuries.[39] It was certainly one of the aspects that patients commented upon, like Edward Trevor who was a son of the controversial Sir John Trevor, a prominent legal and political figure who became Master of the Rolls and Speaker of the House of Commons.[40] Edward claimed that, as a consequence of being 'Barbarously Misused' by his mother, he spent two periods totalling over six years in Mrs Woodford's madhouse near Moorfields, in London, between about 1675 and 1681. He described how, after his second admission, he was 'Chain'd to the Floor, and had only one Arm at liberty for a considerable time'.[41] Some years earlier, George Trosse had been subjected to various instruments of coercion when confined in the Glastonbury madhouse:

> All the while I was full of *Horrour, delusions, Blasphemy, &c*, and all attended with great Temptations to undo my self. Sometimes I continu'd in the Bed all the Day; Sometimes they put Bolts on my Hands and Fetters on my Feet, when I prov'd *violent* and *unruly* (which I often did); for I would often *strive* and *fight*, contending with my *utmost Strength*, to get away from them, and so to free myself from that Place, which I thought to have been *Hell* and from those Persons whom I thought to have been *Tormentors*.[42]

However, Trosse seemingly acknowledged that, in his case, the use of mechanical restraint had been justified.

Others were less accepting than Trosse. Edward Goldney complained that, following his arrival at Joseph Mason's Bristol madhouse in 1745, he was subjected to 'very rough and severe discipline', forcibly detained and kept in irons for several weeks.[43] Alexander Cruden denounced the various forms of restraint to which he was subjected. Soon after admission to Bethnal Green in 1739 he was chained to the bedstead by his leg. After two days he was put into a strait waistcoat, 'made of strong Tick, with long sleeves which came a great way below the ends of his Fingers', and his hands were tied together behind his back. Three days later he was additionally put into handcuffs. Cruden eventually escaped, with a chain fastened to the leg of the bedstead in his hand.[44] Samuel Bruckshaw was reportedly chained to the bed for a month at Scout Mill and then released, but, after criticising his 'cruel usage' and another patient's treatment, he was again chained up in a garret for several weeks.[45]

Allied to criticisms regarding the excessive use of restraint, there were allegations of actual physical assault. Edward Trevor claimed that, during his first period in Mrs Woodford's Moorfields madhouse, he was 'so Ill Used, that he had one of his Fore-Teeth broke out, by forcing things down his Throat'.[46] Alexander Cruden alleged that, at Wright's Bethnal Green madhouse in 1739, a keeper named Davis gave him 'a Blow on the Face, which almost beat out his Eye, and much disfigured his Face, of which he was not recovered for some weeks'. Although Davis apologised the following day, Cruden was far from mollified.[47] He allegedly endured more violence at Inskip's Chelsea madhouse in 1754, sustaining several beatings and a partial smothering, at the hands of various keepers and even Inskip himself.[48] Samuel Bruckshaw made various accusations regarding his time at Scout Mill. He asserted that the proprietor John Wilson had on one occasion lunged at him with a large knife, and on another Mrs Wilson had furiously threatened to hit him on the head with a poker if he repeated any complaints of ill-treatment to a visitor.[49]

The medical and surgical treatment received in madhouses provoked a certain amount of comment. Alexander Cruden noted, without making particular criticism, that he had received 'physick', vomits and been bled from the foot at Bethnal Green, in 1739, under the instructions of Dr James Monro.[50] At Chelsea, in 1754, Cruden was bled and purged on the prescriptions of his son Dr John Monro, without much protest, though he did resent being forcibly fed. On one occasion he and Monro 'conversed together in a very friendly manner', Cruden considering him to be 'a very valuable gentleman, of good capacity and genteel behaviour'. He even continued to take the 'purging draught' prescribed by Monro after escaping from the madhouse a few days later.[51] Others, however, were rather less complimentary about similar medical treatment. For example, Edward Goldney complained that, whilst at Joseph Mason's madhouse in 1745, Mason 'Drenched and Poured nauseous medicines down his Throat, frequently Vomiting Bleeding and Purging him'.[52]

One apparently common complaint among patients was that medicines or other drugs were surreptitiously hidden in their food. Honoria Lady Willoughby, who spent a period in James Newton's Clerkenwell madhouse, alleged in 1694 that 'I had poysonous powders given me unknown to me in my spoone meat to make me mad'.[53] The unfortunate Dorothea Fellowes, sister of a Norfolk landowner and MP, who was committed in

1791 to Dr Samuel Foart Simmons's Fisher House in Islington,[54] became increasingly convinced that she was being poisoned by drugs hidden in her food and drink.[55] She complained to the government in July 1799:

> my Butcher's Meat is Musted, Tarts are Musted, Puddens mix'd with something that makes them unwholsome. A variety of unwholsome Drugs in my milk, & unless I get a little Plain Water, I cannot get any that has not must, or something pernicious in it, as to make me ill.—The quantity of Food that is brought me, is sufficient; but the adulteration makes me fearful of eating it, the salmon particularly; so that I am starving as well as slow poison'd—[56]

However, despite her apprehensions, Dorothea's general physical health reportedly remained 'extremely good'.[57]

Richard Meux was another who made numerous complaints about his food and drink being adulterated with drugs. In 1806, when first in lodgings arranged by Thomas Warburton, he became convinced that laudanum 'was given to me in my porter', and that it was subsequently mixed with his food. He later decided that it was not laudanum, but 'some other medicine, which as I do not know the name of it, I can only describe to you as having the tendency to make me impotent'. After he was transferred into Whitmore House in Hoxton, 'medicine was almost daily given to me in my food'. He was later moved to Sir Jonathan Miles's Hoxton House, where medicines were again 'frequently mix'd with my food and forced down my throat'.[58] It is, of course, a distinct possibility that such complaints of food adulteration had some basis in reality, as a means to ensure that resistant patients took their medicines.

Perceptions of the Proprietor

Where there were active psychological, relational or spiritual aspects to treatment, these were normally undertaken by the madhouse proprietor or under his (or her) direction. Such methods were occasionally alluded to in patients' writings, usually with approbation. George Trosse recalled how Mrs Gollop, the proprietor of the Glastonbury madhouse, was of great assistance in his recovery. She was a deeply religious woman, who would pray each evening with the 'Family' in the madhouse: 'She had great Compassion upon me; would many times sit and discourse with me; would give me good Directions, and offer me considerable Encouragements.' However, 'all was, for some Time, lost upon me, who understood *little* or *nothing* of what was said to me'. Eventually, however, Mrs Gollop became influential in bringing about Trosse's 'Conversion'. As his reason returned, assisted by '*Physick*, a *low Diet* and *hard Keeping*', he turned more to religion and regularly prayed with 'the Gentlewoman in her Family'.[59]

Christian spiritual counselling also proved to be of great value for the poet William Cowper, who spent from December 1763 until June 1765 in Dr Nathaniel Cotton's madhouse at St Albans. He arrived in a tormented, suicidal state, which persisted for several months before his condition began to improve.[60] Cowper attributed much of his recovery to Cotton's close observation, supervision and empathic counselling.[61] He elaborated in a letter to his cousin Lady Hesketh, a month after leaving St Albans:

> I was not only treated by him with the greatest tenderness while I was ill, and attended with the utmost diligence, but when my reason was restored to me, and I had so much need of a religious friend to converse with, to whom I could open my mind on the subject without reserve, I could have hardly found a fitter person for the purpose ... The doctor was as ready to administer relief to me in this article likewise, and as well qualified to do it, as in that, which was more immediately his province.[62]

Interestingly, and in contrast to the common tendency to denigrate the subordinate staff of madhouses, Cowper also gave much credit to his devoted keeper, Sam Roberts, who left the house with him and remained as his personal servant for many years.[63] For Cowper, Cotton's madhouse was nothing less than 'the place of my second nativity'.[64]

Even Alexander Cruden had some positive things to say about the madhouse proprietors he encountered, and their wives. He conceded that, after two weeks in the Bethnal Green madhouse in 1738, he was taken next door to the White House, where he was 'civilly received by *Wright* and his Wife, which Change in their Carriage made him somewhat astonished', especially as Wright 'carried him into the Garden, and gave him a book to read in his parlour, a paraphrase of the Gospels and Epistles', and Mrs Wright 'shewed him several books'.[65] In 1754, whilst at Peter Inskip's Chelsea madhouse, Cruden observed that Mrs Inskip 'seemed to be a sensible woman'. She allowed him to walk in the garden, 'where he diverted himself with her youngest child, a girl of about a year and a half old, drawing her up and down the walk in her wheeled chair for a great while'.[66] As he recovered, he was allowed regular walks in the gardens and the surrounding area, and dined in the parlour with Mr and Mrs Inskip and other selected patients.[67] Generally, however, Cruden's views on the proprietors were much less positive. He spoke of Mrs Wright's '*wheedling Pretences*', and derided her and Mr Wright for being motivated by 'an insatiable thirst after Money'.[68] As for Peter Inskip, his involvement in Cruden's alleged violent maltreatment revealed him as 'barbarous' and guilty of 'cowardice'.[69]

Several other reluctant patients expressed less than complimentary views regarding the madhouse proprietor. In 1694, Lady Willoughby described James Newton's madhouse as the 'English Inquesistion'. She claimed that murders were 'dun in ye house' and that the body of 'one old Gentlewoman Mrs Rockliff', who was 'beat to Death there', was buried 'in his Gardin at Clerkenwell, where was a heap of Earth at one End like such a place'.[70] Samuel Bruckshaw parodied the Yorkshire dialects and rough manners of John Wilson, his wife and son, construing them as ignorant upstarts who had risen from pauperism, took money under false pretences, and displayed outright cruelty.[71] When Reverend Robert Hall emerged from Thomas Arnold's Leicester madhouse in 1804, he 'looked pale and emaciated. His eye had lost its brilliancy, his spirits were broken by severity and harshness'. Although Hall did not blame Arnold directly for the treatment meted out by his 'lazy' keeper, he did resent the 'severity' to which he had been subjected. He made his family and friends promise that, in the event of a relapse, he would not be returned to Leicester.[72] When Hall did indeed relapse a few months later, an unsuccessful attempt was made to confine and care for him at home, before he was placed in Joseph Mason Cox's madhouse near Bristol. Here he gradually recovered under the 'mild and kind treatment practised by Dr. Cox at the Fish Ponds', subsequently referring in warm terms to 'the superiority of that institution'. Cox 'gave him some directions calculated to prevent a return of the complaint', which Hall adhered to, and he never experienced a major recurrence of his madness.[73]

One of the most outspokenly hostile critics was Richard Brothers, who published various attacks on Dr Samuel Foart Simmons, the co-proprietor of Fisher House. He accused Simmons of blatant self-interest in declaring him insane and incarcerating him in the madhouse where he had direct financial involvement.[74] Simmons was, he suggested, 'decrepid in his judgment', 'weak in his intellect', 'ruffian-like' in his behaviour, and guilty of 'arrogant treatment'.[75] Brothers lambasted his gentlemanly and professional pretensions, represented in his status as physician to St Luke's Hospital and his F.R.S.:

> A man, under the appellation of a Fellow of the Royal Society, may be as ignorant as a Goth, yet he will be looked upon as a Colossus of learning; he may be as unfeeling as a Vandal, yet he will be counted as humane as an Apostle. To complain against a man who is shielded by a fellowship, and so powerful by being physician to a charitable institution, would not only be useless, but actually I should be accused of fresh insanity to do it.[76]

Brothers' hostility did relent somewhat. In 1802 he wrote personally, as 'King of the Hebrews', to Simmons with a 'friendly disposition to do you a benefit'. He offered to 'save you from impending ruin … For die you must surely, unless I interpose by divine power to save you'. If Simmons would not release him, 'I am sure your house, business and property will go to ruin'.[77] However, the grim prophecies had little effect and Brothers was kept in the madhouse for some years longer.[78]

Conclusions

These disparate voices provide us with glimpses into the complex world of the late seventeenth- and eighteenth-century madhouse. The material cited illustrates that the authors were, alongside their troubled circumstances and psychological distress, in many respects intelligent, able people, well able to describe their situations, express their views and articulate their grievances. Although, in a few instances, they could acknowledge the benefits of the management and treatment they received, the general tenor was largely critical of the madhouse itself, the proprietor and those regarded as responsible for their committal and incarceration. There is a certain inevitability to this, as the more complimentary or acquiescent patients were far less likely to leave written records than those who were disgruntled or antagonistic. The more favourable perspectives of people like George Trosse and William Cowper were notable exceptions, and they contribute to the depiction of a more rounded view of the operation of these formative institutions.

From the various patient testimonies we learn more about the circumstances that led to people's committal to a madhouse, the means adopted to take them there, the physical conditions they might experience, the measures deployed to contain them, and the treatment methods applied. We also can appreciate something of the diverse attitudes, dispositions and approaches of the madhouse proprietors themselves. The distinct imbalances of power between patients, albeit educated, wealthy or aristocratic, and even the most enlightened of proprietors are clearly confirmed. As is still the case to this day, the patient voice reveals the institution as a locus of control as well as care, of containment as well as therapy, and of resentment as well as appreciation.

Notes

1. Roy Porter, 'The Patient's View: Doing Medical History From Below', *Theory and Society* 14, no.2, March 1985, 175–198; Alexandra Bacopoulos-Viau and Aude Fauvel, 'The Patient's Turn: Roy Porter and Psychiatry's Tales, Thirty Years On', *Medical History* 60, no.1, January 2016, 1–18.
2. Roy Porter, *Mind Forg'd Manacles: A History of Madness in England From the Restoration to the Regency* (London: Athlone, 1987).
3. Richard Hunter and Ida Macalpine, *Three Hundred Years of Psychiatry 1535–1860* (London: Oxford University Press, 1963); William Ll. Parry-Jones, *The Trade in Lunacy: Private Madhouses in England in the Eighteenth and Nineteenth Centuries* (London: Routeldge and Kegan Paul, 1972).
4. Porter, *Mind Forg'd Manacles*, 175, 206–222; Roy Porter, 'Was There a Moral Therapy in Eighteenth-Century Psychiatry?', *Lychnos*, 1981–1982, 12–26; Roy Porter, 'In the Eighteenth Century Were English Lunatic Asylums Total Institutions?', *Ego: Bulletin of the Department of Psychiatry, Guy's Hospital*, Spring 1983, 12–34; Roy Porter, 'Madness and Its Institutions', in Andrew Wear (ed), *Medicine in Society: Historical Essays* (Cambridge: Cambridge University Press, 1992), 277–301; Roy Porter, 'Shaping Psychiatric Knowledge: The Role of the Asylum', in Porter (ed), *Medicine in the Enlightenment* (Amsterdam: Rodopi, 1995), 255–273.
5. Charlotte Mackenzie, *Psychiatry for the Rich: A History of Ticehurst Private Asylum* (London: Routledge, 1992, 2013); Jonathan Andrews and Andrew Scull, *Undertaker of the Mind: John Monro and Mad-Doctoring in Eighteenth-Century England* (Berkeley and London: University of California Press, 2001); Jonathan Andrews and Andrew Scull, *Customers and Patrons of the Mad-Trade: The Management of Lunacy in Eighteenth-Century London* (Berkeley and London: University of California Press, 2003); Chris Philo, *A Geographical History of Institutional Provision for the Insane From Medieval Times to the 1860s in England and Wales: The Space Reserved for Insanity* (Lampeter and New York, 2004), ch.5; Akihito Suzuki, 'The Household and the Care of Lunatics in Eighteenth-Century London', in Peregrine Horden and Richard Smith (eds), *The Locus of Care: Families, Communities, Institutions and the Provision of Welfare Since Antiquity* (London: Routledge, 1998); Peter Carpenter, 'Thomas Arnold: A Provincial Psychiatrist in Georgian England', *Medical History* 33, 1989,

199–216; L.D. Smith, 'Eighteenth-Century Madhouse Practice: The Prouds of Bilston', *History of Psychiatry* 3, 1992, 45–52; Leonard Smith, '"God Grant it May Do Good Two All": the Madhouse Practice of Joseph Mason, 1738–79', *History of Psychiatry* 27, 2016, 208–219; Leonard Smith and Timothy Peters, 'Details on the Establishment of Doctor Willis, For the Cure of Lunatics (1796)', Classic Text No.111, *History of Psychiatry* 28, 2017, 365–377.

6. Parry-Jones, *The Trade in Lunacy*, 7–9; Philo, *A Geographical History*, 309–312; Leonard Smith, *Private Madhouses in England: Commercialised Care for the Insane* (Palgrave Macmillan, Cham, Switzerland, 2020), 19–36.
7. Philo, *A Geographical History*, 322–325, 340–345; Andrews and Scull, *Undertaker of the Mind*, 153–189; Smith, *Private Madhouses in England*, 47–57, 92–99.
8. Elaine Murphy, 'Mad Farming in the Metropolis. Part 1: A Significant Service Industry in East London', *History of Psychiatry* 12, 2001, 245–282.
9. Philo, *A Geographical History*, 325–348; Smith, *Private Madhouses in England*, 103–114, 144–145.
10. Porter, *Mind Forg'd Manacles*, 261–270; Allan Ingram (ed), *Voices of Madness: Four Pamphlets 1683–1796* (Stroud: Sutton, 1997); Allan Ingram, *Patterns of Madness in the Eighteenth Century: A Reader* (Liverpool: Liverpool University Press, 1998).
11. Ingram, *Voices of Madness*, 11–17; Katharine Hodgkin, *Madness in Seventeenth-Century Autobiography* (Basingstoke: Palgrave, 2007), 28–30, 52–53, 105–110, 113–117, 145–146, 152–153, 170–173.
12. J. Hallet (ed.), *The Life of the Reverend Mr Geo. Trosse, Late Minister of the Gospel in the City of Exon, Who Died January 11th, 1713, In the Eighty Second Year of His Age, Written by Himself, and Publish'd According to His Order* (London: Joseph Bliss, 1714), 53–55.
13. Ingram, *Patterns of Madness*, 93–97; Porter, *Mind Forg'd Manacles*, 149–150, 159, 262–263, 269–270; Andrews and Scull, *Undertaker of the Mind*, 93–116.
14. Alexander Cruden, *The London-Citizen Exceedingly Injured; Or a British Inquisition Display'd* (London: T. Cooper, 1739), 5.
15. Alexander Cruden, *The Adventures of Alexander the Corrector. Wherein is given an Account of his being unjustly sent to Chelsea,.... With An Account of the Chelsea-Academies, or the Private Places of Confinement of such as are supposed to be deprived of the Exercise of their Reason* (London: For the Author, 1754), 7–9.
16. Bristol Archives, Jefferies Collection, 44784/19, 169; H. Temple Phillips, 'The History of the Old Private Lunatic Asylum at Fishponds, Bristol 1740–1859' (University of Bristol, M.Sc Dissertation, 1973), 37–40; Smith, '"God Grant it May Do Good Two All"', 210.

17. Porter, *Mind Forg'd Manacles*, 260–262; Ingram, *Patterns of Madness*, 1998, 156–163; Ingram, *Voices of Madness*, 75–126; Dale Peterson (ed.), *A Mad People's History of Madness* (Pittsburgh: University of Pittsburgh Press, 1982), 57–73.
18. Samuel Bruckshaw, *One More Proof of the Iniquitous Abuses of Private Madhouses* (London: For the Author, 1774a), 15–36.
19. Ibid., 37–38.
20. Ibid., 38–42.
21. Royal College of Physicians Archives, RCP – LEGAC/ENV 391, 30 May 1809, Richard Meux to Sir Lucas Pepys and the Commissioners in Lunacy.
22. *A Full and True Account of the Whole Tryal, Examination, and Conviction of Dr. James Newton, Who Keeps the Mad House at Islinsston, for Violently Keeping and Misusing of William Rogers* (London: J. Benson, 1715), 1.
23. Bruckshaw, *One More Proof*, 15–27; Samuel Bruckshaw, *The Case, Petition and Address, of Samuel Bruckshaw, Who Suffered a Most Severe Imprisonment for Very Nearly a Whole Year, Loaded With Irons, Without Being Heard in His Defence, Nay Even Without Being Accused, and At Last Denied an Appeal to a Jury. Humbly Offered to the Perusal and Consideration of the Judicious and Humane Public* (London: 'Printed and Sold for the Sufferer', 1774), 9–17, 26.
24. Peter Leach, 'Miller, Sanderson (1716–1780), Architect', *Oxford Dictionary of National Biography* (henceforth *ODNB*), http://www.oxforddnb.com.ezproxyd.bham.ac.uk/view/article/37767, accessed 30/10/17; Lilian Dickins and Mary Stanton (eds), *An Eighteenth-Century Correspondence; Being the Letters of Deane Swift – Pitt – The Lytteltons and the Grenvilles ... to Sanderson Miller, Esq. of Radway* (London: John Murray, 1910), 2.
25. Warwickshire County Record Office, CR 611/725/9, 27 December 1759, Talbot to Newsham; CR 611/726/11, 1 July 1760.
26. William Hawkes (ed), *The Diaries of Sanderson Miller of Radway* (Stratford on Avon: Dugdale Society, XLI, 2005), 329, 372–374.
27. Hawkes, *The Diaries of Sanderson Miller*, 46, 328, 383; *Morning Post and Daily Advertiser*, 26 April 1780.
28. Clarke Garrett, *Respectable Folly; Millenarians and the French Revolution in France and England* (Baltimore and London: Johns Hopkins University Press, 1975), 181–205; E.P. Thompson, *The Making of the English Working Class* (London: Pelican, 1968), 127–129; John Barrell, *Imagining the King's Death; Figurative Treason, Fantasies of Regicide 1793–1796* (Oxford: Oxford University Press, 2000), 504–537; J.F.C. Harrison, *The Second Coming: Popular Millenarianism, 1780–1850* (London: Routledge and Kegan Paul, 1979), 57–85; Timothy C.F. Stunt, 'Brothers, Richard

(1757–1824), Self-Styled Prophet', *ODNB*, http://www.oxforddnb.com.ezproxye.bham.ac.uk/view/article/3573, accessed 30/10/17.

29. Richard Brothers, *Wrote in Confinement. An Exposition of the Trinity. With a Farther Elucidation of the Twelfth Chapter of Daniel: One Letter to the King: And Two to Mr Pitt, &C. By Richard Brothers, The Descendant of David, King of Israel, Who Will Be Revealed to the Hebrews as Their Prince, Deliverer and King* (London: 1796).
30. James Carkesse, *Lucida Intervalla: Containing Divers Miscellaneous Poems, Written at Finsbury and Bethlem by the Doctors Patient Extraordinary* (London, 1679), 6; Hunter and Macalpine, *Three Hundred Years of Psychiatry*, 214–215; Porter, *Mind Forg'd Manacles*, 97–98; Andrews and Scull, *Undertaker of the Mind*, 193, 203, 274–275.
31. *A Full and True Account*, 1.
32. Bruckshaw, *One More Proof*, 42–43; Bruckshaw, *The Case, Petition and Address*, 21.
33. *London Evening Post*, 7 April 1772; *Public Advertiser*, 9 April 1772; *Daily Advertiser*, 10, 18 April 1772; *Gentleman's Magazine* XLII, April 1772, 195–196.
34. *Gentleman's Magazine*, April 1772, 195; *The English Law Reports*, Vol. 98, King's Bench, Michaelmas term, 12 Geo 3, 1772, 'The King Against Coate, the Keeper of a Madhouse', 540–542.
35. Cruden, *The London-Citizen Exceedingly Injured*, 8–9.
36. Ibid., 13. The 'White House' catered primarily for pauper lunatics.
37. Susan Tyler Hitchcock, *Mad Mary Lamb; Lunacy and Murder in Literary London* (New York and London: W.W. Norton, 2005); Edwin Marrs Jr (ed), *The Letters of Charles and Mary Lamb*, Vol. II, *1801–1809* (Ithaca and London: Cornell University Press, 1976), 185–186, 9 November 1805, Mary Anne Lamb to Sarah Stoddart.
38. John Greene, *Reminiscences of the Rev. Robert Hall, A.M. Late of Bristol and Sketches of His Sermons Preached at Cambridge to 1806* (London: Frederick Westley and A.H. Davies, 1834), 47–48; Carpenter, Thomas Arnold', 211.
39. Porter, *Mind Forg'd Manacles*, 10, 124–126, 214–217; Jonathan Andrews, Asa Briggs, Roy Porter, Penny Tucker and Keir Waddington, *The History of Bethlem* (London: Routledge, 1997), 214–217, 423–431; Leonard Smith, *Lunatic Hospitals in Georgian England, 1750–1830* (London: Routledge, 2007), 156–163; Smith, *Private Madhouses in England*, 217–219.
40. Kathryn Ellis, 'Trevor, Sir John (c1637–1717), Judge and Speaker of the House of Commons', *ODNB*, http://www.oxforddnb.com.ezproxye.bham.ac.uk/view/article/27729, accessed 31/10/17.

41. Edward Trevor, *A Breif Account of the Severe Usage of Sir John Trevor to his Eldest Son* (c1705).
42. Hallet, *The Life of the Reverend Mr Geo. Trosse*, 55–56.
43. Bristol Archives, Jefferies Collection, 44784/19, 169.
44. Cruden, *The London-Citizen*, 6–9, 35–36.
45. Bruckshaw, *One More Proof*, 42–44; Bruckshaw, *The Case, Petition and Address*, 21–22.
46. Trevor, *A Breif Account.*
47. Cruden, *The London-Citizen*, 24–25.
48. Cruden, *The Adventures of Alexander the Corrector*, 12–13; Andrews and Scull, *Undertaker of the Mind*, 108–109.
49. Bruckshaw, *One More Proof*, 21–22.
50. Cruden, *The London-Citizen*, 7, 10, 12.
51. Cruden, *The Adventures*, 14, 17–19, 22; Andrews and Scull, *Undertaker of the Mind*, 108–111.
52. Bristol Archives, Jefferies Collection, 44784/19, 169.
53. Lancashire Archives, DDKE/HMC/892, 23 November 1694, Lady Willoughby to Roger Kenyon.
54. Huntingdonshire Archives, Fellows MSS, R32/7, 11 September 1791.
55. Norfolk County Record Office (henceforth CRO), FEL 656/554, 3 May 1799, Dorothea Fellowes to 'the Legislature'.
56. Norfolk CRO, FEL 656/554, 6 July 1799, Dorothea Fellowes to 'the Legislature'.
57. Norfolk CRO, FEL 656/554, 24 April 1800, Simmons to William Fellowes.
58. Royal College of Physicians Archives, RCP – LEGAC/ENV 391, 30 May 1809.
59. Hallet, *The Life of the Reverend Mr Geo. Trosse*, 58–59, 63; Hodgkin, *Madness in Seventeenth-Century Autobiography*, 107–109, 172.
60. William Cowper, *Memoir of the Early Life of William Cowper, Esq. Written By Himself. And Never Before Published. With An Appendix, Containing Some of Cowper's Religious Letters, and Other Interesting Documents, Illustrative of His Memoir* (London: R. Edwards, 1816), 60–72, 82; Porter, *Mind Forg'd Manacles*, 265–266; Ingram, *Patterns of Madness*, 137–142.
61. Cowper, *Memoir of the Early Life*, 73–74, 79–80; William Hayley, *The Life and Letters of William Cowper, Esq. With Remarks on Epistolatory Writers* (London: J. Johnson and Co., 1812), 96–98, 109–112 – 4 July 1765, Cowper to Lady Hesketh.
62. Hayley, *The Life and Letters of William Cowper*, 111–112.

63. Cowper, *Memoir of the Early Life*, 83–84; Hayley, *Life and Letters*, 105–106, 24 June 1765, Cowper to Joseph Hill; Parry-Jones, *The Trade in Lunacy*, 185.
64. Cowper, *Memoir*, 83.
65. Cruden, *The London-Citizen*, 12.
66. Cruden, *The Adventures*, 11–12.
67. Ibid., 14, 20–23.
68. Cruden, *The London-Citizen*, 12.
69. Cruden, *The Adventures*, 12–13.
70. Lancashire Archives, DDKE/HMC/892, 23 November 1694. James Newton was author of *The Complete Herbal* and noted for his botanic garden – Anita McConnell, 'Newton, James (1664–1750), Physician and Botanist', *ODNB*, http://www.oxforddnb.com.ezproxyd.bham.ac.uk/view/article/20060, accessed 1/11/17.
71. Bruckshaw, *One More Proof*, 38–40, 43–46.
72. Greene, *Reminiscences of the Rev. Robert Hall*, 45–49.
73. Ibid., 57–60.
74. Richard Brothers, *A Letter From Mr Brothers to Miss Cott, the Recorded Daughter of David, and Future Queen of the Hebrews, With an Address to the Members of His Britannic Majesty's Council, and Through Them to All Governments and People on Earth* (London: G. Riebau, 1798), vii. For Simmons see Smith, *Lunatic Hospitals in Georgian England*, 79–80, 91, 98–99.
75. Brothers, *A Letter From Mr Brothers to Miss Cott*, 14, 21, 23.
76. Ibid., 23.
77. *Copy of a Letter From Mr. Brothers, Who Will Be Revealed to the Hebrews, as Their King and Restorer to Dr Samuel Foart Simmons, M.D. Islington, Jan, the 28th, 1802* (London: A. Seale, 1802), 1–2.
78. Garrett, *Respectable Folly*, 197.

CHAPTER 7

"Tells his Story Quite Rationally and Collectedly": Examining the Casebooks of the Grahamstown Lunatic Asylum, 1890–1910, for Cases of Delusion Where Patients Voiced their Life Stories

Rory du Plessis

Roy Porter observed that "there is no more splendid cache of psychopathological material than the delusions recorded over the centuries by the insane".[1] A growing body of scholarship in the history of psychiatry has aimed to identify, explore, and analyse, both how the content of delusions reflects the sociocultural context and is a product of the beliefs of the time, and also how the content is influenced by a patient's gender and race.[2] While this scholarship has primarily focused on psychopathological content recorded in an asylum's casebooks, there is a dearth of research that examines the casebooks for content that relates to patients'

R. du Plessis (✉)
University of Pretoria, Pretoria, South Africa
e-mail: rory.duplessis@up.ac.za

R. Ellis et al. (eds.), *Voices in the History of Madness*, Mental Health in Historical Perspective,
https://doi.org/10.1007/978-3-030-69559-0_7

articulation of their life stories and personal accounts of institutionalisation.[3] In short, the research has focused on delusions as recorded from a medical perspective, rather than on the voice of the patient giving their own account of themselves. This chapter seeks to address the gap in understanding through an exploration of the casebooks of the Grahamstown Lunatic Asylum (GLA), South Africa, from 1890 to 1910, to identify and examine instances in which patients diagnosed as delusional articulated their life story and gave their personal accounts of institutionalisation.

As the chapter is primarily concerned with investigating the casebooks, it is important to underscore that a patient's life story, testimony, and confessions that are contained in the casebooks are mediated accounts of the patient's voice, in that they are "filtered" by an alienist's "diagnostic and therapeutic monoculars".[4] Even though the casebooks offer a mediated account of a patient's voice, for Hilary Marland they are "as close as historians can come to hearing the stories of [...] asylum patients":[5]

> given the rarity of patients' accounts, it could be argued that we would poorly serve the majority of nineteenth-century psychiatric patients [...] if their case histories were ignored, for we have little else to work with.[6]

To this end, this chapter does not claim to offer an authoritative and comprehensive account of the voice of any particular patient but aims to develop an awareness, an understanding, and a sense of the life stories of the patients.

The GLA (currently known as Fort England Hospital) was established in 1875 in Makhanda, formerly known as Grahamstown. The GLA was part of the Cape Colony's asylum network, which was underpinned by policies and practices of racial discrimination, in which black patients were segregated from white patients and received limited provisions, a severely reduced diet, and a regimen of physical labour in the guise of occupational therapy.[7] Dr Thomas Duncan Greenlees (1858–1929), a Scot who had previously worked in a number of British asylums, was appointed as the medical superintendent of the GLA from 1890 to 1907. During Greenlees's tenure, the asylum consisted of a heterogeneous patient body of different races, languages, nationalities, and genders, as well as different forms and stages of mental illness. By 1908, the GLA was reserved for white patients only. Thus, by broadly delimiting the study to the period of Greenlees's tenure, the chapter is able to include an examination of the life stories articulated by black subjects, which have largely been omitted from and silenced in the asylum's annual reports and scientific articles authored by Greenlees.[8]

The Life Stories and Testimonies of Sanity Given by the Patients

Steven J. Taylor provides useful context for this chapter's agenda in an examination of child insanity at five pauper lunatic asylums in England from 1845 to 1907, in which he highlights how the representation of the children in the admission documents is at odds with the way their behaviour was described in the asylum.[9] For example, "the children described as dangerous often did not display the same characteristics inside the asylum as those that featured on their certificates of insanity".[10] Although Taylor's article focused on children, the findings of his research can be seen as a call for scholars to consider the way an asylum's casebooks contain multiple representations of a patient:

> A reliance on diagnoses taken from Medical Certificates and asylum admission documents by scholars means that the experience of patients goes unnoticed [...]. Rather, the function of asylums must be evaluated using representations of patients prior to, during and after admission.[11]

The content of the GLA's casebooks that is derived from the medical certificates provides a record of a patient's delusions, formed by observations made by the certifying doctors. By following Taylor's advice and turning to the casebook entries for an investigation of a patient's stay at the GLA, it can be seen that there are several cases where there is a disjuncture between the way the medical certificates represented the patients as harbouring delusions and how they were portrayed in the asylum as being free from delusions. The following discussion seeks to explore these cases as a potentially rich site for explaining how the alienists of the GLA came to their findings through engaging with the testimonies of the patients. The admission interviews and the cross-examining conducted by the alienists can perhaps be regarded as a crucial moment, where the patient was presented with an opportunity to offer an account of their committal, their life story, and a personal testimony of the soundness of their mind.

In the casebooks for black patients, there are numerous cases where the certifying doctors—who were "almost always a white, male, British-trained doctor"[12]—declared a patient to be insane on the basis that they presented with a delusion; yet on the patient's admission to the asylum the alienist documented that they were no longer delusional but were considered to be sane. These cases fall into two main groups. In the first group, while the patients were under the influence of alcohol or were suffering from a severe fever, they made an outlandish claim or were struck by a passing delusion. Adesh was admitted to the asylum on 20 December 1892, with medical certificates exclusively citing delusions as evidence of psychopathology.[13] The certificates indicated that Adesh saw snakes and monkeys in the air, and that Satan was tempting him. From Adesh's first day at the asylum, Greenlees deemed him to be "perfectly rational", and he observed that he "expressed no delusions". By 30 December, Greenlees concluded that Adesh's bout of delusions and his attack of insanity was attributed "purely and simply to drink", and he proceeded to discharge him. The medical certificates for Keabetswe certified him to be insane on the grounds that he thought someone was going to cut off his head.[14] On admission to the asylum, Keabetswe admitted to "being off his head from drinking habits". Keabetswe showed no signs of insanity, and his discharge followed soon.

Henriette was represented in the medical certificates as restless, violent, and delusional.[15] Yet, on admission to the asylum on 4 December 1901, she was portrayed as calm and rational. She informed the alienists that she had been very ill and was unable to provide an account of the past two weeks. The alienists agreed that she was sane, and after receiving the testimony of two consulting doctors, Henriette was discharged from the asylum on 11 December 1901 as "not insane". Madalitso was said to have become maniacal and to have professed to be Christ.[16] On admission to the asylum, Dr Leslie—the assistant medical officer at the GLA from 1903 to 1907—indicated that Madalitso had no delusions, could "give a good account of himself", and was "bright and intelligent". Madalitso testified that his attack of insanity was the result of drink, and he was discharged after less than two weeks at the asylum.

The second group of patients were erroneously certified as insane as they were unable to correctly answer the questions posed by the certifying doctors. These patients lacked access to basic schooling and were illiterate, and were thus unable to pass the interrogations presented by the certifying doctors.[17] By way of example, an emaciated man in his early twenties, Dibata, came to the attention of the colonial authorities for being in a cadaverous condition while he wandered about in search of his father's house.[18] Dibata was brought before a doctor, who declared him to be delusional, as he "says he is centuries old". On Dibata's admission, Dr Adam—the assistant medical officer at the GLA from 1894 to 1896—diverged from the certifying doctor by claiming that Dibata expressed no delusions and answered questions in a rational manner. Dr Adam asserted that "I presume his ignorance regarding his age is solely due to the fact that his education has been so limited he has never been taught the value of figures". Dibata was discharged from the asylum, and as his father's whereabouts could still not be ascertained, he was admitted to the Chronic Sick Hospital, an institution that offered welfare support for destitute individuals.

The certifying doctors' representation of the black patients can be regarded as one of the "problematic effects" of using medical certificates derived from Britain,[19] which were

> designed to describe generic forms of insanity, divorced from particular social, economic, gender, race, and class contexts. [...] In a colonial context characterized by little understanding of or sympathy for colonized peoples, the medical certificates were an inevitably inaccurate portrayal of complex intersubjective situations.[20]

The medical certificates completed by the certifying doctors were not the only inaccurate representation of black subjects. In general, the Cape Colony's alienists knew very little about the lives of the black patients in their care, and this resulted in the casebooks having a paucity of entries, as well as very few details about the interactions of the alienists with the patients.[21] In this regard, the cases presented here are of significance, as they offer us a glimpse of the GLA's alienists engaging with a black patient's testimony, as well as an enquiry into the history of each case. By listening to the patients and engaging with their life story, it is possible to argue that the GLA's alienists accepted—albeit only in a minority of cases—black subjects to be "legitimate storyteller[s] about their own [lives]".[22]

The discussion has highlighted the cases where the content of the medical certificates did not correspond with the representation of the black subject who was admitted to the GLA. During the interviews and cross-examining conducted by the alienists, the black subject's speech, conversation, and thoughts were discerned to be devoid of delusions. It would, however, be erroneous to claim that the interviews and questioning done by the asylum's alienists was always able to instantly and conclusively discern patients who were sane from those who were insane. To cite a case in point, the medical certificates for Lindie portrayed an individual who was incoherent in her speech and was plagued by delusions of persecution.[23] Lindie, on admission to the asylum on 25 June 1903, was described by Greenlees as a "[s]tolid looking woman; talks silly at times". On 8 July, Greenlees testified to the Solicitor-General that Lindie "suffers from mania. Talked foolishly on admission". Yet, in the course of a few days, Lindie was described as quiet, rational, and free from delusions. On 24 July, Greenlees submitted a further report to the Solicitor-General that Lindie was "ready for discharge". Lindie was subsequently discharged as "Not Insane".

In the casebooks for white patients, the careless way in which the certifying doctors identified a patient as delusional is in stark contrast to the approach of the asylum's alienists. The casebooks reveal that the alienists deliberated over the statements presented by the patients, rather than summarily labelling them as delusional. Likewise, the alienists' decision to discharge a patient was based on acceptance of the testimony presented by the patient regarding their life story and mental health. Ruan entered the asylum with medical certificates that reported delusions of grandeur related to an inflated sense of his wealth and property.[24] In contrast to the picture of delusions presented in the certificates, on admission to the asylum Greenlees pronounced that Ruan gave a "connected and rational account of himself", and he did not believe that Ruan presented with any delusions. Even though Ruan informed Greenlees that Paul Kruger—the president of the South African Republic from 1883 to 1900—"is a relation and is willing to assist him with money", Greenlees responded by saying that it "may be true". In cases like that of Ruan, where Greenlees found himself unable to distinguish fact from fiction, he opted to resist labelling a patient's statement as delusional.[25] After less than a month since admission, Greenlees declared that Ruan "exhibited no further symptoms of insanity", and he was subsequently discharged.

The case of Sebastian also illustrates the hasty and injudicious manner in which medical doctors labelled an individual's thoughts as an expression of a delusion, and how this led to their rash decision to certify the individual as insane.[26] Sebastian's medical certificates are surprisingly brief, and they provide the following symptoms of insanity: "refusal to work—extravagant ideas as to his wealth and position". On admission to the asylum, the cross-examination conducted by the alienist indicated how he presented with no form of exaltation or delusion. Instead, the casebook contains comments on how he related his story "quite rationally and collectedly", and how he could "tell all his history and recent movements". Owing to the "insufficient evidence of insanity", he was deemed "not insane" and was discharged from the asylum.

Overall, the simplistic and sketchy representation of the patients by the certifying doctors may be indicative of their "rudimentary knowledge of insanity".[27] For Greenlees, an understanding of "psychological medicine" was not only evidenced in avoiding errors in the completion of the medical certificates,[28] but more fundamentally was demonstrated by recognising that insanity is an "extremely difficult thing to define".[29] Greenlees held that "insanity varies in its definition according to the individual concerned, the race to which the individual belongs, and the person who is attempting to make the definition".[30] Thus, only by examining an individual's "social and other surroundings" would it be possible to determine if they are sane or insane.[31]

Drawing on Greenlees's insights, it is reasonable to suggest that the certifying doctors did not seek to consider a patient's account of the context and circumstances of their committal, or to cross-examine whether a patient's speech and thoughts did present a bona fide delusion.[32] To substantiate by reviewing the cases for the black patients, if the certifying doctors had engaged with the life story of these patients, they would have understood that the observed delusions were due to a temporary eclipse of a patient's consciousness, induced by alcohol or a severe fever, or that the fanciful expressions of a patient were not a delusion but evidence of limited schooling. It is also plausible to suggest that if the certifying doctors had visited the patients more than once, they would have witnessed the wearing off of the influence of drink or fever on the minds of the patients, and, consequently, restoration of their sound mind. In sum, the observations made by the asylum's alienists may be regarded as evidence of a sustained interest that they had in engaging with the testimonies and life stories presented by the patients under discussion.

Cross-examination of a Patient's Personal Account of Restored Sanity

For the patients who entered the asylum exhibiting delusions, Greenlees embarked upon a therapeutic regimen that sought to offer labour duties and amusements as a means of "diverting the mind from its insane notions and giving it a new and healthy direction".[33] Accordingly, the casebooks provide a disproportionate focus on the patients' performance at work duties and their engagement with the recreational offerings of the asylum. Nevertheless, the decision to discharge a patient was not solely dependent on these criteria. Significantly, the following discussion reveals that for both black patients and white patients, a confession that an expressed idea was a delusion, followed by the alienists conducting a cross-examination of their personal account of restored health, was an integral factor in obtaining a discharge from the asylum.

In general, willingness of a black patient to work and participate in the labour and ward duties of the asylum was held by the alienists to be a sign of restoration of mental health, and it thus featured significantly in the alienists' decision to discharge black subjects from the asylum as "cured".[34] For the black patients who professed to harbouring delusions, a notable feature in several cases is that their discharge from the asylum as recovered was also informed by the findings of a cross-examination. Regina entered the asylum on 19 April 1902 harbouring a delusion that she was burnt by a fire from heaven.[35] On 23 May 1902, she was discharged recovered from the asylum. Greenlees's decision to discharge Regina was based on the following findings: "converses quite rationally [...]. She has been [...] cross examined today and appears to me quite well. She admits she was insane before she came here".

Phindiwe's path to discharge started when she informed Greenlees that she "feels better".[36] Soon thereafter, Greenlees proceeded to cross-examine her, and he came to the conclusion that she was "quite rational, working well and expresses no delusions. As far as can be ascertained she is quite well mentally now". Nqobile's discharge was initiated once it was concluded that he was "free from delusions, rational in conversation".[37] The medical certificates for Banele record how he believed the Lord told him to strip naked and to dress in his employer's clothes, which he accordingly did.[38] Soon after admittance to the asylum, he was quiet and well behaved and would "laugh" when referring to the beliefs that he formerly held. Banele's recognition that he had harboured a delusion was met by the alienists granting him a period of parole followed by discharge from the asylum. Tiyiselani had delusions that God appeared to him at night and told him that he "was a great saviour".[39] Tiyiselani's discharge was authorised once he acknowledged that his thoughts were "all nonsense". On admittance to the asylum, Kefilwe was burdened by thoughts that people wanted to kill her.[40] A few months later, after cross-examining her,

Greenlees mentioned how Kefilwe "is quite rational, has no delusions, indeed laughs at them, and converses perfectly".

For the white patients who acknowledged that a professed idea was a delusion, the alienists regarded this to be an important sign of a patient's path towards recovery and their being ready to be discharged from the asylum. In a few instances, on cross-examining the patients, the alienists determined that although a patient was no longer delusional, the personal account of recovery that they presented did not provide conclusive evidence of restored mental health, and there were indications that their character was eccentric. Stated differently, although a patient's delusions ceased, there were still indications of underlying mental instability, or a patient's so-called natural disposition was regarded as eccentric. Despite the alienist's identification and awareness of these two facts, the patient was still discharged. For example, Craig claimed to be outrageously wealthy and so incredibly strong that he could lift a house.[41] His delusions soon ceased, but Dr Adam also noted that Craig "shows a gradual obliteration of his higher mental faculties, has considerable difficulty in expressing his ideas properly". Although Craig showed "evidence of motor and mental enfeeblement", he was capable of exercising self-control, and his discharge was thus processed. Terence entered the asylum with ideas of conspiracies and persecution.[42] After a week at the asylum, he informed Dr Leslie that his ideas were delusions. Terence was discharged a month after admission. The concluding entry indicated that Terence had improved mentally, but his character and work conduct were not above reproach:

> In his work he is very dilatory and careless [...]. He has a somewhat exaggerated opinion of his powers and position and is rather given to talking big but otherwise is quite well mentally.[43]

There is also evidence that Greenlees directly intervened to protect a recovering patient from executing business ventures that were "flights of fancy". James entered the asylum with various melancholic delusions and felt that there was "no hope" for him.[44] On admission, he was placed on a suicide watch list, but a few weeks later he was removed from the list, as he had become "quite a different person: cheerful, tidy and active". His improvement continued, and James was eventually granted parole. James spent his parole "going in for business" to town and returning to the asylum for meals. During one of his trips, he attended a sale and secured the purchase of a house costing £1150 by paying a deposit of £100. Once

Greenlees got wind of James's actions, he proceeded to go to town to cancel the purchase. Greenlees then advised James to cease going into town, but the advice fell on deaf ears, as James was "very enthusiastic and believes he has a 1000 things 'on'" in the town. Nevertheless, this incident did not prolong James's institutionalisation, as a few weeks later Greenlees discharged him, as he had "kept quite well" and had shown no further "symptoms of mental disease".

Over the course of this discussion, the cases illustrate willingness of the patients to engage in exchanges with the alienists, make confessions, and submit to cross-examinations. There are also several cases that record patients who resented entering into such dialogue. Georgina harboured a delusion that she was 10 months pregnant.[45] Georgina loathed the interviews and questioning conducted by Greenlees. During these encounters, she never mentioned her delusions, but was "very pompous", and at times Greenlees noted that she "will not speak to me, turning her back on me when I question her". She remained "reticent" towards Greenlees and would quickly run away when he attempted to speak to her. It was only when she wished "to get away" from the asylum that she engaged with Greenlees. However, her decision to communicate with Greenlees and the staff of the asylum did not result in a change in her interpersonal relations with them. She annoyed everyone, until her discharge was consented to.

Personal Accounts of Institutionalisation

There are a few cases where Greenlees attempted to counsel patients out of a delusion. For Maryke, Greenlees mentioned that "I have done my utmost to convince her that her opinions and ideas of persecution are wrong and that she has no enemies",[46] and for Bridgett, who was plagued by delusions of persecution, Greenlees requested that she "write down her thoughts and […] forget them".[47] Once a patient was deemed to be suffering from a chronic form of insanity, it appears that Greenlees was not overly concerned with trying to counsel the patients. Damien would burst into song, singing a rollicking jingle "of his own composition" whenever grace was sung and during all of the asylum's concerts and entertainments.[48] Greenlees noted that whenever Damien was reprimanded for singing, he "drops into a prophetic vein, glaring at one, and using language which is in imitation of the prophetic writings of the Old Testament". Damien continued to sing and prophesy, and he was eventually transferred to the Port Alfred Asylum, an institution reserved for the care of chronic patients. Mitchell spent his time at the GLA writing poetry and sermons, which he considered to be the result of direct inspiration from God.[49] Greenlees considered the writings "a lot of perfectly incoherent nonsense of a religious nature", and Mitchell was recommended for transfer to the Port Alfred Asylum.

Thomas Clouston explains that in cases of delusional insanity, "[h]alf the discipline of asylums is directed against insane appearances, habits, and ways. By suggestion those would daily strengthen delusions and confirm evil habits if uncorrected".[50] In the cases scrutinised, it appears that Greenlees was not overly concerned with discouraging manifestations of delusions in the patients who were suffering from chronic forms of insanity. Although this meant that the patients were mostly unhindered in expressing their delusions and acting on them, the asylum did in most cases opt to relegate their care to the Port Alfred Asylum.

Many chronic patients spent their days writing letters to various individuals. Greenlees considered the letters written by the insane as a means of offering "insight to the morbid mind that we might not otherwise experience", and thus a considerable number of the letters were attached to the casebooks as an indication of a patient's mental state.[51] The letters composed by the chronic patients were dismissed by the alienists as containing "absurd, abusive or lewd" content,[52] and were thus of very little value apart from providing "proofs, or illustrations, of madness".[53] In contrast to the alienists' sole interest in the psychopathological content of the letters, the following discussion, much like the chapters authored by Leonard Smith and Tomas Vaiseta in this volume, seeks to explore how the letters can be interpreted as "patient testimony"[54] of their experiences and responses to long-term institutionalisation.[55]

Branden entered the asylum at the age of 51 as a non-paying patient, and for the remainder of his life he was confined to its walls. Branden spent his time writing letters signed as the prophet Elijah. In the casebook, the alienists disparaged his epistolary output: "writes long letters to Government officials making difficult complaints about the [GLA's] staff. He says the day will come when we will all be severely punished for the way we treat him".[56] By engaging with Branden's letters, it is possible to view his contempt for the staff in response to the personal indignities that he suffered while institutionalised. By way of example, Branden complained that

> I've washed my own under garments, such as shirts, singlets, draws, and handkerchiefs, to ensure wearing raiment, which others, possibly affected with venereal disease, such as syphilis, or other contagious affections have used; for during my natural life, have not, by the Grace of God, been in such dire necessity as to wear cast-off garments or such as already worn by others.[57]

Branden's letter indicates how he experienced the asylum's practice of recycling clothes amongst the non-paying patients as an act that degraded his sense of self.[58] Along these lines, the letter can be interpreted as a protest against the "physical contamination" Branden endured by having to wear clothes considered tainted by disease, and consequently, how his self-image was degraded.[59]

Emily was admitted to the asylum as a paying patient at the age of 33. The casebook entries are dominated by the alienists lamenting Emily's resistance to their instruction and discipline. Emily professed that she was the Goddess Mizpah, and she would demand a great deal of attention from the nurses. Emily frequently erupted into relentless fits of excitement and rage when her demands were not met. During these fits, she offended the staff, "as she finds the weak points in most people's armour", and she was frequently confined to the asylum's strongroom.[60] For several years, Emily was pronounced the "most trying patient in the Asylum", and her frequent sentences of confinement to the strongroom did not result in a change in behaviour, but rather saw her decorating the room with magazine pictures and writing letters to occupy herself.[61] Thus, it is not surprising that a recurrent theme in her letters was protest at being confined to the strongroom:

> I wish to draw your attention to the fact that I am kept here, and actually compelled to stay night and day in a horrible single room […] and shutter closed from 6 pm to 6 am next morning, no ventilation, just inhaling the same air over and over again—why it is slow poison. […] [T]his life I am compelled to endure here is enough to make a Saint from heaven curse and swear and to tear her hair. […]
>
> [The asylum's doctors have] put me here to be abused and insulted as I've never been insulted before, amongst all the mixed pickles. […]
>
> I am compelled to stay night and day in a horrible […] single room laying on a mattress on the floor, while he lets murderesses, liars and thieves have more freedom than me.[62]

Emily's letters are a protest against the physical indignity that she endured while confined to the strongroom, but they also express how her sense of self was "contaminated by contact with undesirable inmates".[63] To substantiate, Emily abhorred being in the company of the asylum's "mixed pickles"—the murderers, the criminals, and the paupers—and it is a reasonable assumption that as a paying patient she expected to be kept apart from such individuals.[64] Thus, the letters record the physical indignities that she underwent while in the strongroom, and when outside of the room the frustration that she experienced in being exposed to people that she did not wish to be associated with.

The epistolary outputs of Branden and Emily contain substantial sections of lucid and coherent content, but they are also riddled with "inconsistencies, omissions and imponderables".[65] Although the incompleteness of the letters poses "problems of interpretation", this should not deter one from the key significance of the letters in providing the researcher with an awareness of and an appreciation for a patient as a subject with a personal account of institutionalisation.[66] Accordingly, the letters can be regarded as an aid that prevents the researcher from viewing the narratives contained in the casebooks as the sole evidence of the subject's experiences of institutionalisation and of their personality and behaviour. Said differently, while the casebook entries chart a patient's institutionalisation in terms of a "clinical narrative",[67] and they present a negative portrayal of a patient's behaviour and personality, the letters offer a counterbalance, by bringing into view the individuality and the humanity of the patients. To this end, while the casebooks portray Branden as a "general nuisance"[68] and Emily as "emotional, hysterical" and "a child of impulse",[69] the letters highlight their humanity and their desire to preserve their personal sense of self.

Conclusion

In the cases of delusion investigated in this chapter, there are two main approaches in the way the alienists of the GLA engaged with the life stories and testimonies given by the patients. First, it is evident that for certain groups of patients their testimonies and confessions were instrumental in their pathways out of the asylum. To elucidate further, in the group of patients who were represented in the medical certificates as delusional, the casebooks reveal that the interviews and cross-questioning conducted by the alienists offered the patient an opportunity to provide an account of their life story and a personal testimony of the soundness of their mind.

The alienists accepted the patient's testimony and proceeded to discharge them from the asylum. In the group of patients who were recovering from insanity, a confession that an expressed idea was a delusion was an integral factor in the patient receiving a discharge from the asylum. Second, for patients suffering from chronic forms of insanity and who remained delusional, their letters and the personal accounts of institutionalisation that they contained were dismissed by the alienists. An investigation of a selection of the letters reveals the turmoil, indignities, and dissatisfaction that the patients experienced at the asylum. The letters testify to the denial of personal dignity that the patients experienced from an asylum regimen that ignored their pleas for clothes, interpersonal relations, and spaces in the asylum that might preserve rather than taint their sense of self.

Notes

1. Roy Porter, *The Faber book of madness* (London: Faber & Faber, 1991), 131.
2. For a review of the studies, see Rory du Plessis, "A hermeneutic analysis of delusion content from the casebooks of the Grahamstown Lunatic Asylum, 1890–1907", *South African Journal of Psychiatry* 25 (2019).
3. See also Rafael Huertas, "Another history for another psychiatry. The patient's view", *Culture & History Digital Journal* 2, no. 1 (2013): 1–11, 8.
4. Sally Swartz, "Can the clinical subject speak? Some thoughts on subaltern psychology", *Theory & Psychology* 15, no. 4 (2005): 505–525, 513.
5. Hilary Marland, *Dangerous motherhood: Insanity and childbirth in Victorian Britain* (Houndmills: Palgrave Macmillan, 2004), 96.
6. Ibid., 101.
7. See Rory du Plessis, "Photographs from the Grahamstown Lunatic Asylum, South Africa, 1890–1907", *Social Dynamics* 40, no. 1 (2014): 12–42.
8. Rory du Plessis, "Pathways of patients explored hermeneutically in the casebooks from the Grahamstown Lunatic Asylum between 1890 and 1907", PhD diss., University of Pretoria (2017).
9. Steven J. Taylor, "Depraved, deprived, dangerous and deviant: Depicting the insane child in England's county asylums, 1845–1907", *History* 101, no. 347 (2016): 513–535.
10. Taylor, "Depraved, deprived, dangerous and deviant", 534.
11. Ibid., 535.
12. Sally Swartz, "'Work of mercy and necessity': British rule and psychiatric practice in the Cape Colony, 1891–1910", *International Journal of Mental Health* 28, no. 2 (1999): 72–90, 79.

13. Western Cape Archives and Records Service (Henceforth WCARS), Grahamstown Lunatic Asylum Casebooks (Henceforth HGM), HGM 3, 76.
14. WCARS, HGM 5, 157.
15. WCARS, HGM 18, 230.
16. WCARS, HGM 15, 102.
17. Du Plessis, "Pathways of patients", 103–107.
18. WCARS, HGM 3, 128.
19. Swartz, "Work of mercy and necessity", 79.
20. Ibid., 80.
21. Ibid., 84.
22. Akihito Suzuki, "Framing psychiatric subjectivity: Doctor, patient, and record-keeping at Bethlem in the nineteenth century", in *Insanity, institutions, and society, 1800–1914: A social history of madness in historical perspective*, eds. J. Melling and B. Forsythe (New York: Routledge, 1999), 115–136, 132.
23. WCARS, HGM 20, 30.
24. WCARS, HGM 4, 70.
25. H. H. Newington, "Certificates, medical", in *A dictionary of psychological medicine*, Volume 1, ed. D.H. Tuke (Philadelphia: Blakiston, 1892), 189–195, 193.
26. WCARS, HGM 7, 193.
27. Thomas Duncan Greenlees, "Medical, social, and legal aspects of insanity", *South African Medical Record* 1, no. 8 (1903): 121–125, 121.
28. Thomas Duncan Greenlees, "An address on the ethics of insanity", *British Medical Journal* 2 (1910): 301–303, 302.
29. Thomas Duncan Greenlees, *The nursing of nervous and mental diseases* (Grahamstown: Asylum Press, 1896), 15.
30. Thomas Duncan Greenlees, *On the threshold: Studies in psychology. A lecture delivered to the Eastern Province Literary and Scientific Society, Grahamstown* (Grahamstown: Asylum Press, 1899), 34.
31. Ibid., 33.
32. See also E. Mendel, "Diagnosis", in *A dictionary of psychological medicine*, Volume 1, ed. D.H. Tuke (Philadelphia: Blakiston, 1892), 372–382, 375.
33. WCARS, CO 7170, Government Notice No. 267 of 1892.
34. Du Plessis, "Photographs from the Grahamstown Lunatic Asylum".
35. WCARS, HGM 18, 253.
36. WCARS, HGM 20, 24.
37. WCARS, HGM 15, 56.
38. WCARS, HGM 2, 191.
39. WCARS, HGM 5, 166.
40. WCARS, HGM 21, 20.

41. WCARS, HGM 4, 55.
42. WCARS, HGM 8, 167.
43. WCARS, HGM 8, 167.
44. WCARS, HGM 4, 67.
45. WCARS, HGM 22, 89.
46. WCARS, HGM 18, 50.
47. WCARS, HGM 17, 143.
48. WCARS, HGM 5, 30.
49. WCARS, HGM 4, 211.
50. Thomas S. Clouston, *Clinical lectures on mental diseases* (London: J. & A. Churchill, 1892), 247.
51. Thomas Duncan Greenlees, *Notes on some forms of mental disease* (Cape Town: Townshend, Taylor & Snashall Printers, 1907), 3.
52. WCARS, HGM 8, 201.
53. Jonathan Andrews, "Case notes, case histories, and the patient's experience of insanity at Gartnavel Royal Asylum, Glasgow, in the nineteenth century", *Social History of Medicine* 11, no. 2 (1998): 255–281, 277.
54. Ibid., 269.
55. Michael Barfoot and Allan W. Beveridge, "Madness at the crossroads: John Home's letters from the Royal Edinburgh Asylum, 1886–87", *Psychological Medicine* 20, no. 2 (1990): 263–284; Michael Barfoot and Allan W. Beveridge, "'Our most notable inmate': John Willis Mason at the Royal Edinburgh Asylum, 1864–1901", *History of Psychiatry* 4, no. 14 (1993): 159–208; Allan Beveridge, "Voices of the mad: Patients' letters from the Royal Edinburgh Asylum, 1873–1908", *Psychological Medicine* 27, no. 4 (1997): 899–908; Allan Beveridge, "Life in the Asylum: Patients' letters from Morningside, 1873–1908", *History of Psychiatry* 9, no. 36 (1998): 431–469; Allan Beveridge and Morag Williams, "Inside 'The Lunatic Manufacturing Company': The persecuted world of John Gilmour", *History of Psychiatry* 13, no. 49 (2002): 19–49; Jade Shepherd, "'I am very glad and cheered when I hear the flute': The treatment of criminal lunatics in late Victorian Broadmoor", *Medical History* 60, no. 4 (2016): 473–491.
56. WCARS, HGM 7, 238.
57. WCARS, CO 7800, 31 January 1909.
58. Erving Goffman, *Asylums: Essays on the social situation of mental patients and other inmates* (Harmondsworth: Penguin, 1968), 30.
59. Goffman, *Asylums*, 33.
60. WCARS, HGM 22, 264
61. WCARS, HGM 22, 240.
62. WCARS, CO 7800, 4 November 1910.
63. Goffman, *Asylums*, 36.

64. Rory du Plessis, "The principles and priorities of Dr T.D. Greenlees, medical superintendent of the Grahamstown Lunatic Asylum, 1890–1907", *Historia* 60, no. 1 (2015): 22–46, 33.
65. Barfoot and Beveridge, "Madness at the crossroads", 282.
66. Ibid., 282.
67. Rory du Plessis, "Beyond a clinical narrative: Casebook photographs from the Grahamstown Lunatic Asylum, c. 1890s", *Critical Arts* 29, supl (2015): 88–103, 91.
68. WCARS, HGM 7, 264.
69. WCARS, HGM 22, 263.

CHAPTER 8

Dehumanizing Experience, Rehumanizing Self-Awareness: Perception of Violence in Psychiatric Hospitals of Soviet Lithuania

Tomas Vaiseta

"I, V. V., am at the T.B.C. department of Žiegždriai hospital. On April 9, [...] I heard a noise in the corridor and someone shouting 'don't hit'. I went out into the corridor and saw orderly J. S. with some man [...]. At that moment, he [...] slammed the patient against a wall. He saw me, probably got scared and led the patient into a room. After a little [while], shouts and moans started again. I went out to see what was happening. I saw the orderly beating patients with a rubber hose. Then it got quiet and I fell asleep. At 3 o'clock, J. S. [came into] my room N6 and started beating patient B., asleep, with the same rubber hose".[1]

This letter, written in first person singular, was sent to a Kaunas newspaper by two patients at Žiegždriai Psychiatric Hospital in 1964. The letter made its way to the Ministry of Health of the Lithuanian Soviet Socialist Republic [SSR], which appointed a commission to investigate the complaint. When members of the commission came to the hospital, one of the

T. Vaiseta (✉)
Vilnius University, Vilnius, Lithuania

R. Ellis et al. (eds.), *Voices in the History of Madness*, Mental Health in Historical Perspective,
https://doi.org/10.1007/978-3-030-69559-0_8

letter's two authors denied the information and the other one was nowhere to be found. He had escaped from the institution. According to the commission's report, "other patients could not say anything due to their mental condition". However, the allegations in the letter proved to be correct: two night-shift orderlies had been drinking, then got hold of a rubber hose, went into wards, pulled blankets off sleeping patients and hit them without any apparent reason. At least seven patients were hurt, one suffered a nosebleed.

Such brutal and pointless outbursts of violence were quite rare in the psychiatric hospitals of Soviet Lithuania (1944–1990). But pettier psychological and physical violence, as well as use of coercion, were everyday occurrences. The letter quoted above and the story it narrates provide a window into the culture of violence that prevailed in mental institutions and how easily this culture could have been disguised in bureaucratic documents. Commissions charged with investigating complaints would rarely be as thorough as in the case above. But the most interesting part of the story, though, is the complaint letter itself. The letters like this written by the patients is a unique source, yet very rarely quoted in Soviet psychiatry research. They could give us a glimpse into how patients experienced not just violence, but being in a psychiatric hospital in general: how they made sense of the experience, how they felt, and how they wanted to tell others about it. In this sense "the voices" in this chapter will be understood as this expression of experience of mental patients by their self. And the complaint letters will be considered as a written form of these voices.

These letters should be discussed in a context of the concept of "narrative of illness". But they are not a traditional form of this narrative. Their primary purpose was not to speak about illness experience or describe the patients' inner states of being, but rather by a purposeful act of communication to draw the attention of the addressees to a problem they had the power to solve. Thus complaint letters always employed a certain communicative tactic. For a historian, primarily, they are a source of information about what the writer wanted others to see and think that he thought and felt. The purpose of being heard and receiving assistance may come before openness and sincerity. Complaint letters can be manipulative and naive or direct in equal measure. It means, for example, a patient may exhibit greater trust in the institution or its agents than he actually feels. So meaning-making, normally seen as the purpose of narratives of illness,[2] is in this case rather a side effect. However, what links complaint letters and the more traditional forms of narratives of illness is not just the desire "to be in communication even if from the margins",[3] but also an authentic voice of mental patients. The letters are not a direct product of the institution and its medical discourse, unlike patients' case histories or other institutional documents about them[4] (for wider discussion see Chap. 7). Patients' letters can be inflected by the institutional discourse and later be absorbed into it, processed, assessed, but they maintain a degree of autonomy.

Mental patients' voices were largely absent from what went for the Soviet public space. Nor have any non-public testimonies of patients survived from Soviet Lithuania. Therefore, besides official case history files, complaint letters are essentially the only surviving sources one can draw on to try to reconstruct mental patients' narratives and understand their experiences captured in the present tense. The Ministry of Health of the Lithuanian SSR archive, held by the Lithuanian Central State Archive, contains at least several hundred complaint letters written between 1951 and 1989 by patients of Soviet psychiatric hospitals or their families and addressed to the ministry, the press, public prosecutors, or Communist Party institutions. Not all of them describe violence or only violence. Yet violence from the staff of mental institutions directed at patients was a recurring theme.

In this chapter, by analysing the complaint letters written by mental patients, I will seek to explore the voice of mental patients in a context of violence, that is, how patients would express and make sense of their experience of violence in an institution. It must be stressed that this analysis will not comprehend the whole experience of mental patients in psychiatric hospitals of Soviet Lithuania, but only a small part, which decided to express their voice in a particular situation for a particular addressee.

Before the Soviet Union's collapse in 1991, Western researchers were interested mostly in a dissident experience and stories about how the Soviet regime used psychiatry to deal with its political opponents.[5] More recently, this interest has re-emerged,[6] and the analysts focus again on dissident discourses.[7] It seems that there is no comprehensive study looking into the lives of a seemingly less politically significant, but much bigger group of patients. As if Roy Porter's dictum of three decades ago to take up "patient view"[8] has yet to reach Soviet psychiatry studies. It could be even said that the historiography of Soviet psychiatry continues to favour the system over the people in and affected by that system. Before 1991, the Soviet psychiatric care system had interested Western researchers as a different, ideologically and politically engaged model of psychiatry.[9] In the last ten or fifteen years there has been some renewed interest in socialist psychiatry in general[10] and its Soviet variant in particular.[11]

The Soviet psychiatric model that emerged in the middle of the twentieth century was not radically different from the theories and practices of Western psychiatry, although it did move in its own distinctive direction. The Soviet state's materialist ideology rejected "idealist theories" like psychoanalysis and, for some time, relied dogmatically on Ivan Pavlov's teaching. The dominant psychiatric discourse was expert-led by psychiatrists and consumer discourse never emerged to question it. Psychiatrists had a limited range of options and patients, especially in the periphery of the USSR, essentially none at all. But arguably the most important feature was the immense significance of institutional treatment: despite developing and expanding a network of dispensaries, the Soviet psychiatric system remained mostly hospital-centred until the very end (1991). During the 1950s–1970s when strong criticism of psychiatric hospitals in the West led to partial deinstitutionalisation, the number of hospitals in the USSR steadily grew. For example, in the early 1950s Great Britain had eight times as many psychiatric hospital beds per capita as the USSR, but by the early 1980s the numbers were equal.[12] The tiny Lithuanian SSR with a population of between 2.5 and 3 million operated two psychiatric hospitals in the 1940s and eight in the 1980s. Hospital, therefore, was an essential part of the experience of a person whom Soviet psychiatry would declare its patient.

Patient View and Medical Gaze

Violence experienced by patients in psychiatric hospital relates not just to the institution itself. It also relates to the discourse of modern medicine represented by the institution, practically realized within its premises, created and reproduced in it. After all, the violence a person is subjected to in psychiatric hospital essentially and fundamentally contradicts the explicit promise formulated by the medical discourse to care and to help, that is, to return him or her to a "normal" and "ordinary" state. Therefore the question of how a person perceives and expresses his or her experience of violence in psychiatric hospital allows one to consider not just a time- and space-specific (Soviet) case, but a more universal issue: the relation between a human being and medical discourse.

Medical discourse is a result of a modern process that historiography has come to call medicalization.[13] It allowed for the medical profession's dominance, while the newly defined role of the "patient" was ascribed qualities like helplessness, need of assistance, and incompetence to help oneself.[14] The "disease" diagnosed by doctors is seen as an objective fact or a problem whose identification and solution requires their expert, that is, exclusive, knowledge and competence. The patient's own narrative about how he or she feels is of secondary importance, in fact, an obstacle for knowing the "real condition". For this reason, as the historian of medicine Mary E. Fissell argues, from about the mid-eighteenth century, narratives of the ailing about themselves and their illness in Western Europe were gradually pushed out by a disease-oriented diagnosis of the modern medical discourse, eventually rendering the patient's narrative of illness "utterly redundant".[15]

The story of the medical discourse's rise to dominance thus conceived and narrated has led to a view, popular among sociologists and anthropologists of medicine, that the sick individual has been deprived of the right to speak in their own voice and be heard, becoming merely an object for medical professionals, stripped of all power. The medical discourse, sometimes designated as a hegemonic meta-narrative or a totalizing ideology,[16] thus effects the patient's victimization through the suppression of their voice. When the patient's narrative of illness became an object of active interest in the 1980s, the patient's relation to the medical discourse was initially and mainly defined through the binary opposition of the "medical gaze" and the "patient view". Scholars who studied narratives of illness and underlined their significance would justify their interest in them by arguing that these narratives "empower[ed] the user"[17] or could be "emancipatory".[18] That is to say, they could counter the medical discourse and help de-victimize patients, give them back their voice and the power of their subjectivity.[19] In general, this view owes to the Foucauldian tradition. The latter holds that the modern subject is shaped and objectified by biopolitical power discourses. Then the individual subject can gain some autonomy and define him- or herself only in resistance to these truth regimes.[20] However, one can wonder whether this explanation allows to appreciate the full spectrum of complicated and nuanced discursive techniques through which people make sense of and express their experience of being ill, being a patient, or being in a medical institution.

Without denying the constitutive role of discourses, the sociologist Anthony Giddens criticizes Foucault for seeing the process of discursive impact as a fixed and one-way intrusion of "power knowledge" into social organization. He proposes instead the concept of institutional reflexivity.[21]

According to this, the reflexive relation between a person and discourses allows to see him not just as a passively shaped object, but also as an acting—albeit within a predefined framework—subject. This subject self-reflects by reacting to, or even using, categories suggested by discourse, without necessarily identifying with them when his everyday experience contradicts them. More than passively adopting categories of the medical discourse, he can lean on them or question them critically to raise issues existentially important to him. He can not only resist the medical discourse, but also use the opportunities it opens up or manipulate it for his own benefit. Furthermore, the conceptions of what it means to be a patient are influenced not just by the medical discourse, seemingly the one in control, but also by other public (traditional communal attitudes or popular culture, like films, books, the media) and private (generated in the family or close environment) discourses.[22] As Kerry Davies, who explored how patients' oral testimony can contribute to and challenge the history of mental illness, puts it, mental patients within a single account "negotiate and utilize the various different languages of madness and mental illness available in order to establish meaning—to re-construct and to narrate their experiences".[23]

Finally, in the medical discourse the promise to care and to help the ailing is programmed and openly proclaimed. This promise itself is one of the main sources of empowerment for more active and reflexive relations between the patient and the medical discourse. From the point of view of the patient, this promise has gradually become a more or less conscious expectation to get care and help, to at least make all possible effort toward recovery if not complete recovery. During the twentieth century, with the rise and entrenchment of the human rights discourse, this expectation was gradually articulated and eventually enshrined as patients' rights. In the Soviet system, the "universally accessible and free treatment" was part of its ideological programme and was formally delivered, albeit with serious defects and problems.[24] Therefore it could be claimed that the promise articulated by the medical discourse formally was fulfilled. Although patients' expectations in the West and the Soviet Union could and did differ greatly, it does not diminish the fact that the formulation itself of these expectations could enable patients to conceive of their special status not just in negative terms (being helpless, suffering, rendered incompetent object) but in positive terms as well (able to act: expect, ask, demand, sometimes decide). In other words, expectations could determine self-conception as a patient: what I am, what I can expect, what I can.

The Hidden Power of Medical Discourse: The Externalization of the Self

The most characteristic motif of violence experienced in psychiatric hospitals is the sense of powerlessness and dehumanization. It is expressed in complaint letters through narratives of self-victimization and being an object under someone else's power. The letters suggest that direct violence and other circumstances (overcrowded patient wards, bad sanitary conditions, bad diet) make the status of a psychiatric hospital patient feel akin to standing on the lowest step of social hierarchy, where the only way to be heard is by begging, pleading, using strong rhetorical figures to appeal on the grounds of one's hopeless condition.

"We are writing from pazasliu hospital that they hurt us without mercy beat and torture [...] don't give a drop of water if patients ask, sometimes beat to death, no one's paying any attention [...]," two patients from Pažaislis Hospital wrote in 1962.[25] From the patient's perspective, being subjected to violence by hospital staff (usually orderlies) or witnessing acts of violence directed at another patient would not so much create as reaffirm the culturally dominant "mental patient" stigma. This stigma would disqualify one from the community of "normal", "full" humans. Helplessness and disqualification is often consolidated not just by violence itself, but by the accompanying sense of loneliness, isolation, and abandonment. Complaint letters, like the one quoted above, contain recurring motifs of failing to receive help, being ignored by the staff, inability to report violence and other problems. All of this is usually linked to the psychiatric patient status: "[Orderlies] come to work drunk, fierce men not afraid of nothing, they can beat patients because they brainless got no word to say".[26] The violence is the physical expression of stigmatization, causing physical pain and psychological trauma. This sense is reinforced by the public setting of violence which, in patients' eyes, can in a way legitimize it, make it a matter-of-course and unquestioned practice.

The sense of disqualification is so strong in some letters that the patients seemed to feel excluded not just from "normal" people, but from people in general, and that violence erased their humanity. For a person, the measure of his state could be less physical or mental health than the moral category of being "human". Losing one's "humanity" can be the main sign of being "out of one's mind", while preserving it an attribute of health. The violence is precisely what stands in the way of recovery: "Hear this, I want to return to my family and have a human life before I lose my mind. And here they beat all humanity out of you, they call you names and hit whenever and however they want. My health is getting worse and worse every day".[27] Patients express this feeling of forced degradation and dehumanization by comparing themselves to animals or even describing themselves as animals (dogs, pigs, rabbits, etc.) to their intended addressees. For example: "When I warned the senior nurse not to be so tactless towards the patients, I was treated like a dog".[28] Violence may well be the most important dehumanizing experience, but it rarely occurs separately from other circumstances that reinforce dehumanization. An entire set of behaviours is what turns one into an "animal": not being allowed to go out for walks, being fed bad food or having one's food stolen by hospital staff, being arbitrarily punished and called names.

The medical discourse, its vocabulary, categories and images may not even appear on the surface of patients' complaint letters. While their relations with the medical staff are sometimes described in terms of conflict, the staff can often be seen as a threat, the main source of violence, as people not to be trusted because they hold the power that disqualifies patients as humans: "Just like in Chekhov's *Ward No. 6*, they walk drunk from ward to ward […] looking for someone to harass, especially young women, sometimes until morning, and moreover, hit helpless patients. If you want to warn them, they tell you, what you gonna do, it's your word alone against us four or more. When you complain to the senior doctor, they go write false reports about the patient and then laugh how well they played, that is, what a successful show".[29] Patients report that the hospital management control and intercept their letters and punish them for complaining with additional aminazine injections.[30] If a complaint reaches its intended recipient, the investigation is pure imitation. This way, the source of threat becomes identified with the entire institution, not just its lot-level staff. Indeed, complaint investigation reports often use medical vocabulary and medical categories to eliminate the complaint author as a subject. They foreground diagnosis to cast doubt on the witness's reliability, insist on relying on "lucid patients" or put doctors' testimonies above those of patients'. It is reasonable to argue that these complaints show the patients' authentic experience rejecting the medical discourse, which fails to deliver on its promise to care and help, and opting for a different vocabulary that exists beyond it.

But even if the argument is valid, it does not always hold. The absence of the medical discourse from patients' narratives may mean not just their failure to adopt it. It also can mean that it is so strong, albeit implicitly, that the patient refuses to accept their situation or experience as belonging to the imaginary shaped by the medical discourse. The above-noted patients' disappointment is not just with the fact that the stigma disqualifying them as humans exists, but that it crosses into the medical institution as well. It means that the patient brings along not just their experience of previous stigmatization, but also an expectation that it would stop here. The medical discourse itself supplies this expectation. So disappointment also means an inner contradiction. To resolve the conflict between the expectation created by the medical discourse and his or her authentic experience, the patient can use the strategy of externalizing the self and the surrounding reality. For the medical discourse to remain effective, valid, and accepted, the experience of violence in a psychiatric hospital has to be transformed into something outside the world promised by the medical discourse.

Narratively, the externalization is effected by transforming the meaning of hospital as an institution, of its staff, and of oneself. If the hospital is a setting of violence, it is stripped of its status as a "normal" or "real" hospital. In this case it is named something else, often borrowing the strongest symbols for sites of violence that the Soviet ideological culture can offer, for instance, Nazi concentration camp, where millions of people were imprisoned and killed ("Being here makes you lose your patience, brings you to nervous exhaustion, you don't want anything, not even to live. You want to leave this concentration camp as soon as possible"[31]). Equally, the violent staff is held to be something else than "normal" or "real" hospital staff. They are rather "hooligans" and "bandits". In the end, they even invert the roles, starting to regard members of the medical staff as mentally unsound: "Orderly T. is mentally insane and hated by his coworkers, he's been through all the hospital departments. Nurses are aware of his violent actions [...]".[32] The dehumanization motif described above is also could be a part of this externalization, in this case, of oneself: one is not a "real patient", because a patient would not be treated this way.

If we accept this reading, then even those patient narratives that do not seem to explicitly rely on the medical discourse are not necessarily independent from its power to shape or influence these narratives. It can manifest itself through negative externalization forms.

In Alignment with Medical Discourse: Violence as a Result of Disorder

It is not always the case that writers of complaint letters relate to the medical discourse in such concealed forms. Many of the messages establish an active, highly reflexive, even negotiating relation with the medical discourse. Writers borrow its basic ideal images and conceive of psychiatric hospital as a medical institution that has to perform clear therapeutic functions, in other words, as an order structure with necessary elements and procedures. In such cases, patients may exhibit medical knowledge, use medical jargon, and describe the problems they face in a medical institution by contrasting them to the formal set of rules established by the medical discourse. They can discuss, for instance, how doctors should talk to patients versus how they actually do or what the treatment a patient is entitled to versus what he or she gets. This ostensible (demonstrated) understanding of medicine and functioning of medical institutions can, in rare cases, push the writer's self-conception to a sort of intermediary status between patient and medical staff member. Without rejecting their patient status, the letter writers show themselves to be more than just patients. They offer advice to medical staff on how to do their work more efficiently and how to treat other patients. One man from Žiegždriai Psychiatric Hospital wrote in 1968 that "iron bars should be installed on the external side of windows, because patients are jumping through the windows and running away".[33]

The narrative in these letters, it seems, completely conforms to the medical discourse and their authors are conditioned by it. Though in fact, complete congruence is made impossible by the patients' authentic experience, namely, problems they face daily in a hospital and, most significantly, violence. The way they reflect on most of their problems still exhibits a strong influence of the medical discourse. The patients describe their hardship through this discourse and explain the causes within its logic. So rather than externalizing, the letter writers opt for particularization. They assume that the problem lies in a particular hospital not functioning the way it should, that it is not programmed into the nature of the medical institution per se, but is a dysfunction caused by the management or staff of a particular hospital not performing their duties or breaking the rules. Violence, in this view, is seen as arising less from the order in the psychiatric hospital (which would be the explanation of some in the anti-psychiatry movement) than from disorder. Some letters make references to a lack of order: "A lot of mess can be observed in the hospital".[34] Likewise, hospital workers that abuse and mistreat patients are still seen as members of the medical staff, but ones who "discredit the honourable medical profession",[35] that is, as deviating from the norm.

However, the understanding of violence—more concretely, what is to be regarded as violence and what is maintenance of order—is where the narrative in these letters stray most markedly from the medical discourse. Formally, physical and psychological abuse against patients would not be tolerated in psychiatric hospitals, but restraining and immobilization (methods of coercion) were seen as necessary to maintain institutional order. And this is where institutional practices could clash with patients' views. Reports of inspections conducted by psychiatric specialists following patients' complaints would state: "The treatment of patients by the medical staff is not rough. Although individual patients have stated that they are sometimes beaten, there is no such practice in the hospital: what they see as beating is the constraining of restless patients while shaving, putting them to sleep, tying to the bed if they are restless and so on".[36] The patients, however, saw such coercion practices as another form of violence against them and their use as upsetting order rather than upholding it. The highly disciplining Soviet psychiatric hospital environment did not fit with how the patients defined themselves and their freedom (what I can do, what others can do to me). For example, one man from Pažaislis Psychiatric Hospital wrote a letter to the newspaper *Tiesa* (the local equivalent of Moscow's *Pravda*) in 1960, opening with a rather typical declaration: "This is to inform you that our hospital is in complete disorder". He reports having been beaten up by nursing assistants in August that year: "Three of them grabbed me in the ward, threw to the bed and started strangling, I almost suffocated. Then they hit me in the chest and hurt my leg and my side." He concludes the letter by pleading to bring order to the hospital "with the help of Medical authorities". The man makes no secret that he was beaten because he had a "small knife".[37] However, the official inspection report reveals very well the logic of the Soviet medical discourse. It interprets the situation differently: the patient has "paranoid schizophrenia" (therefore, can be dangerous) and was carrying a knife and a door handle to open doors. The orderlies admitted that they had used force to take these things from the man, but denied that they had strangled or beaten him.[38] The report recommends taking note of orderlies' rough treatment of patients. But at the same time it concludes that their actions were aimed at maintaining order (safety). So the author can invoke the medical discourse in ways, to the extent that, and as long as it suits his purposes. Even though he sees himself as a patient, he can maintain a reflexive relation with this discourse. He uses it to interpret reality, but not necessarily identify completely with it; uses it manipulatively, simultaneously negotiating what a particular rule or norm defined by the medical discourse means or should mean.

Shelter of Medical Discourse: Violence as an Enforcement of Madness

As the medical discourse developed, it redefined people hitherto treated as mad. A separate sociocultural type characterized by deviant behaviour became the sick individuals, that is, people like everyone else, except with a mental condition. Formally, the transformation of the "madman" into the "patient" should have alleviated stigmatization. The medical discourse, by turning madness into a disease, in a way normalized it, rendered it a "normal abnormality", that is, a disease like any other.

The most significant distinction between disease and madness lay in the medical discourse's promise that a disease can be treated. In practice, however, even as psychiatric therapy advanced, the realization of this potentiality depended a lot on a person's mental state, that is, the type of disease. Some experienced greater or weaker effects (identified as "improvement" or "recovery"). Others remained immune to any treatment. Therefore, as is evident in the complaint letters, even though the medical discourse and psychiatric practices essentially treated all as psychiatric patients, they themselves saw that there were two distinct groups. The first consisted of more or less sane patients, sick but able to recover, the "normally abnormal". The second consisted of the insane, the so-called chronic patients, the "abnormally abnormal". By this distinction, only the first group belonged to the world conceived and governed by the medical discourse where mental patients were exactly or almost like any other person. The second group were still in the older pre-modern world of madmen where their humanity was in doubt.

Essentially all the writers who invoke this distinction put themselves in the first group, insisting emphatically they do not belong with the "madmen". They use the culturally typical us–them opposition whose concrete content may vary: "fake" versus "real" invalids, "nerve" versus "mind" patients (although both are diagnosed with psychiatric conditions), "temporary" versus "chronic" patients. The time dimension is a significant criterion. Being sick is a temporary status and being mad, a permanent, unchanging one. It means that the possibility of returning to the community of "normal people" remains open for the former, but not the latter group. This group is condemned to a non-quite-human situation: "I ask dear comrade Minister to take my statement into consideration and issue an order that I be transferred to a nerve hospital and not be left among completely crazy people whose fates are settled, for I want to recover and work, be of use to myself and the society".[39]

This effort to put oneself into the temporarily sick group has to do with the desire to escape stigmatization as much as possible. The medical discourse's patient category offer a hope to accomplish this. Hence from the point of view of the patient, the medical discourse does not drown out or displace their authentic perception of the self. It acts as a shelter from the prejudice against people with psychiatric conditions who are still seen as mad and not belonging to the community of "normal people". Therefore the relation between the writers of these letters and the medical discourse should be described not in terms of resistance or submission but as instrumental cooperation. Even if the patient category offered by the medical discourse deprives one of subjectivity and assigns stigmatized qualities, it can still be seen by patients as a lesser evil or even salvation from the premodern madman prejudice.

On the other side, violence suffered at the hands of medical staff can be a factor threatening to end this cooperation. Such actions can be seen not so much as discrediting the institution and the discourse but as an attack on the patient status, a refusal to treat him as temporarily sick, an attempt to tear him out of the world of the medical discourse and throw into the dehumanized world of the mad. In short, violence can appear as a move to turn a patient into a madman. For instance, a letter written by a woman to a prosecutor's office of the Lithuanian SSR in 1973 describes the violence she experienced (actions she herself perceives as violence) in almost symbolic terms. Force was used against the woman when she resisted being moved from a ward for mild patients to one for serious patients, that is, from the "temporarily sick" group to the "mad": "I refused to move to Ward 1, because my health had not deteriorated. But despite my objections, the ward nurse called in an orderly from Ward 1 and two from Ward 2, they twisted my arms, dragged me out of bed and kicked me while dragging through the room".[40]

In such cases, essentially the only way to defend oneself from violence and from being put into the world of the "mad" was still an appeal to the patient category within the medical discourse and the "patient's rights" arising from therein. The latter not only fostered expectations of help (what I can expect as a patient) but also offered discursive protection (what cannot be done to me): "I think that medical workers on duty are there to help patients when help is needed, but they have no right to threaten, terrorise, punish them. In the end, the psychiatric ward is an institution for treatment, for treating certain illnesses, and it is unacceptable to use it, forgetting its purpose, as a jail or a lockup".[41] True, the letters sent to government or other institutions represent the voice of only a small fraction of those who experienced or witnessed violence. This part did not capitulate and kept fighting, if only by pleading, to remain and be seen as patients rather than "madmen". But in general, these examples show how significant cooperation with the medical discourse could have been for people facing violence. This did not necessarily protect them from violence or help restore justice in its wake, but it could have helped to draw their own trajectory of consciousness.

Conclusions

By drawing a sharp opposition between medical gaze and patient view, the historiography of illness narratives blinds itself to the full scope of possible relations between the medical discourse and the person-turned-patient. Such a view neglects and undervalues his or her personal, authentic narrative that may well defy the medical discourse and its rules. And, vice versa, a person's narrative signifies more than just resistance to the suppressive power of the medical discourse. The reading of the complaint letters written by patients of psychiatric hospitals in Soviet Lithuania confirms the argument that these people, regarded as "mental patients", and their narratives, have long been pushed out of the public space and ignored by the society. Their complaints, which would almost invariably circulate only inside the bureaucratic machine, without reaching the wider public, serve as emerging narratives and a means of emancipation for the patients. The medical discourse, however, emerges not just as a discursive force to free oneself from, but also as a discursive instrument enabling the emancipatory action.

By concentrating not on narratives of illness in general but on one particular element, the experience of violence, we see that the bipolar opposition between patient view and medical gaze turns into something closer to a three-way relation of patient, medical discourse, and violence. The medical discourse then shows itself to be operating even in those patient narratives where it is not readily apparent. It acts as a force that motivates patients to externalise the self and the surrounding reality in the face of violence, as I have attempted to demonstrate. In other cases, the medical discourse's effect on the patient's self-perception appears strong and self-evident, but there remains some scope for subjectivity vis-a-vis this discourse. The patient relies on it to interpret reality, but does not necessarily fully identify with it, and at times even uses it manipulatively. Finally, the medical discourse can act as a defensive shield for the self, a tool to protect oneself from hostile, alien, dangerous reality. The medical discourse can objectify and infantilize the patient, but still be seen as an opportunity rather than a threat. This opportunity was offered by the expectations programmed into the patient category which would sometimes evolve into and be understood as rights.

The role of patients' rights that emerged within the medical discourse is important. The notion of rights implies not just moral, but also legal and, consequently, political power of appeal. It could enable patients to speak out, not to be afraid, not to give in. The experience of violence—painful, traumatizing, humiliating as it was—would at times activate this notion of patients' rights. Some would resign to passive nothingness when faced with marginal situations, but others might be encouraged to look for solutions. In this case the conception of self as a patient would point in the possible directions. Granted, in Soviet reality, institutional power would often use the same medical discourse to frustrate and eliminate these efforts. But looking at patients' letters from a temporal distance, we can see clear attempts to define and enable the self in relation, of one kind or another, to the medical discourse. Patients' complaint letters are significant not just for their content but also for how and why they were written. The content reveals a world of dehumanization, helplessness, disqualification, and fear. But their narrative form and the very fact of their existence testify to the patients' efforts to constitute themselves as human beings like everyone else. These letters tell us about dehumanizing experiences and rehumanizing self-awareness.

Notes

1. Lithuanian Central State Archive (further—LCSA), f. R-769, op. 1, d. 2554, l. 171.
2. Bruce MZ Cohen, *Mental Health User Narratives: New Perspectives on Illness and Recovery* (Basingstoke, New York: Palgrave Macmillan, 2008), 38; Lars-Christer Hydén, Jens Brockmeier, "Introduction: From the Retold to the Performed Story", in *Health, Illness and Culture: Broken Narratives*, eds. Lars-Christer Hydén, Jens Brockmeier (New York, London: Routledge), 2.
3. Cheryl Mattingly, *Healing Dramas and Clinical Plots: The Narrative Structure of Experience* (Cambridge: Cambridge University Press, 1998), 1.
4. Guenter B. Risse, John Harley Warner, "Reconstructing Clinical Activities: Patient Records in Medical History", *Social History of Medicine* 5, no. 2 (1992): 183–205.
5. For example, Sidney Bloch, Peter Reddaway, *Russia's Political Hospitals: The Abuse of Psychiatry in the Soviet Union* (London: Gollancz, 1977); Sidney Bloch, Peter Reddaway, *Soviet Psychiatric Abuse—The Shadow over World Psychiatry* (London: Gollancz, 1984); Harvey Fireside, *Soviet Psychoprisons* (New York, London: W. W. Norton & Company, 1979).
6. Robert van Voren, *On Dissidents and Madness: From the Soviet Union of Leonid Brezhnev to the "Soviet Union" of Vladimir Putin* (New York, Amsterdam: Rodopi, 2009).
7. Rebecca Reich, "Inside the Psychiatric Word: Diagnosis and Self-Definition in the Late Soviet Period", *Slavic Review* 73, no. 3 (2014): 563–584; Rebecca Reich, *State of Madness: Psychiatry, Literature, and Dissent After Stalin* (DeKalb: Northern Illinois University Press, 2018).
8. Roy Porter, "The Patient's View: Doing Medical History from Below", *Theory and Society* 14, no. 2 (1985): 175–198.
9. Joseph Wortis, *Soviet Psychiatry* (Baltimore: Williams & Wilkins, 1950); Paul Calloway, *Soviet and Western Psychiatry: A Comparative Study* (Keighley: The Moor Press, 1992).
10. Greg Eghigian, "Care and Control in a Communist State: The Place of Politics in East German Psychiatry", in *Psychiatry and Mental Health Care in the Twentieth Century: Comparisons and Approaches*, eds. Marijke Gijswijt-Hofstra, Harry Oosterhuis, Joost Vijselaar, Hugh Freeman (Amsterdam: Amsterdam University Press, 2005), 183–199; Mat Savelli, Sarah Marks, eds., *Psychiatry in Communist Europe* (Basingstoke, New York: Palgrave Macmillan, 2015).
11. Benjamin Zajicek, *Scientific Psychiatry in Stalin's Soviet Union: The Politics of Modern Medicine and the Struggle to Define 'Pavlovian' Psychiatry, 1939–1953: A Dissertation* (Chicago: The University of Chicago, 2009);

Benjamin Zajicek, "Soviet Psychiatry and the Origins of the Sluggish Schizophrenia Concept, 1912–1936", *History of the Human Sciences* 31, no. 2 (2018): 88–105; Irina Sirotkina, *Diagnosing Literary Genius: A Cultural History of Psychiatry in Russia, 1880–1930* (Baltimore, London: The Johns Hopkins University Press, 2002); Grégory Dufaud, Lara Rzesnitzek, "Soviet Psychiatry through the Prism of Circulation: The Case of Outpatient Psychiatry in the Interwar Period", *Kritika: Explorations in Russian and Eurasian History* 17, no. 4 (2016): 781–803.

12. Calloway, *Soviet and Western Psychiatry*, 64.
13. Nikolas Rose, "Beyond medicalisation", *Lancet* 369 (February 24, 2007): 700.
14. Talcott Parsons, *The Social System* (London: Routledge, 1991), 296–298.
15. Mary E. Fissell, "The disappearance of the patient's narrative and the invention of hospital medicine", in *British Medicine in an Age of Reform*, eds. Roger French, Andrew Wear (London, New York: Routledge, 1991), 93.
16. Jurate A. Sakalys, "The political role of illness narratives", *Journal of Advanced Nursing* 31, no. 6 (2000): 1470.
17. Bruce MZ Cohen, *Mental Health User Narratives*, 2.
18. Jurate A. Sakalys, "The political role of illness narratives", 1472.
19. Claudia Malacrida, "Contested memories: efforts of the powerful to silence former inmates' histories of life in an institution for 'mental defectives'", *Disability & Society* 21, no. 5 (2006): 400.
20. Joseph D. Lewandowski, "Rethinking Power and Subjectivity after Foucault", *symploke* 3, no. 2 (1995): 221.
21. Anthony Giddens, *The Transformation of Intimacy: Sexuality, Love and Eroticism in Modern Societies* (Stanford: Stanford University Press, 1992), 28–29.
22. Mike Bury, "Illness narratives: fact or fiction?", *Sociology of Health & Illness* 23, no. 3 (2001): 269–271.
23. Kerry Davies, "'Silent and Censured Travellers'? Patients' Narratives and Patients' Voices: Perspectives on the History of Mental Illness since 1948", *Social History of Medicine* 14, no. 2 (2001): 274.
24. Mark G. Field, "In Sickness and in Health", *The Wilson Quarterly* 9, no. 4 (1985): 46–60.
25. LCSA, f. R-769, op. 1, d. 2034, l. 27.
26. Ibid., d. 4953, ll. 197–197v.
27. Ibid., d. 2827, l. 22.
28. Ibid., d. 9286, l. 117.
29. Ibid., d. 2038, l. 60v.
30. Ibid., d. 7013, ll. 108–109.
31. Ibid., d. 7013, l. 109.

32. Ibid., d. 4545, l. 174.
33. Ibid., d. 4155, l. 100.
34. Ibid., d. 2033, l. 154v.
35. Ibid., d. 6611, l. 97.
36. Ibid., d. 503, l. 94.
37. Ibid., d. 1699, l. 231.
38. Ibid., d. 1699, ll. 230–230v.
39. Ibid., d. 1834, l. 38v.
40. Ibid., d. 7010, ll. 231–231v.
41. Ibid., d. 2556, l. 67.

CHAPTER 9

"I Like My Job because It Will Get Me Out Quicker": Work, Independence, and Disability at Indiana's Central State Hospital (1986–1993)

Emily Beckman, Elizabeth Nelson, and Modupe Labode

Indiana's Central State Hospital (CSH) in the USA provides a case study for understanding the relationship between labour and independence for psychiatric inpatients with intellectual disabilities. This study focuses on the years leading up to the hospital's 1994 closure, examining work as a part of institutional life and as part of the process of deinstitutionalization.

"I'm Working at the Workshop," *DDU Review*, September 1989, Indiana Medical History Museum (IMHM) archives, Indianapolis, Indiana. We have omitted the last names of patient-authors who wrote in the DDU Review because we have not been able to obtain the permission to identify individuals with their writings.

E. Beckman (✉) • E. Nelson
Indiana University–Purdue University Indianapolis, Indianapolis, IN, USA
e-mail: embeckma@iupui.edu

R. Ellis et al. (eds.), *Voices in the History of Madness*, Mental Health in Historical Perspective,
https://doi.org/10.1007/978-3-030-69559-0_9

Labour conditions shifted significantly in 1992, when, in preparation for the hospital's closing, a work program at the hospital switched from an on-site sheltered workshop model to a framework of supported employment. We argue that the changing work policies during the process of the hospital's phase-out and closure had inadvertent negative effects on patient perceptions of, and abilities to realize, their goals. In common with other authors in this volume, we analyse previously overlooked sources to uncover patients' experiences of the asylum. More specifically, we rely on several narrative sources to reconstruct patient experiences within rehabilitative vocational programs. Of these sources, the most relevant is the *DDU Review*, a newsletter produced by patients in the Dual Diagnosis Unit (DDU) from 1986 through 1993. This newsletter consisted of brief articles, updates, and illustrations authored by the patients themselves as part of a recreational therapy program.[1] The monthly newsletter provides a detailed view, from the perspective of the patients, of everyday life on the DDU wards, evoking the daily routines of a long-stay state psychiatric institution and making visible the dynamics of the DDU community. Most importantly, the newsletters provide access to often under-represented patient voices, a rare and valuable resource as we attempt to consider new ways of thinking about life within and outside of a state psychiatric institution. In addition to the *DDU Review*, oral history interviews conducted with former hospital staff, along with newspaper articles and administrative records, help define the patient work experience and provide insight into how those who worked closely with patients understood the hospital's policies around work.

Work played many roles in patients' lives at CSH: as part of rehabilitative programming intended to prepare patients for fully or semi-independent lives in the community; as a way to earn money; and as part of patients' daily routines, self-conceptions, and expectations for the future. As revealed in the *DDU Review*, CSH patients with intellectual disabilities often believed they had the potential to gain privileges and, ultimately, release from the hospital through consistent work and other forms of "good behaviour." Sustained employment, moreover, would prepare patients for the job they desired after release. Patients imagined their post-release work life as an essential part of independent life in the community. The 1992 announcement that the hospital would close, and the concurrent shift from sheltered work to the supported employment model, led many

M. Labode
National Museum of American History, Washington, DC, USA

patients to imagine that their dreams of living independently and working in the community might soon become a reality. With supported employment, patients began to take jobs in the community rather than labouring in more controlled conditions at the hospital worksite, the APS Workshop. However, the promises of supported employment were not realized. Few discharged patients would experience the level of freedom and self-sufficiency that they had imagined while living within the hospital, though some did find some measure of stability.

While well-intentioned, the switch to supported employment depended on, but did not adequately consider, the patient–staff relationships that would have been the key to its success. Interviews with former staff reveal the extent to which, even in a resource-poor institution on the brink of closure, daily life at CSH was characterized by intimate dynamics of care. Despite the exploitative nature of the sheltered workshop model, dedicated staff built intimate relationships with patients within this space, seeing the work as a way to reinforce, at the very least, interpersonal skills such as cooperation, manners, and emotional control. These were not only useful skills for holding down a job, but part of a more staff-driven holistic approach to encouraging self-realization and better mental health.[2] During the transition to supported employment, policy makers assumed that patient–staff relationships, built on cooperation and trust, would gradually be dissolved. This assumption succinctly captures one of the fundamental problems of deinstitutionalization in the late twentieth century, specifically the lack of recognition of *inter*dependence as a positive value and long-term success strategy for people with mental and intellectual disabilities.

Work and Disability

Disability as a socio-political category has been defined largely in relation to labour. Ever since the nineteenth century, people with disabilities have been constructed as unproductive.[3] The growth of custodial institutions that served people with physical and intellectual disabilities, as well as mental illness, sits in dynamic relation to this particular construction of disability. These institutions provide at minimum, basic support (food, housing) for people labelled as disabled or mentally ill. At the same time, from their origins in the nineteenth century, institutions were financially dependent on the unpaid labour of their residents.[4] Increasingly over the course of the twentieth century, institutions emphasized rehabilitative programs meant to restore their wards to full or partial participation in the community, participation defined largely by workforce participation and self-support.

Whether work performed in institutions by people with disabilities was required to be remunerated, and at what rate, was a matter of intense federal attention in the US from the 1970s. In 1973, the US district court decision *Souder v. Brennan* required that state-run institutions apply minimum wage standards, established by the 1938 Fair Labour Standards Act (FLSA), to patient workers.[5] This decision placed significant financial strain on many institutions, and some disability rights advocates and proponents of vocational rehabilitation argued that the decision had the adverse effect of removing opportunities for employment and work-based rehabilitation for patients with disabilities.[6] Some institutions expanded "sheltered workshop" programs, nonprofit ventures that only employed people with disabilities.[7] A 1986 amendment to the FLSA established a certification process for employers of people with disabilities that continued the longstanding practice of paying these workers a subminimum wage and enabled the growth of sheltered workshops in both community settings and at custodial institutions.[8] Proponents of sheltered workshops at institutions argued that such programs instilled vocational skills that would enable workers to eventually find employment in the communities. Critics have charged that such programs segregate and exploit people with disabilities, and often provide businesses with a way to extract underpaid labour for profit.[9]

Central State Hospital

CSH opened in 1848 as the "Indiana Hospital for the Insane." Originally located two miles west of Indianapolis, a city that would eventually grow to surround the hospital, CSH was the first and largest of the state of Indiana's system of "mental" institutions that, by the 1930s, included psychiatric hospitals, a village for people with epilepsy, and schools for "feeble-minded" adults and children.[10] Like many state-run mental hospitals in the US, CSH experienced cycles of overcrowding, scandal, and reform.[11] Despite legal action and protest, the hospital facilities and care often proved inadequate. As the psychiatric profession shifted toward the reliance on medications and community-based care for all but the most seriously mentally ill, the patient population at CSH declined from over 2200 in the 1950s to fewer than 500 in the 1980s. In 1992, after investigations into the deaths of several patients shed light on the hospital's significant deficiencies, the governor accepted the recommendation of a special commission to close the hospital by 30 June 1994.[12]

From the time of the hospital's founding, medical directors conceived of patients' work in spaces such as the hospital's farm and laundries as both therapeutic and "of profit to the institution."[13] In the 1970s, a department of rehabilitation was established at CSH, comprising vocational, occupational, recreational, music, and speech therapies. These developments were part of the hospital's increased emphasis on rehabilitative programs focused on instilling needed skills for discharge into the community. This period witnessed the creation of specialized units for particular patient populations, as in the DDU (dual diagnosis/developmental disabilities unit) which was founded in the mid-1970s and certified by the federal government as an Intermediate Care Facility/Mental Retardation (ICF/MR) in 1978.[14] The DDU served patients diagnosed with both mental illness and what was called "mental retardation," which was determined by IQ tests and other psychological measures.[15]

As in other hospital units, DDU patients interacted with a team of professionals, including psychiatrists, nurses, psychologists, and social workers, but rehabilitation therapists played an especially large role in DDU patients' day-to-day lives.[16] Rehabilitation programs commanded a significant amount of patients' time and included recreational activities such as sports, ceramics, music appreciation, and camping. In occupational programs, patients learned to cook, sew, do laundry, and navigate public transportation—practical skills that residents needed for life "in the community," that is, outside the hospital.

By 1980, a private, not-for-profit organization called Associated Patient Services (APS) established a sheltered workshop program, staffed by DDU residents, at CSH. The business-friendly aspects of the sheltered workshop may have attracted Indiana legislators when they authorized implementing the program in the state hospital system, as federal rules required that patients be paid, albeit at sub-minimum wage, for their work.[17] A 1985 profile of APS Industries approvingly noted that "the production services of the company is a profitable alternative for the private sector, which seeks competitive bids for contract work."[18]

Methodology

Patients' experiences at the sheltered workshop and in the supported employment programs were recorded in the *DDU Review*. Participants in the "Newspaper Club" produced the newsletter. The club itself was a cross-disciplinary rehabilitative program founded in 1986 by a recreation therapist, an educator, and a speech pathologist.[19] The production of the paper, they asserted, "bolsters low self-esteem, develops conversation skills, sharpens academic skills and increases attention span."[20] Each issue of the newspaper featured around two dozen brief articles that were often illustrated with line drawings by patients in the DDU. Patients reported mainly about events in their lives, including their experiences as workers. A small portion of the newspaper was occupied with articles written by rehabilitation therapists that provided updates and news about programs and recognized the achievements of individual patients.

Although there is an ample literature within disability studies, policy, and the social sciences assessing the impact of deinstitutionalization on people with disabilities, studies that focus on the lived experiences and life-stories of people with disabilities are more rare.[21] While sources such as CSH administrative records, newspaper articles, and policy documents shine some light on the philosophy and economics of work-based rehabilitation, the *DDU Review* allows us to attend to the voices of patients who engaged in these programs. This chapter is a unique resource for building an understanding of institutional labour and deinstitutionalization as lived experiences. Our analysis of the patient-produced newsletter the *DDU Review* can therefore be situated in a historiography that seeks to narrate the psychiatry and mental health care "from below."[22] Much like Tomas Vaiseta's analysis of complaint letters in Chap. 8, we take a narrative approach to the newsletter, examining patient writings in terms of what they revealed about their status, hopes, and expectations, and tracing how those expectations changed in response to changing opportunities, situations, and policies. The periodical form of the *DDU Review* enables the reconstruction of patients' attitudes, perspectives, and experiences in the unfolding of time.

We conducted a narrative study of 42 issues of the *DDU Review* published between September 1988 and September 1993, and took steps to verify information when possible. The specific "contextual focus" of our study is the patient work experience among individuals living at CSH.[23] Clandinin and Connelly suggest that "narrative research is best for capturing the detailed stories or life experiences" and a primary goal of this research is to capture the life experience of the CSH patient as worker.[24] Therefore, we have spent a considerable amount of time with our "field texts," which appear in the form of patient-authored newsletters, as well as supplemental materials that provide context for the *DDU Review*: oral histories, a longitudinal discharge study carried during and after the hospital closure, newspaper articles, and CSH administrative documents.[25] Creswell suggests "narrative researchers situate individual stories within participants' personal experiences …, their culture and their historical contexts (time and place)."[26] Therefore, the additional data help us more clearly define the lived experience of the CSH patients as workers. Finally, we "restory" the information into a framework that "makes sense," which requires us, as researchers, to make connections or provide a "causal link" to show the relationship between ideas and configure the chronology of events which help further define the experience.[27] Central to narrative research is the relationship between the researchers and those being researched.[28] While we have not yet communicated directly with the patients who authored the newsletters, we have done so with former CSH staff. The three investigators of this study represent different disciplinary perspectives, Medical Humanities, History, and Museum Studies, and independently analysed the data before meeting to review and refine final analysis and conclusions.

Results: Patient Goals and Experiences of Work

CSH patients laboured in a number of different contexts, within and outside of hospital grounds. Some patients found jobs at the hospital, for example, cleaning tables and mopping the floors of the canteen known as the Brass Rail, or working in one of the hospital dining rooms.[29] Others worked off grounds at non-profit organizations that aimed to further employment for people with disabilities, such as Goodwill Industries.[30] At CSH, the main workplace for DDU patients was the APS Workshop, founded by 1980 as a sheltered workshop. There, patients engaged in "production work," fulfilling work orders for private corporations.[31]

At the APS sheltered workshop program, Central State patients performed repetitive tasks, such as taking apart and cleaning Chrysler and Navistar helmets,[32] "put[ting] screws and bolts in a bag,"[33] and "recycling plastic, untangling telephone cords or assembling small parts."[34] One worker wrote, "We do all kinds of work. Sometimes we paint park benches.

We strip cassette tapes. We put plastic tapes in a big pile in a box."[35] Patients generally described work in the APS Workshop as "fun" and "easy," though some did note that the pay was low.[36]

Both within and outside CSH, working usually required an evaluation before placement. One patient wrote, "I am going to get a job at the Brass Rail. I took a test yesterday, I put a bag in the trash can and mopped the floor and cleaned out the sink for the test."[37] Another provided a detailed description of going to work at another workshop: "I went to Noble Industries for an evaluation. They tested me to see how I did with putting boxes together, counting out beans and putting them in bags, and about how much strength I had in my hands."[38] At the APS workshop, efficient work was expected and contributed overall to higher production rates, and the promise of paychecks each period: "She [the supervisor] wants me to work faster … I think it is fun to work. I like to make money. I like to do helmets and paper work too."[39] Workers were recognized for highest production and most improved production each month, and parties marked special occasions or fulfilled goals. Occasionally workers were able to hold two jobs. For example, one patient worked part time in a hospital dining room in addition to her regular job at APS.[40]

The pace of work varied; sometimes the workshop could not take on new orders/had to decline orders due to lack of space, while other times there were few orders. During slow times, residents made craft projects, watched movies, and did puzzles.[41] After 1991, however, there was increased emphasis on skills that would help patients to transition to working in the community: "We cannot do arts and crafts anymore … they have new down-time jobs. We talked about how you act on an outside job."[42] In March 1992, workers moved to a new APS work area that provided more space for increased production. Additional jobs came in, such as putting together boxes for Imperial Fireworks. "They are red boxes. We had to fold all of our folds so they will stay closed. There was a sticker that we had to put on the back of them. We also put a cat poster inside the boxes. I enjoyed doing them."[43]

Many patients eagerly sought opportunities to work in order to have funds that they controlled. DDU residents used their wages to buy cigarettes, food, and other items that made their lives more comfortable. Some bought gifts for family and friends, or saved up to make a more significant purchase, such as a radio or television. *DDU Review* writers frequently refer to the hospital bureaucracy of work for pay, such as the "pink slips" patients redeemed for cash and "Patient Accounts," which was a type of savings account for patients. One patient wrote of his plans for wages: "I want to go to Kroger [a local grocer] with my paycheck and buy a carton of cigarettes. I'll put the rest of it in Patient Accounts."[44]

DDU Review reporters referred to the work on their progress toward release from CSH in terms that would make sense to fellow patients who read the newsletter. One woman was relieved that she was now "off of the restrictions," because she could use the phone and go to work. She knew that if she stayed off restrictions, a staff member would "start working on getting me into a group home."[45] At "staffing," regular meetings in which staff, the patient, and sometimes family members reviewed the patient's progress, work performance also featured. Staff advised another patient, for example, that he needed to get to work on time and stop fighting "before I ever can go to a group home."[46] As part of reinforcing self-control and good behaviour, employed patients met weekly at Job Club to discuss individuals' work progress and their feelings about work, including "good or bad things that may have happened at work during the week."[47]

Some patients expressed strong support for individual labour and hard work as virtues in themselves. In this respect, their perspectives corresponded with common American ideas about self-sufficiency where people expect, and are expected, to work hard to support themselves and their families without relying on others, specifically the government, for help. Noting the Labour Day holiday, one man wrote that the "hardest working boys are the one's [*sic*] that get out and make their own living. Same goes the women."[48] Another described a fellow patient who was leaving for a group home as "a good worker. She has two jobs."[49] Even as hard, disciplined work was a marker of independence, some patients appreciated the help that supervisors and others gave them, acknowledging that interdependence was a fact of their work life at work.[50]

Productive work was an important aspect of patients' recollections of their previous experiences outside the hospital. One patient wrote, "I used to work. I worked so many places" and specified that he had worked at a gas station and "put gas in the cans."[51] Another regretted not completing high school, because if he had graduated, he could "get a good job."[52] Even more than a means to achieving independence, the ability to do productive, useful work seemed inherently valuable to many patients.

Correspondingly, paid labour featured in writers' speculations about what life might look like once they were discharged from the hospital. Many patients had detailed plans for where they would live and what type of work they would pursue. One man wanted to emulate his brother and work as a contractor. Another hoped to work at a convenience store "so I can help people put groceries in their car. I want to work to have food in my house," while yet another envisioned working at a service station or as a carpenter, or mechanic.[53]

Ultimately, many patients saw work as a way to leave the hospital and achieve some sort of independence. As one patient stated, "I like my job because it will get me out quicker."[54] These attitudes were reinforced by patients who were moving on to group homes and reported on the process of having their work skills assessed as they received their placement in the community.

Staff Goals and Policy Changes During the Closure

Key staff members who administered the DDU and associated work programs were less convinced that the sheltered workshop was adequate preparation for getting a job in the community. Mike Flores, the director of the DDU who arranged for the sheltered workshop program to be brought to Central State in the late 1970s, recalled the workshop as fundamentally limited. It was merely "someplace for [patients] to go and at least go through some of the structure of employment."[55] Flores emphasized how little work was done between projects, "A lot of it was sitting around and drinking coffee because there wasn't any work and they'd get bored but it was neat for them to go there. It was a place to go."[56] Flores did note that participation in work programs was yet another way for patients to demonstrate their readiness for work in the community. "We didn't have a whole lot of carrots to dangle in front of them, so it was like, well, if you go there on time, plus you go to your other programs on time, you listen, don't do anything that creates all kinds of problems … that is good for when you interview and you get a job."[57] Flores' recollections echo comments made in 1985 by the Central State APS program director Dale Marion, who noted that the workshop program for DDU residents was "largely therapeutic. While the program provides them some income, it also provides a daily activity that is extremely important."[58]

The limits of the sheltered workshop model as a form of training for "outside jobs" were thrown into relief with the decision by Indiana's governor to close the hospital in 1992. The process of closing down the hospital took two years (until the summer of 1994), and it intensified demands on rehabilitation specialists as patients' prospects of release and placement in the community were accelerated. The sheltered workshop model came under scrutiny and policy makers deemed the APS sheltered workshop model inadequate for preparing patients for outside jobs. However, Vickie Cole, who was a floor supervisor for APS in 1992 when the decision was made to close the hospital, believed that her team's approach gave patients important interpersonal skills: "The statistics had shown that the job skills they learned did not transfer out into jobs in the community. Now that made no sense to me, because we worked more on not how you move your fingers, but how you address people, how you cooperate when there is a decision to be made, a lot of those kinds of things."[59] Cole believed the sheltered workshop offered "honest to God work"; the work not only provided job skills, but the wages also built patient's self-esteem and increased general motivation.[60]

Nevertheless, with the imminent closure and deinstitutionalization of patients, in January 1993, the APS workshop program received a complete overhaul, as a $2.4 million-dollar grant from the state government allowed for the expansion of supported employment at various community mental health centres, including CSH. In contrast to the sheltered workshop model, which segregated employed people with disabilities, supported employment allowed patients to work alongside workers without disabilities. These changes were chronicled in the *DDU Review*. One patient wrote, "APS has new rules. The staff at APS are doing a real good job. They are trying to find jobs for us. APS is teaching us the right skills. APS is a training centre."[61] Other patients reported the arrival of several job coaches at APS, new management, and new activity schedules.[62]

Within the first month of supported employment, ten of the twenty patients working at APS had jobs based in the community. Patients working at APS toured potential workplaces and understood that to qualify for this new program they needed to "have good behaviour, be off of restrictions, and get back from breaks on time."[63] Training in these jobs was facilitated by additional job coaches that transported the employees to and from CSH, working alongside them until they were sufficiently skilled to work more independently.[64] Patients were employed at local restaurants, warehouses, and stores, doing jobs such as dishwashing, cleaning, and "folding clothes and putting them on hangers."[65] For example, one patient washed dishes and cleaned at a restaurant, with his job coach helping him get oriented and escorting him to and from work. The goal was for him to become more and more independent, eventually needing the assistance of a coach only occasionally, or not at all.[66]

At the time of the hospital's closure, many observers were positive about the transition to supported employment. Vickie Cole, a former supervisor at the sheltered workshop, noted that many of the patients who were working in the community were more engaged and less guarded. Eighteen months after the hospital closed, at least eight former CSH patients were still at work in Central Indiana under supported employment.[67] It is difficult to account for the long-term effects of the supported employment program given the difficulty of tracking former patients.[68] Cole's perspectives, however, provide important insights into the implementation of supported employment.

With the shift from work in the CSH-sheltered workshop to supported employment in the community, Cole became a job coach, accompanying patients to their jobs off grounds. She maintained that some of the patients may have had more success finding a job in the community because of their previous sheltered workshop experience, though hospital administration denied any real benefit. Cole also emphasized the importance of the relationship between the staff and patients, which allowed her to focus on the needs of each individual patient. However, as the state's model assumed that intensive support, including the job coach, would eventually become less involved in the patient's work life, Cole believed that there was ultimately little success with the transition to supported employment: "either they could make it or they couldn't and if they couldn't there was nowhere to put them."[69] Moving patients into a supported employment environment, Cole explained, required constant assessment from supportive staff. "You don't have any preconceived notions. You start out here and if he can do it, good, you go on up, on up, on up. Maybe he can do it on his own from then on and you're with him with … maybe three weeks until he learns how to do the task, where the bathrooms are, not to go in the women's restroom, where the break room is, when do you get your lunch and all of those kinds of things."[70]

Another former CSH job coach, Doug Crandell, recalled in a 2016 essay how difficult it was to secure positions for patients with disabilities in the community. Crandell describes developing a close relationship with a particular patient called "Riley" as they searched in vain for employment and toured diverse worksites around the city of Indianapolis: "I was trying hard to find him a job, but all the fast-food places weren't interested in hiring someone who didn't speak or hear."[71] Any progress Crandell and Riley made toward securing a job was interrupted when Riley was transferred to a sheltered workshop site in northern Indiana, likely in conjunction with living in another state facility or perhaps a group home. While anecdotal, Riley's story is indicative of broader themes: the job coach program encouraged CSH patients diagnosed with intellectual disabilities and mental illness to imagine a life that included employment in the community; this trajectory was often disrupted by discharge, the severance of supportive relationships, and placement in equally restrictive environments.

According to a study tracking CSH patients more than ten years after the hospital closed, 58.1% of patients classified as "dual diagnosis" were living in semi-independent living programs.[72] At least some of these patients held down jobs in the community and thrived after moving out of CSH. Cole recalled in particular a young woman who was limited in her ability to care for herself inside the hospital who went on to work at a daycare centre after her discharge.[73] However, only 5.8% of patients with dual diagnoses were living in private residences and 8.1% were living in other state-operated facilities.[74] The other surviving/remaining dual diagnosis patients from CSH lived in supervised group living facilities, Medicaid waiver homes, and nursing homes. This study provides some crucial insight into the work lives and living situations of former patients. At the time of the report, moreover, 17 (19.8%) patients with dual diagnosis had died.[75]

The same report noted that almost 20% of patients with dual diagnosis had died within 10 years of the hospital's closing. This corresponds with what former staff reported during the oral history interviews. Cole remembers large numbers of former patients dying soon after the closure, explaining that "they were taken out of their home and placed where they didn't know anybody, they didn't feel safe … it scared them to death."[76] One man attempted to leave his new group home and return to CSH. According to Cole, he filled a grocery cart with all of his possessions and was killed by a car as he walked along a road.[77] Another man drowned in a retention pond near his group home. Cole recalled that she attended 14 funerals for former patients in the two years following the closure of the hospital.[78] When recounting such stories of "people thrown away," in the words of one expert, it is important to emphasize the failures of Indiana's policymakers to ensure adequate supports for people who were fully capable of success, with the proper resources.[79]

Notes

1. Our data set is defined by the holdings of the IMHM and the personal files of former DDU director, Mike Flores. The earliest issues of the *DDU Review* (October 1986–January 1987; March 1987–January 1988; February 1991, June 1991, and July–August 1992) have not been located. All *DDU Review* articles referenced in the present study are housed at the IMHM.
2. Vickie Cole, oral history interview by Emily Beckman, Elizabeth Nelson, and Angela Potter, Indianapolis, May 3, 2018. Recording and transcript currently held at the Medical Humanities and Health Studies Program, Indiana University-Purdue University, Indianapolis (IUPUI), but will be deposited at the IUPUI Ruth Lilly Special Collections and Archives.
3. J.W. Trent, Jr., *Inventing the Feeble Mind: A History of Mental Retardation in the United States* (Berkeley: University of California Press, 1994); S.F. Rose, *No Right to Be Idle: The Invention of Disability, 1840s–1930s* (Chapel Hill: The University of North Carolina Press, 2017).
4. J. Abbas, "A Legacy of Exploitation: Intellectual Disability, Unpaid Labour, & Disability Services," *New Politics* XIV-1, no. 53 (Summer 2012), http://newpol.org/content/legacy-exploitation-intellectual-disability-unpaid-labour-disability-services.
5. University of Michigan Law School: Civil Rights Litigation Clearinghouse, "Souder v. Brennan." Available at: https://www.clearinghouse.net/detail.php?id=15215.
6. D. Safier and R. Barnum, "Patient Rehabilitation through Hospital Work under Fair Labor Standards," *Hospital and Community Psychiatry* 26, no. 5 (May 1975): 299–302.
7. D.B. Schwartz, "Expanding a Sheltered Workshop to Replace Nonpaying Patient Jobs," *Hospital and Community Psychiatry* 27, no. 2 (February 1976): 98–101.
8. United States Department of Labor: Wages and Hour Division, "Fact Sheet #39: The Employment of Workers with Disabilities at Subminimum Wages," https://www.dol.gov/whd/regs/compliance/whdfs39.htm.
9. Abbas, 2012; M. McDonald and S. Herr, "Case Studies: Which Clients Should a Sheltered Workshop Serve?" *The Hastings Center Report* 14, no. 5 (October 1984): 52–54. For a recent overview of this topic see, R. Beckwith, *Disability Servitude: From Peonage to Poverty* (New York: Palgrave Macmillan, 2016).
10. "Statistical Survey of Public Assistance in Indiana: Special Study, Establishment and Growth of the State Institutions" (April 1938). Indiana Clipping File, Indiana State Library. By the 1930s, along with eight institutions for "mental cases," Indiana also administered several prisons and

reform schools, a veteran's home, an orphanage, a tuberculosis sanatorium, and schools for Deaf and blind children.

11. E. Dwyer, "Mental Health Care in Early Twentieth Century Indiana and the Limits of Reform," *Indiana Medical History Quarterly* 9 (1983): 23–27.
12. E.C. McDonel, E.C., Meyer, L. and R. Deliberty, "Implementing State-Level Mental Health Policy Reforms in Indiana: Closing a State-Operated Psychiatric Hospital and Passing Major Mental Health Reform Legislation," *International Journal of Law and Psychiatry* 19, no. 3&4 (1996): 239–264.
13. L. Dunlap, J.S. Bobbs, J. Blake, E.J. Peck, J. Wilkins, and S. Major, *Report to the General Assembly of the State of Indiana. General Assembly of Indiana at Thirty-Third Session Commencing December 3, 1849, Part Second* (Indianapolis: John D. Defrees, 1849).
14. Mike Flores, "Employment Narrative: Central State Hospital," Mike Flores, Personal Files. As of 2010, these facilities are called Intermediate Care Facilities for Individuals with Intellectual Disabilities (ICF/IID), https://www.cms.gov/Regulations-and-Guidance/Legislation/CFCsAndCoPs/Intermediate-Care-Facilities-for-Individuals-with-Intellectual-Disabilities-ICF-IID.html.
15. Central State Hospital, *139th Annual Report*, 1986–1987.
16. Central State Hospital, *142nd Annual Report*, 1989–1990.
17. D.B. Schwartz, "Expanding a Sheltered Workshop to Replace Nonpaying Patient Jobs," *Hospital and Community Psychiatry* 27, no. 2 (February 1976): 98–101; M. McDonald and S. Herr, "Case Studies: Which Clients Should a Sheltered Workshop Serve?" *The Hastings Center Report* 14, no. 5 (October 1984): 52–54; United States Department of Labour: Wages and Hour Division, "Fact Sheet #39: The Employment of Workers with Disabilities at Subminimum Wages," https://www.dol.gov/whd/regs/compliance/whdfs39.htm.
18. Rex Redifer, "Special Hospital Program Provides Useful Lives for Mental Patients," *Indianapolis Star*, September 19, 1985, 27.
19. Terry Duwe, Lisa Freeman, and Bonnie O'Connor, oral history interview by Emily Beckman, Modupe Labode, Elizabeth Nelson, and Angela Potter, Indianapolis, August 2017. Recording and transcript currently held at the Medical Humanities and Health Studies Program, Indiana University-Purdue University, Indianapolis (IUPUI), but will be deposited at the IUPUI Ruth Lilly Special Collections and Archives.
20. Kathy Whyde, "Capturing Pride in Print," *The Indianapolis Star*, April 9, 1988, p. 37.
21. L. Ben-Moshe, "The Contested Meaning of 'Community' in Discourses of Deinstutionalization and Community Living in the Field of Developmental Disability," *Disability and Community* 6 (2011): 241–264; Research and Training Center on Community Living, "Behavioral Outcome of

Deinstitutionalization for People with Intellectual and/or Developmental Disabilities: Third Decennial Review of U.S. Studies, 1977–2010," *Policy Research Brief* 21, no. 2 (2011): 1–11; K. Johnson, R. Traustadóttir, C.M. Bigby, and K. Kristiansen, *Deinstitutionalization and People with Intellectual Disabilities: In and Out of Institutions* (London: Jessica Kingsley Publishers, 2005).

22. R. Porter, "The Patient's View: Doing Medical History from Below," *Theory and Society* 14, no. 2 (1985): 175–198; A. Bacopoulos-Viau and A. Fauvel, "The Patient's Turn: Roy Porter and Psychiatry's Tales, Thirty Years On," *Medical History* 60, no. 1 (January 2016): 1–18.
23. J. O. Ollerenshaw and J.W. Creswell, "Narrative Research: A Comparison of Two Restorying Data Analysis Approaches," *Qualitative Inquiry* 8, no. 3 (2002): 329–347.
24. D. J. Clandinin, F. M. Connelly, *Narrative Inquiry: Experience and Story in Qualitative Research* (Hoboken, NJ: Wiley, 2000).
25. J.H. McGrew, E.R. Wright, B.A. Pescosolido, "Closing of a State Hospital: An Overview and Framework for a Case Study," *Journal of Behavioral Health Services & Research* 26, no. 3 (August 1999): 236–245; J.H McGrew, E.R. Wright, B.A. Pescosolido, E.C. McDonel, "The Closing of Central State Hospital: Long-Term Outcomes for Persons with Severe Mental Illness," *Journal of Behavioral Health Services & Research* 26, no. 3 (August 1999): 246–261; B.A. Pescosolido, E.R. Wright, K. Lutfey, "The Changing Hopes, Worries, and Community Supports of Individuals Moving from a Closing Long-Term Care Facility," *Journal of Behavioral Health Services & Research* 26, no. 3 (August 1999): 276–288; A. H. Lawson, E. R. Wright, S. Jaegber, J. McGrew, B. Pescosolido, *The Central State Hospital Discharge Study: Tracking Report* (Bloomington: Indiana Consortium for Mental Health Services Research, 2005).
26. Creswell, J. W., *Qualitative Inquiry & Research Design: Choosing among Five Approaches*, 3rd ed. (Thousand Oaks, CA: Sage, 2013).
27. J. O. Ollerenshaw, J.W. Creswell, 2002, 329–347.
28. J. O. Ollerenshaw, J.W. Creswell, 2002, 329–347.
29. "The Brass Rail Job I am Getting," *DDU Review*, December 1988; "Job at Brass Rail," *DDU Review*, February 1989; "I Have Two Jobs," *DDU Review*, May–June 1992. The restaurant/canteen was named for an antique brass rail salvaged from one of the hospital's historic buildings ("The Brass Rail," *The Indianapolis News*, November 12, 1985, 6).
30. "What Happened to Vicki at APS," *DDU Review*, April 1989.
31. "Sheltered Work New Years [*sic*] Party," *DDU Review*, January 1989; Vickie Cole, "APS News," *DDU Review*, September 1989.
32. "[Redacted Name]'s New Job," *DDU Review*, June 1989.
33. "My New Job," *DDU Review*, March/April 1992.

34. J. Fahy, "APS Industries Befriends Mentally Ill," *The Indianapolis Star*, December 24, 1995, A7.
35. "My New Job at APS," *DDU Review*, May–June 1992.
36. "Rushing at Work," *DDU Review*, July 1991; "APS News," *DDU Review*, November/December 1991.
37. "The Brass Rail Job I am Getting," *DDU Review*, January 1989.
38. "Darin Goes to Noble," *DDU Review*, April 1990.
39. "Rushing at Work," *DDU Review*, July 1991.
40. "I Have Two Jobs," *DDU Review*, May–June 1992.
41. "APS," *DDU Review*, November 1988; Vickie Cole, "APS News," *DDU Review*, September 1989.
42. "APS News," *DDU Review*, September 1991.
43. "News at APS," *DDU Review*, March/April 1992.
44. "Working at the Brass Rail," *DDU Review*, February 1989; "I'm Working at the Workshop," *DDU Review*, September 1989; "Rushing at Work," *DDU Review*, July 1991.
45. "Back to Work," *DDU Review*, March 1990.
46. "Me Getting Better," *DDU Review*, June 1990; "My Staffing," *DDU Review*, July 1991.
47. "What do You All Think About Job Club?" *DDU Review*, April 1989.
48. "Labor Day," *DDU Review*, September 1988.
49. "Barbara Leaves," *DDU Review*, May–June 1992.
50. "Job at Brass Rail," *DDU Review*, February 1989.
51. "Labor Day," *DDU Review*, September 1988.
52. "Back to School," *DDU Review*, August 1989.
53. "Reporter of the Month," *DDU Review*, October 1988; "Reporter of the Month," *DDU Review*, November 1988; "Reporter of the Month," *DDU Review*, May 1989; "My Future," *DDU Review*, November–December 1990.
54. "I Like My Job Because It Will Get Me Out Quicker," *DDU Review*, September 1989.
55. Mike Flores, oral history interview by Emily Beckman, Elizabeth Nelson, and Angela Potter, Indianapolis, May 16, 2018, and May 21, 2018. Recording and transcript currently held at the Medical Humanities and Health Studies Program, Indiana University-Purdue University, Indianapolis (IUPUI), but will be deposited at the IUPUI Ruth Lilly Special Collections and Archives.
56. Flores, oral history interview.
57. Flores, oral history interview.
58. Dale Marion, quoted in Redifer, 1988.
59. Vickie Cole, oral history interview.
60. Vickie Cole, oral history interview.

61. "Rules are Changing at APS Workshop," *DDU Review*, 1st Quarter 1993.
62. "New Staff at APS," *DDU Review*, 1st Quarter 1993; "New Boss at APS," *DDU Review*, 2nd Quarter 1993; "New Schedules on Ward 37," *DDU Review*, 1st Quarter 1993.
63. "APS Moved," *DDU Review*, Holiday Edition.
64. Joe Fahy, "Program Provides Ex-Mental Patients a Working Solution," *Indianapolis Star*, December 24, 1995, A1, A7; Fahy, "APS Industries Befriends Mentally Ill," *Indianapolis Star*, December 24, 1995, A7.
65. "[Name Redacted] is Working at Fridays," *DDU Review*, 2nd Quarter 1993; "[Name Redacted]'s New Job," *DDU Review*, 2nd Quarter 1993; "A Job at Galayan's," *DDU Review*, 2nd Quarter 1993; "We Work at Galayan's," *DDU Review*, 2nd Quarter Edition, 1993; "My Boss is Going to Get Me a New Job Off Grounds," 2nd Quarter 1993; "Supportive Employment," *DDU Review*, 2nd Quarter, 1993.
66. "[Name Redacted] is Working at Fridays," *DDU Review*, 2nd Quarter Edition, 1993; Fahy, "APS Industries Befriends Mentally Ill," A7.
67. Fahy, "APS Industries Befriends Mentally Ill," A7.
68. Fahy, "Program Provides Ex-Mental Patients a Working Solution," A7.
69. Vickie Cole, oral history interview.
70. Vickie Cole, oral history interview.
71. Doug Crandell, "Activities Of Daily Living," *The Sun*, November 2016. Online: https://www.thesunmagazine.org/issues/491/activities-of-daily-living.
72. Central State Hospital Discharge Study Tracking Report, Indiana Consortium for Mental Health Services Research, Institute for Social Research at Indiana University, 2005.
73. Vickie Cole, oral history interview.
74. Central State Hospital Discharge Study Tracking Report, Indiana Consortium for Mental Health Services Research, Institute for Social Research at Indiana University, 2005.
75. Central State Hospital Discharge Study Tracking Report, Indiana Consortium for Mental Health Services Research, Institute for Social Research at Indiana University, 2005.
76. Vickie Cole, oral history interview.
77. Vickie Cole, oral history interview.
78. Vickie Cole, oral history interview.
79. Gary Bond, psychologist and specialist in the assessment of supported employment programs, personal communication, 2019.

CHAPTER 10

"More than Bricks and Mortar": Meaningful Care Practices in the Old State Mental Hospitals

Verusca Calabria, Di Bailey, and Graham Bowpitt

Introduction

Former patients' perspectives on institutional care practices remain marginalised in the history of mental health care.[1] The focus of this chapter centres on the dynamic interplay between people who provided care, both formally and informally, and those who received it in the now-closed mental hospitals in Nottinghamshire, UK. It echoes the call made by Roy Porter more than 30 years ago to research the experiences of those who received care in order to challenge conventional documentary history, which tells us very little about the patients' experience and even less about the interactions between patients and staff.[2] The oral histories discussed in this chapter are based on Calabria's doctoral research.[3] The empirical study aimed to understand what has been lost through the modernisation

V. Calabria (✉) • D. Bailey • G. Bowpitt
Nottingham Trent University, Nottingham, UK
e-mail: verusca.calabria@ntu.ac.uk

R. Ellis et al. (eds.), *Voices in the History of Madness*, Mental Health in Historical Perspective,
https://doi.org/10.1007/978-3-030-69559-0_10

of mental health services, where the relationships between staff and patients are typically short-term and veer towards crisis management.[4] The research broadly represents the voices of people who have been inpatients of mental hospitals in one district of England and the staff who worked there over a period of 50 years of living memory. The significance of patient voices in the study of healthcare systems in interdisciplinary contexts offers the potential for more nuanced understanding of the changing meanings of inpatient care from asylum to community care.

The involvement of and co-production with people with lived experience of mental ill health and significant others such as carers have become increasingly important to contemporary mental health research and policy.[5] This research has taken a multidisciplinary approach by combining two distinct yet complementary methodologies, namely participatory action research (PAR) and oral history, with the intention of making visible the experiences of those who received and delivered care in the now-closed psychiatric asylums in Nottinghamshire, UK.[6] The oral histories, which form the primary source of data in the research, were collaboratively produced with ex-patients who received care from two mental hospitals and retired staff who worked there between 1948 and 1994, and were collected 30 years after the hospitals' closure. Twenty people with first-hand experience were interviewed multiple times. The study is located within the defined geographical area of Nottinghamshire, which has a long-established tradition of innovation in mental health services such as early community care through the introduction of extra-mural services, therapeutic community (TC) principles and an open-door policy from the 1940s onwards.[7]

Background

The negative perception of care provided in institutions in Britain was fuelled by a number of influential studies from the 1960s onwards, which were referred to as the 'literature of dysfunction' for their anti-institutional stance.[8] Besides the economic and political forces that led to the closure of asylums, the damning critiques of institutional care that emerged from the anti-psychiatric movement from this period onwards have been credited for changing public perceptions of residential care, including the care provided in the now-closed large state mental hospitals.[9] This in turn led to deinstitutionalisation and the new policy of care in the community in the UK in the 1990s.[10] The main premise within the literature of dysfunction rests on the assumption that care provided in the community was superior and preferable to care within institutional settings. Goffman's *Asylums* highlighted the extent of institutionalisation within psychiatric institutions; 'total institutions' were characterised by the loss of freedom of the patients and the social control exercised over them. He likened the institutions to prison environments on account of the barriers to social relations, such as locked wards, high walls and the isolated geographical locations. This portrayal has had a profound effect on institutional care in the western world.[11] His work on the pathology of institutional life details the dynamics that shaped staff–patient relationships through common institutional practices in closed institutions; institutionalisation was revealed through the paternalism in clinician–patient relationships, identified as a key feature of psychiatry in the nineteenth and twentieth centuries and a main characteristic of psychiatric institutionalisation to this day.[12] The dynamics that shaped relationships between doctors, nurses and patients in mental institutions were seen as solely defined by the exercise of control, understood to be the essential feature of staff–patient interactions, commonly reported in accounts of institutional life.[13] Goffman painted a pessimistic picture of the role of the medical hierarchy, whose sole purpose was to strip individuals of their own social identities and replace them with diagnostic labels; the imposition of the 'career of the mental patient' as a form of social control was viewed as part of the 'cure' from the medico-psychiatric perspective.[14]

The arguments of the anti-institutional movement, which were based on the dehumanising and depersonalising practices within the mental hospitals as a result of the routinisation and deprivation of meaningful roles, were substantiated by a series of scandals in the 1960s and 1970s that exposed the abuse of patients that took place in some long-stay hospitals as a direct consequence of their highly controlling environments.[15] The failure to provide adequate care was attributed to the closed systems of the mental hospitals, which were unchecked by external corrective feedback, thus confirming Goffman's notion of 'total institutions.'[16]

The anti-institutional literature such as Goffman's *Asylums* failed to take into account the rise of social psychiatry from 1940s onwards, influenced by the principles of therapeutic communities.[17] The advent of the pharmacological age gave impetus to a community-oriented psychiatry that adopted an open-door system and played an important role in deinstitutionalisation and in shaping early care in the community policies; as a result, mental hospitals experienced changes that countered their totalising characteristics.[18] The resulting 'social turn' shifted the focus from the medical model based on reducing symptoms to an emphasis on prevention focusing on the effects of environmental stresses on wellbeing.[19]

The literature of dysfunction helped to influence a turn against residential care and the eventual closure of the mental hospitals with the move to community-based services. However, closing the mental hospitals was largely based on the assumption that, once patients were freed from the damaging effects of institutional life, community care would automatically be beneficial and that people with long-term mental health needs could just help themselves. The choice and personal autonomy born out of consumerism can be a form of neglect, as the recovery model can be seen to deny the need for inpatient care to those that need it; for people vulnerable to mental health crisis, the therapeutic environment of the psychiatric hospitals could offer a safe place to recover in situations where caring for oneself is not an option; current mental health services are largely fragmented, which in turn negatively impacts on the quality of services available to those in need.[20] Moreover, the overemphasis on the totalising features of hospital environment had the effect of overlooking the importance of support structures therein. In particular, the value of the long-term interpersonal staff–patient relationships within the mental hospital for vulnerable individuals in need of care has not been widely researched, as Beckman et al. argue in this volume and Calabria has highlighted elsewhere.[21]

Methodology

The doctoral research discussed in this chapter employed participatory action research (PAR) as an overall framework and oral history as a data collection method, which are both interpretative and grounded mainly in the lived experiences of individuals.[22] The main aim of adopting a PAR-led oral history approach was to facilitate the active participation of research subjects, who usually occupy a passive role in traditional research, in all aspects of the research process. The choice of mixed methods was influenced by the desire to reverse the marginalisation of service users in mental health research, whose voices, involvement and co-production have become increasingly important in the debates and planning relating to current approaches to prevention, care and treatment in mental health.[23] The terms used to describe individuals receiving psychiatric treatment have been contested and have evolved as a result across the history of psychiatry and mental health care. The relatively modern term 'service user', which is used to describe individuals at the receiving end of psychiatric treatment, originates from the rise of the patients' movement in Britain from the post-war period onwards. This group exposed ill treatment in psychiatric institutions and campaigned for patients' rights.[24]

PAR differs from other approaches to health and social care research as it seeks the active involvement of service users with the aim of improving care and reducing inequalities.[25] It is an applied and cyclical research process that invites all interested stakeholders who have a vested interest in knowledge constructed about them to produce action towards social change; the goal is to uncover different kinds of realities from those limited by conventional inquiry, which privileges the knowledge of experts.[26] PAR makes valuable theoretical and practical contributions when undertaking research with mental health service users whose voices have generally been ignored both in the history of psychiatry, as du Plessis and Smith argue in this volume, and in mental health policy.[27]

Oral history was used as a data collection method as it holds the potential to balance the documentary evidence by giving those who are less socially powerful a central place in the creation of their own histories.[28] The method is intrinsically collaborative, in that the researcher shares authority within the dialogical nature of the oral history encounter through the collaborative generation of meanings.[29] Oral history is a unique source of history in which the interview becomes the primary instrument in researching the past.[30] It draws on memory and testimony to gain a more complete or different understanding of the past, experienced both individually and collectively. What makes oral history different is that it allows a window into the realm of subjectivity and the emergence of a multiplicity of standpoints about particular experiences.[31] This PAR-led oral history study made it possible to examine the relationship between personal and collective experiences of living and working in the Nottinghamshire mental hospitals while harnessing the stakeholders' knowledge by experience. The mixed methods approach challenged the dominant perception of mental hospitals as outmoded and total institutions, which tends to exclude the often-contradictory meanings of the hospitals both as closed depersonalising environments and as healthcare systems that could function as sanctuaries and places of respite.[32]

The staff sample consists of individuals at every level of the institution: nurses, casual staff and their children. Service users were all short-term patients in the mental hospital for a maximum of six months and all are long-term users of mental health services. Retired staff recalled their experiences of major policy changes, including the impact of the social turn in psychiatry from the 1950s onwards and early care in the community. Ex-patients filtered memories of their time at the mental hospital in light of the shortcomings of care in the community they experienced or witnessed; their testimonies were coloured by the structural inequalities they share in common, namely chronic unemployment, abject isolation and social stigma.

Contested Meanings of Institutional Care

Through a PAR-led oral history approach, ex-patients and former staff challenged the dominant overall perception of the psychiatric asylums as undesirable and outmoded institutions. They provided alternative interpretations of aspects of care they found meaningful for recovery and also criticised some aspects of care as unhelpful and depersonalising. The themes that emerged from participants' oral histories centred on some aspects of institutional care as forms of social control, while others were perceived to be based on relational care; participants expressed ambivalent experiences of care in the community, presenting seemingly conflicting meanings of care practices in institutional and community settings. The institutional characteristics such as the regimentation of everyday life that survived the rehabilitation turn were still present in the Nottingham mental hospitals up to their closure, resembling the general characteristics and common features of Goffman's 'total institutions.'[33] Some patients recalled being dismissed by staff and some recalled instances of psychological and physical abuse, a common occurrence in mental institutions as Vaiseta points out in this volume. Misuse of power by staff through forced treatment and the dismissal of patients' own views, for example, has been a common feature reported in the literature.[34] However, through the iterative phases of PAR, ex-patients and staff steered the research agenda to include topics that were relevant to them. Former staff from the Nottingham mental hospitals recalled being deeply influenced by the 'social turn' in psychiatry, reporting its significant impact in terms of ameliorating the provision of care with a definite change of focus from custodial to social rehabilitation from the 1950s onwards. Ex-patients discussed the importance of relational care, including their experiences of therapeutic relationships that were central to their recovery, which was provided in the mental hospitals but is perceived to have been lost in the current system of care. Both ex-patients and former staff who took part in this study expressed a sense of loss of a community of belonging after the closure of the hospitals. All recounted experiencing or witnessing neglect for people with long-term mental ill health in the community after the closure of the hospitals due to a lack of adequate access to relational care in the current system.

Community Psychiatry at the Nottingham Mental Hospitals

Former patients and nurses recalled the influence of the therapeutic community (TC) movement on the provision of care. TC principles were part of the care provided at Mapperley hospital in the form of group therapy from 1950s onwards, placing emphasis on therapeutic staff–patient relationships as well as putting patients in decision-making positions across 50 years of service. Despite some experiences of bullying and excessive use of force by staff, ex-patients' memories relating to staff during their hospitalisation tended to be mostly positive. Patients recalled experiencing supportive and helpful relationships, helped by having continuity with the same nurse and by staff making an effort to form positive and long-lasting relationships with patients, involving them in their care, and encouraging them to develop new interests. Albert, ex-patient (1971, 1981, 1990), took part in group therapy at Mapperley hospital during his hospitalisations. He described sessions that were helpful in his recovery, such as learning coping techniques from other patients. He set up his own anxiety self-help group in the community as a result of the help he got from the hospital's therapy group. Jane, inpatient at Mapperley hospital in the 1990s, was encouraged by "her" psychiatrist to talk to the nurses to help with her recovery while an inpatient in the 1990s, "because they can be very helpful, and they were." As an inpatient, Jane had positive experiences of receiving support from a nurse:

> I remember this staff nurse, she would come and pull up a chair beside me, she'd say well, we can talk or not talk, it's up to you, if you don't want my company you tell me... It was very sensitive of her and her just sitting there sometimes in silence was enough to be helpful, so she was excellent, didn't impose herself on me.

Jane learnt some coping techniques from the nurses who cared for her, which she used to support a friend she made on her ward when she experienced a panic attack:

> I thought distraction was a good thing because I can remember talking to her and trying to get her to look around, I did this because that's what the nurses did for me, this is what they used to do in those days, I knew she was really in a bad place. I just knew the nurses had done that for me.

All the former nurses described developing relationships with patients by building rapport and trust, by forming and maintaining genuine, respectful and authentic relationships that would aid recovery, and by encouraging choice for patients within what was available in terms of psychosocial approaches to treatment and rehabilitation. Raymond, nurse (1948–1993), remembered that there was a basic form of group therapy at Mapperley hospital in 1950s in which staff and patients would discuss the running of the ward in open meetings. Moreover, Sean, nurse (1968–1979), who began working at Mapperley hospital in 1968, recalled the importance of forming and maintaining close relationships with patients, an essential part of the role even when he worked in a mental hospital in Ireland at the end of the 1950s: "You worked towards building close relationships with patients." He remembered the value of fostering therapeutic staff–patient relationships in defusing patients' aggressive behaviours; building trust and rapport was vital to reducing incidents of violence:

> In all my time there I was only attacked once, and I would like to think that was because I learnt the proper way to approach clients, so they trusted and formed a relationship, so they trusted you.

Andrew, nurse (1968–1979), was in charge of a mixed admission ward that ran on TC principles; he maintained that psychiatric care at the hospital had been influenced by Dingleton hospital, Scotland.[35] He referred to Mapperley hospital as "an early adopter of modern treatments" for introducing the open-door policy in 1952. He recalled efforts made to encourage patients' active involvement in their own care:

> We ran on therapeutic community lines, the ward ran as a community and we encouraged patients to make decisions about how the ward ran, the staff and the patients became a team together in a way and we spent an awful lot of time with the patients, we'd have group therapy, nobody's contribution was any more or less valuable.

The nurses involved in providing group therapy recalled that patients were actively encouraged to openly talk about their needs and to offer support to one another through group therapy. Andrew remembered fostering therapeutic relationships in the admission wards in the 1970s: "We sat with the patients, watched telly and made cups of tea and lived like a community." He stressed the importance of involving patients in decision-making:

> A lot of the interactions would be between nurses and patients on a day-to-day basis and that's the therapeutic community, everything was aimed towards therapy and helping the patients improve to make decisions for themselves and to get better.

Kathryn, nurse (1978–1995), recalled that her main job was to spend time talking to the patients, partaking in rehabilitation activities. She stressed that treating patients with respect and dignity was a central part of her core duties; she recollected that "we were looking at everybody as an individual, we valued them." She remembered forming long-lasting relationships with returning patients: "You got to know your patients quite well. I think it brought them some comfort that they knew you when they came back."

The testimonies suggest that, although routine and medication controlled the rhythm of everyday life, from the 1950s onwards a more enlightened and humanitarian pattern of care emerged as a result of the influence of social psychiatry introduced by Duncan Macmillan, which contributed to the shift from custodial to therapeutic care.[36] TC principles embraced at Mapperley hospital influenced the power relations among staff and patients, encouraging more equal relationships to foster recovery,[37] helping to shed light on the impact of TC principles on mental health recovery, a subject that remains under-researched.[38] Gaining a better understanding of the impact of TC principles in the provision of mental health care could significantly improve inpatient care in current mental health settings. Although the system of care in acute units differs significantly from that within mental hospitals in terms of length of stay and the focus on medication rather than interpersonal relationships, the introduction of TC elements as a form of care in acute units has been found to be successful in improving patient autonomy, with direct positive effects in terms of improving personal recovery in the areas of involvement in treatment and planning for discharge.[39]

The oral histories point to the importance of communal relationships that existed within the hospitals for increased sense of wellbeing, reflecting on how nurses could take an active role in forming positive relationships with patients that promoted recovery by fostering therapeutic alliances within these relationships.[40] Similarly, ex-patients recounted forming therapeutic relationships with staff, which helped them develop coping skills. The intersubjective features of the relationship between client and professional play an important role in determining outcomes.[41] Research suggests that the core features of a helping relationship for service users when engaging in services are feeling safe, accepted and understood, and that the quality of the relationship with staff and their availability, consistency and unconditional respect are effective indicators that personal recovery will likely have a positive outcome. Despite their effectiveness in mental health recovery, therapeutic alliances have largely been unattainable in community care settings, where staff–service user relationships are typically short-term and veer towards crisis management.[42] The most recent independent review of the Mental Health Act 1983 for England and Wales has highlighted the chronic lack of therapeutic benefit in inpatient environments; one of its recommendations rests on improving the social environments of inpatient wards to aid recovery.[43]

Fragmentation of Services in Community

Former patients in this study, all of whom continue to use psychiatric services, reported the absence of long-standing relationships with staff and others in the community and a lack of appropriate support in the provision of current mental health services. They reported feeling safer in the environment of the old mental hospital and recalled a high level of staff numbers, which in turn allowed for a higher level of staff–patient interaction; crucially, all agreed that there were sufficient beds to cope with demand in the old system. Staff and ex-patients felt that the social fabric of the mental hospital has been lost in community care, resulting in the fragmentation of staff–patient relationships.

James, who has been using mental health services since 1976, attributed the loss of quality and continuity of staff–patient relationships over the years to the gradual cuts to services. Reflecting on the level of support available at Saxondale hospital, James recalled that "we didn't know that we had it so well-staffed and well-funded in those days." For James, the deep social connections formed at the hospital were lost: "You knew people around you, you trusted them, they trusted you, it's all gone now." He felt the key element of care lost with the hospitals' closure was the formal social support available from staff: "We haven't really got that listening ear support really now, which we would have done in the old days." He lamented the effects of cuts to services that had the result of reducing the number of experienced staff available, which had previously helped him regain independence during a long spell of mental ill health. The services he had access to in the community over time have closed down as a direct result of the dwindling mental health support in the age of austerity.

The social networks and community that existed within the hospital provided the context of building and maintaining long-lasting friendships. The consensus among ex-patients and staff was that the hospitals' closure meant the loss of friendships and social networks therein, which fostered reciprocity and kinship among the different groups. Michael, who has been receiving mental health care since 1968, felt that the hospital gave him access to communal relationships with staff and others:

> The staff were quite pleasant and would talk to you, nowadays they are too busy with the paperwork, lots is going wrong, back then they had time.

Rodney has relied on inpatient and outpatient mental health services in Nottingham since 1975. He similarly felt that staff in the current system are not easy to relate to as "they have not enough time to get to know you and support creative activities," effectively signalling the loss of professional specialised interpersonal knowledge available in the old system. He bemoaned the loss of the hospital community:

> It was a community that was there and available for us, it has never been replaced, we were promised wonderful care, claiming we needed our freedom, but they never gave it to us.

Jonathan, the son of a consultant psychiatrist at Mapperley, grew up on the hospital site (1940s–1950s). He has a son with serious mental health problems living in the community. He reflected on the fact that the current mental health recovery model's imperative to rely on peer support was a direct result of the fragmentation of therapeutic relationships in the old system:

> There are no peer-support workers in the community, for people with mental health problems that is the problem, that hasn't been happening so the hospital was helping people out that way.

Louise, nurse at Saxondale (1979–1988), felt that "with the closure of Saxondale a sense of community for patients has been lost." Kathryn was a nurse at Mapperley hospital (1978–1995). She now works as a nurse in a local mental community health team and has stayed in touch with some former long-stay residents from Mapperley; she compared the rehabilitation available under the old system to current services:

> The rehabilitation in the old days was good, you could give a lot of time to people and got to know the patients very well, now there is so much paperwork and no time to talk to the patients.

Similarly, Mark, nurse (1980–1995), felt that the closure of the hospitals overlooked the importance of the close-knit communities and that the social aspect of hospital life was lost in the process of modernising services, which disappeared in the 1990s. He recalled how the hospital provided a strong source of social support for long-term service users who tended to be isolated: "I think it meant a hell of a lot to patients, I think it was community, and identity, friendships."

The excerpts above illustrate the loss of therapeutic relationships in terms of reduced access to trained staff, who have limited time available to offer support to service users; this in turn has affected the quality of relationships in the current provision of services when compared to their experiences in the mental hospital, despite evidence that the quality of relationships in mental health is a strong predictor of recovery.[44] The testimonies point to the level of social isolation experienced by ex-patients living in the community who still rely on services, with them reporting feeling uncared for and neglected due to the short-term nature of interventions in community care. The decline in kinship and social contact in the twenty-first century has had a particularly significant impact on people affected by long-term mental health problems, who are likely to experience isolation, exclusion and loneliness as a result of their condition coupled with self and social stigma.[45] Research on the value of social support in mental health points to the paramount importance of friendship. Although this term is difficult to define, regardless of the level of relationship, understanding the social elements that affect patterns of friendships can help inform factors that help or hinder social support during periods of mental health distress.[46] The availability and continuity of staff–patient relationships coupled with access to structured social rehabilitation within the context of the kinship that existed within the hospital environment appear to have been key to fostering social support in the now-closed mental hospitals.

A direct consequence of community care was the loss of long-term employment for staff, which had the adverse effect of fragmenting staff relationships; staff recounted the loss of friendships and camaraderie, signified by memories of reduced collaboration and peer support from each other as staff were less likely to show mutuality to other staff they had no connection to in the new care system. Linda was employed long-term as a hairdresser at Mapperley hospital (1973–1995). Following the hospital's closure, she went on to work as a freelance contractor in local secure mental health units, where she still works. She remarked that the biggest loss that came with the hospitals' closures was the mutual informal support provided by staff to one another. She observed that staff relationships have been difficult to foster in the new system of inpatient care. Linda felt that the essence of caring through the long-lasting relationships formed and fostered in the hospitals has gone; she has not been able to build long-term connections with staff in current inpatient settings, as "I am never in the same place for long enough, before I worked at Mapperley Monday to Friday and got to know everyone." Similarly, for Roger, a porter (1982–1988) who grew up on the Saxondale hospital estate, the impact of closing the hospitals was the loss of kinship between staff and between staff and patients. He felt that the rich social environment of the hospital was lost with its closure: "The big thing at Saxondale was, from the patients to the staff, you knew their sons, you knew their daughters, fathers or mothers."

The above oral history extracts point to two key elements affecting professional relationships in mental health policy in the context of community care services. Firstly, the changing nature of employment has fragmented staff relationships, impacting on the quality and longevity of the relationships that were formed and fostered in the mental hospital and in turn engendered high levels of informal support among clinical and non-clinical staff. Secondly, the lack of continuity of working patterns and location has affected the relationships staff are able to form and foster with service users, which are crucial for the creation of therapeutic alliances. These oral histories suggest that staff in the mental hospitals were able to foster long-lasting therapeutic relationships with patients as a result of the extended time spent interacting with them, a form of relational care crucial to recovery within inpatient and outpatient services.[47]

Experiencing Neglect in Community

Former patients, all of whom are still dealing with long-term mental health problems, expressed a strong sense of dispossession in terms of the removal of and their inability to access adequate rehabilitation services, and the loss of both formal social support and a community of belonging. The sense of loss among ex-patients and staff was expressed in terms of the fragmentation of relationships amongst staff and patients and the effect this has had on care practices, combined with recollections of instances of neglect in the community. Ex-patients who still rely on mental health services expressed their sense of loss of a place of safety, the social support provided therein in terms of the availability of time on the part of staff and others, and the perceived neglect of people with long-term mental health needs since the advent of community care. Rodney, service user (1975–present), expressed a strong feeling of loss with the hospital's closure; he felt that the ideals of community care never materialised: "Saxondale hospital was taken away from us and nothing put in its place." For Rodney, the legacy of the mental hospitals was the economy of scale that could provide regular, large-scale access to rehabilitation facilities and the availability of staff who aided the recovery process. He felt that the consequences of closing the large mental hospitals were for people with long-term needs like himself to remain "untreated, neglected and completely forgotten." He referred to the closure of the mental hospitals as "mass land-grab" by the state and as having an "earth-shattering effect" on people with long-term mental health conditions in need of a place of safety and sanctuary. He compared deinstitutionalisation to a form of "daylight robbery," as "the resources [that] were all there and [that were] made available to patients are gone." Rodney offered a damning critique of community care policies: "There's just a skeleton of mental health services left and I'm afraid people are left to their own devices."[48] He was critical of the Recovery College in Nottingham, located on the same site as the now-closed Mapperley hospital.[49] Rodney equated the service as a form of neglect due to the short nature of the interventions, based on self-help, highlighting the gaps to services for people with the need for continuing care:

> We all yearn to actually have a part in society, you don't get this by claiming that educating us in a recovery college will be the answer to everybody's problems.

For Rodney, the need for longer-term rehabilitation, namely adequate support between the hospital and returning to the community, is key to personal recovery:

> What you swept away by putting a recovery college at the site of the old mental hospital was what was needed; the services that were for people in continuing care restored people to the right stepping stones between hospital and illness and a place back into society.

Similarly, Jane, service user (1994-present), felt that the closure of the hospital was misjudged:

> The propaganda that was put around about these buildings were old Victorian institutions, in actual fact they had moved with the times like any other institution and they were much more progressive that anybody was prepared to concede, mentally ill people were being robbed of the facilities that they had.

She explained the importance of having access to the safe environment at Mapperley hospital during her mental health crisis in the early 1990s:

> There was an awful lot that was good and that was necessary, care in the community often doesn't work because the community is where everything goes wrong, what Mapperley hospital did for me was relieve the situation that had caused me to have a breakdown.

James, patient and service user (1968–present), felt he lost the choice to be a voluntary patient due to the lack of available inpatient beds: "You could admit yourself into a hospital then, the option is no longer there." He reflected on the impact of losing the mental hospital in terms of the absence of a place of sanctuary during crisis in the current system:

> That's a big loss to me, in terms of a place for recovering from illness, it was all just money and business and one fell swoop and they call it care in the community.

Service users and staff alike pointed to the lack of rehabilitative services as a stepping stone between crisis and recovery; there was a consensus that the environment of the mental hospitals provided a more welcoming and relaxing atmosphere conducive to recovery, which was perceived as lacking in current inpatient settings. Crucially, service users felt that they lost the choice to access a place of safety and sanctuary, a choice that is no longer available under the current crisis in the provision of mental health inpatient services due to the pernicious effects of steady cuts in funding. Service users of adult acute inpatient care have consistently reported that the care provided in acute mental health units was anti-therapeutic for the lack of safety, privacy, comfort and meaningful activity to foster recovery.[50] Acute units have been reported as difficult places to work and to recover due to the concentration of people who are most unwell that cannot be treated in community,[51] coupled with the often inadequate staffing levels and overreliance on medication as the preferred mode of treatment at the expense of psychosocial interventions.[52] One of the unforeseen problems with the provision of acute inpatient care in general hospitals has been the blocking of beds by what has been termed as the new 'long-stay patients,' which has been compounded by the steady reduction of hospital beds.[53] The current crisis in availability of acute beds is increasingly leading to long-distance placements, causing a great deal of hardship to people in crisis, which in turn increases their likelihood of suicide, removed from family and friends.[54]

Conclusion

The oral histories reported here represent the vantage points of those that gave and received care in the now-closed mental hospitals. The voices of both ex-patients who rely on current mental health services and professionals help to understand experiences that have not been widely researched. These collaboratively produced oral histories bring to the fore a novel dimension to care practices within the old state mental hospitals as relational environments within which therapeutic relationships were formed and fostered. The narratives challenge the official memory of the all-pervasive power and totality of the institution postulated by Goffman and others. The loss of a place of refuge points to how care in the community policies had the effect of putting an end to the hospital communities that had offered asylum, a sense of belonging and a web of social networks for many. For service users, sense of belonging was inextricably linked to being connected to a group of people in a particular place, an experience not readily available in the community; the social and interpersonal factors of the care available therein fostered a sense of belonging that was perceived to improve wellbeing. Importantly, the findings from Calabria's study evidence a humanistic culture of caring within the Nottingham mental hospitals, albeit combined with aspects of institutionalisation, which contrast significantly with the evidence portrayed in the official narrative of mental hospitals as 'total institutions.'[55] Hospital care practices were influenced by reforms introduced by pioneering psychiatrists from the 1950s onwards, which had a dramatic impact on care provided at the Nottingham hospitals by promoting positive attitudes towards patient rehabilitation, marking the rise of the traditional recovery model, which is not widely reported in the literature.[56] Nurses recounted playing an active role in ameliorating institutional care practices by influencing positive changes in the everyday care of patients and their treatment, as they were best placed to develop interpersonal knowledge and therapeutic relationships with patients. This points to the nature of doctor–nurse relationships as being much more fluid and permeable than reported in the literature, which in turn challenges the traditional hierarchy so often associated with the historiography of psychiatric institutions.[57]

The oral histories of people who worked and lived in institutions have the unique potential of giving voice to previously inaccessible knowledge that has the power to create new paradigms, disrupting the dominant public discourse of mental hospitals in the late twentieth century as custodial institutions solely dominated by discipline and punishment. Overall, the experience of being an inpatient held positive meanings—despite some negative experiences therein. Critiques of institutional care overlooked the relevance of residential care for people undergoing crisis who were in need of a place of respite; residential provision may be the preferred choice for some who may need time out from environments not conducive to their recovery, as service users in this study and others pointed out.[58]

There are some limitations to the qualitative research under discussion. Firstly, the small sample of participants has been largely self-selective. This may reflect involvement of service users and staff with more positive experiences of care practices in the old mental hospitals. In addition, the service users who took part were all short-term patients in the mental hospital with stays of no longer than six months. Some had been sectioned and others were voluntary patients, and some had repeated hospitalisations. However, all are long-term users of mental health services, with an average of 36 years' experience of the psychiatric system; thus, all were able to compare the nature of the care they received in the mental hospitals with care in the community. Importantly, the service users who took part in this study brought to light that voluntary admission was perceived to no longer be an option in the current system due to lack of resources, contributing to their sense of neglect.

Service users felt that the project of care in the community failed them by the degrees of oversight and neglect in the current system. Their experiences of community care require a consideration of the social and cultural costs associated with the closure of the hospitals in terms of the loss of symbolic identity linked to the hospital location and the communities therein. This collaborative oral history research allowed for alternative representations of care practices to emerge through the multiplicity of standpoints, offering a much more nuanced understanding of the fluid and permeable environment of the mental hospitals that bears on current mental health provision. These substantive findings evidence the potential significance of psychiatric hospitals in the provision of stability, safety and social connectedness against a backdrop of perceived isolation and neglect for people with long-term mental health issues. Participants' situated knowledge helps establish an evidence base for positive change in mental health provision by providing new insights into the value of relational care through interpersonal and therapeutic relationships that existed therein and into how these have been affected in the shift away from institutional care.

Data Access Statement

The oral histories cited in this chapter are copyrighted to Verusca Calabria. Informed consent was sought from participants to take part in Calabria's study and to deposit the interviews in a public archive. The transcripts are available to bona fide researchers from the Local Studies, Nottingham Central Library, Angel Row, Nottingham. The catalogue number of this collection is L36.48.

Notes

1. Roy Porter, "The Patient's View: Doing Medical History from Below." *Theory and Society* 14, no. 2 (1985): 175–198.
2. Ibid.

3. Verusca Calabria. *Oral Histories of the Nottinghamshire Mental Hospitals: Exploring Memories of Giving and Receiving Care*, PhD Thesis (Nottingham Trent University, April 2020).
4. Stefan Priebe, "Do Long-Term Hospitalised Patients Benefit from Discharge into the Community?," *Social Psychiatry and Psychiatric Epidemiology* 37, no. 8 (2002): 387–392; Care Quality Commission, The State of Care in Mental Health Services 2014 to 2017 (2017). https://www.cqc.org.uk/sites/default/files/20170720_stateofmh_report.pdf. Accessed 1 January 2019.
5. Department of Health, Best Research for Best Health: A National Health Research Strategy, (London: Department of Health, 2006); UK Mental Health Research Network, Good Practice Guidance for Involving People with Experience of Mental Health Problems in Research (National Institute of Health Research, 2011).
6. The research has focused on exploring the experiences of giving and receiving care at Mapperley hospital and Saxondale mental hospitals, Nottinghamshire. Both hospitals were built in the Victorian period Hester Parr and Chris Philo, *A Forbidden Fortress of Locks, Bars and Padded Cells?, The Locational History of Nottingham's Mental Health Care* (Historical Geography Research Studies Group series 32, 1996); David Lowe, *Saxondale Memories: Personal History Of A Nottinghamshire Hospital 1902–1988* (Nottingham Health Authority, 1988).
7. Hester Parr and Chris Philo, *A Forbidden Fortress of Locks, Bars and Padded Cells?, The Locational History of Nottingham's Mental Health Care* (Historical Geography Research Studies Group series 32, 1996); David Lowe, *Saxondale Memories: Personal History of A Nottinghamshire Hospital 1902–1988* (Nottingham Health Authority, 1988).
8. Kathleen Jones and A. J. Fowles, *Ideas on Institutions: Analysing the Literature on Long-term Care and Custody* (London: Routledge: 1984); Raymond Jack, *Residential Versus Community Care: The Role of Institutions in Welfare Provision* (Palgrave Macmillan, 1998).
9. The drive to close the mental hospitals and move its former inhabitants to the community was driven not only by the ideology of normalisation but also by the by the neo-liberal government's agenda in the 1980s to reduce public spending in the face of fiscal crisis; see Anne Rogers and David Pilgrim, *Mental Health Policy in Britain* (Palgrave Macmillan, 2006).
10. House of Commons, National Health Service and Community Care Act (1990); Jones and Fowles, *Ideas on Institutions*; Andrew Scull, *Museums of Madness: The Social Organization of Insanity in Nineteenth-century England* (Viking: 1979); Julia Johnson, Sheena Rolph, and Randall Smith, *Residential Care Transformed: Revisiting The Last Refuge* (Basingstoke, Hampshire: Palgrave Springer, 2010); Despo Kritsotaki, Vicky Long, and

Matthew Smith, (eds.) *Deinstitutionalisation and After: Post-War Psychiatry in the Western World* (Springer, 2016).

11. Ervin Goffman, *Asylums: Essays on The Social Situation of Mental Patients and Other Inmates* (Harmondsworth: Penguin, 1961): 76.
12. Rogers and Pilgrim, *Mental Health Policy in Britain*; Nick Crossley, *Contesting Psychiatry: Social Movements in Mental Health* (Routledge, 2006); Winnie Chow and Stefan Priebe, "Understanding Psychiatric Institutionalization: a Conceptual Review." *BMC Psychiatry* 13, no. 1 (2013): 169.
13. Russell Barton, *Institutional Neurosis* (Butterworth-Heinemann, 2013); John Wing and George Brown, *Institutionalism and Schizophrenia: A Comparative Study of Three Mental Hospitals: 1960–1968* (Cambridge University Press, 1970).
14. Goffman, *Asylums.*
15. The Aid to the Elderly in Government Institutions pressure group was instrumental in leading the collection of evidence of ill treatment of patients that led to a national investigation. Barbara Robb, its founder, published *Sans Everything* in 1967, exposing the undignified treatment of elderly patients in long-stay wards in seven hospitals; J. P. Martin documented 15 major scandals in mental and learning disabilities hospitals that led to a series of official inquiries; TV programmes and press campaigns encompassing the period 1968–1979.
16. J.P. Martin, *Hospitals in Trouble* (Oxford: Basil Blackwell, 1984).
17. Catherine Fussinger, "Therapeutic community, Psychiatry's Reformers and Anti-Psychiatrists: Reconsidering Changes in the Field of Psychiatry After World War II." *History of Psychiatry* 22, no. 2 (2011): 146–163.
18. Kathleen Jones, *Asylums and After: A Revised History of the Mental Health Services: From the Early 18th Century to the 1990s* (London: The Athlone Press, 1993).
19. The historiography of psychiatry has traced the development of therapeutic communities in Britain as early attempts to rehabilitate patients in 1940s and 1950s in the form of separate units within larger hospitals run by reformists, such as Duncan Macmillan at Mapperley hospital, Nottingham. See Shulamit Ramon, *Professional Theories and Value Preferences in the 50s.*
20. Barbara Taylor, "The Demise of the Asylum in Late Twentieth-century Britain: A Personal History," *Transactions of the Royal Historical Society* 21 (2011): 193–215; Barbara Taylor, *The Last Asylum: A Memoir of Madness in Our Times* (University of Chicago Press, 2015). Care Quality Commission, "The State of Care in Mental Health Services 2014 to 2017."

21. Verusca Calabria, "Insider Stories from the Asylum: Peer and Staff-Patient Relationships," in *Narrating Illness: Prospects and Constraints*, eds. J. Davidson and Y. Saber, (Oxford: Interdisciplinary Press, 2016), 3–12.
22. Calabria, *Oral Histories of the Nottinghamshire Mental Hospitals.*
23. Ada Hui and Theodore Stickley, "Mental Health Policy and Mental Health Service User Perspectives on Involvement: A Discourse Analysis," *Journal of Advanced Nursing* 59, no. 4 (2007): 416–426; Mental Health Taskforce, *Implementing the Five Year Forward View for Mental Health* (London: NHS England, 2016); Mike Slade, Lindsay Oades, Aaron Jarden, *Wellbeing, Recovery and Mental Health* (Cambridge University Press, 2017).
24. The rise of consumerism in health and social care in the 1980s redefined the role of mental patients as passive to active consumers of services, expressed in some key policy papers such as Working for Patients White Paper (Department of Health 1989) and the Patients' Charter. Nick Crossley, *Contesting Psychiatry, Social Movements in Mental Health.*
25. It is part of a growing trend of action-oriented research in health and social care in the UK for its empowering and inclusive features; see James Ward and Di Bailey. "At Arm's Length: the Development of a Self-injury Training Package for Prison Staff through Service User Involvement." *The Journal of Mental Health Training, Education and Practice* 6, no. 4 (2011): 175–185; James Ward, Di Bailey, and S. Boyd, "Participatory Action Research in the Development and Delivery of Self-harm Awareness Sessions in Prison: Involving Service Users in Staff Development, " *Prison Service Journal* 202 (2012): 20–25; James Ward, J., Di Bailey, "A Participatory Action Research Methodology in the Management of Self-Harm in Prison, *Journal of Mental Health* 22, no. 4 (2013): 306–316.
26. Fran Baum, Colin MacDougall, Danielle Smith, "Participatory Action Research," *Journal of Epidemiology and Community Health* 60, no. 10 (2006): 854–857; Stephen Kemmis, Robin McTaggart, and Rhonda Nixon, "Introducing Critical Participatory Action Research," in *The Action Research Planner* (Singapore: Springer, 2014), 1–31.
27. Porter 1985, "The Patient's View;" Peter Campbell, "The History of the User Movement in the United Kingdom," In *Mental Health Matters: A Reader* (Macmillan Education UK, 1996). 218–225; Anne Borsay and Pamela Dale, "Mental Health Nursing: The Working Lives of Paid Carers from 1800 to the 1990s," (Manchester University Press, 2015); Niall McCrae and Peter Nolan, *The Story of Nursing in British Mental Hospitals: Echoes from the Corridors* (Routledge, 2016).
28. Paul Thompson, *The Voice of The Past: Oral History* (Oxford: Oxford University Press, 2017); Alessandro Portelli, "What Makes Oral History Different," in *The Oral History Reader*, eds. Robert Perks and Alistair Thomson (Routledge, 2015), 48–58.

29. Alistair Thomson, "Introduction: Sharing Authority: Oral History and the Collaborative Process," *The Oral History Review* 30, no. 1 (March 2003): 23–26; Michael Frisch, "Commentary: Sharing Authority: Oral History and the Collaborative Process," *The Oral History Review* no. 30, 1 (2003): 111–113.
30. Perks and Thomson, 2015. *The Oral History Reader*; Thompson, *The Voice of The Past.*
31. Alessandro Portelli, "What Makes Oral History Different"; Alistair Thomson, "Four Paradigm Transformations in Oral History," *Oral History Review* 34, no. 1 (2007): 49–70.
32. Calabria. "Insider Stories from the Asylum," 3–5.
33. Ex-patients and staff alike recalled institutional practices such as the regulation of daily living in the presence of large numbers of people and the consequent enforced lack of privacy, the gender divisions and the strict routines that curtailed freedom. Goffman, *Asylums*; Diana Gittins, *Madness in its Place*; Louise Hide, "From Asylum to Mental Hospital: Gender, Space and the Patient Experience in London County Council Asylums, 1890–1910," in *Residential Institutions in Britain, 1725–1970*, eds. Jane Hamlett, Lesley Hoskins, Rebecca Preston (Routledge, 2015), 51–64.
34. Donald Johnson, *The Plea for the Silent* (Johnson and Norman Dodds, 1957); Robb, *Sans Everything*; Martin, *Hospitals in Trouble*; Ramon Shulamit, *Beyond Community Care: Normalisation and Integration Work* (Macmillan International Higher Education, 2016).
35. Dingleton was the first hospital in Britain to be run on therapeutic community principles; see Jones, *Asylums and After.*
36. Macmillan, "Mental Health Services of Nottingham;" Duncan Macmillan, "Community Mental Health Services and the Mental Hospital," in *Trends in the Mental Health Services*, eds. Macmillan (London: Pergamon, 1963), 226–237.
37. Participants' narratives corroborate Diana Gittins' findings about the dual system of care available at Severrals hospital, both medical and social, under reformer psychiatrist Russell Barton. See Gittins, *Madness in its Place.*
38. David Veale, Paul Gilbert, John Wheatley, Iona Naismith, "A New Therapeutic Community: Development of a Compassion-Focussed and Contextual Behavioural Environment," *Clinical Psychology & Psychotherapy* 22, no. 4 (2015): 285–303.
39. James Hansen, Christopher Slevin, "The Implementation of Therapeutic Community Principles in Acute Care Psychiatric Hospital Settings: an Empirical Analysis and Recommendations to Clinicians," *Journal of Clinical Psychology* 52, no. 6 (1996): 673–678.
40. The concept of therapeutic alliance refers to the therapeutic relationship between staff and service user, based on empathic connection through rap-

port building, common understanding and bonding and engendering hope, which has been found to be a successful predictor of recovery in mental health. See David Pilgrim, Anne Rogers, Richard Bentall, "The Centrality of Personal Relationships in the Creation and Amelioration of Mental Health Problems: The Current Interdisciplinary Case," *Health* 13, no. 2 (2009): 235–254; Priebe and Mccabe. "The Therapeutic Relationship in Psychiatric Settings;" Peter Huxley, Sherrill Evans, Peter Beresford, "The Principles and Provisions of Relationships: Findings from an Evaluation of Support, Time and Recovery Workers in Mental Health Services in England," *Journal of Social Work* 9, no. 1 (2009): 99–117.

41. Hugh Middleton, Rebecca Shaw, Ron Collier, Aimie Purser, Brian Ferguson, "The Dodo Bird Verdict and the Elephant in the Room: A Service User-led Investigation of Crisis Resolution and Home Treatment," *Health Sociology Review* 20, no. 2 (2011): 147–156.
42. Care Quality Commission, "The State of Care in Mental Health Services 2014 to 2017."
43. Department of Health and Social Care, Modernising the Mental Health Act—Final report from the independent review (December 2018).
44. Helen Gilburt, Diana Rose, Mike Slade, "The Importance of Relationships in Mental Health Care: A Qualitative Study of Service Users' Experiences of Psychiatric Hospital Admission in the UK", *BMC Health Services Research* 8, no. 1 (2008): 92; Middleton, *The Dodo Bird Verdict and the Elephant in the Room*; Jerry Tew, Shula Ramon, Mike Slade, Victoria Bird, Jane Melton, Clair Le Boutillier, "Social Factors and Recovery from Mental Health Difficulties: A Review of the Evidence," *The British Journal of Social Work* 42, no. 3 (April 2012): 443–460; Verity Chester, Regi T. Alexander, Wendy Morgan, "Measuring Relational Security in Forensic Mental Health Services," *The British Journal of Psychiatry Bulletin* 41, no. 6 (December 2017): 358–363.
45. Jonathan Leach, *Improving Mental Health through Social Support: Building Positive and Empowering Relationships* (London: Jessica Kingsley Publishers, 2015); R. Forrester-Jones, John Carpenter, P. Coolen-Schrijner, P. Cambridge, A. Tate, A. Hallam, J. Beecham, M. Knapp, D. Wooff, "Good Friends are Hard to Find? The Social Networks of People with Mental Illness 12 Years After Deinstitutionalisation," *Journal of Mental Health* 21, no. 1 (2012): 4–14; Patrick W. Corrigan, Deepa Rao, "On the Self-stigma of Mental Illness: Stages, Disclosure, and Strategies for Change," *The Canadian Journal of Psychiatry* 57, no. 8 (2012): 464–469.
46. Allen, Jessica, Reuben Balfour, Ruth Bell, Michael Marmot, "Social Determinants of Mental Health," *International Review of Psychiatry* 26, no. 4 (2014): 392–407.

47. S. Akther, E. Molineaux, R. Stuart, S. Johnson, A. Simpson, S. Oram, "Patients' Experiences of Assessment and Detention under Mental Health Legislation: Systematic Review and Qualitative Meta-Synthesis," *BJPsych Open* 5, no. 3 (2019): 1–10.
48. Not only patients but also relatives' associations were opposed to the closure of the mental hospitals for fear of safety and neglect of former patients in community. Another concern for relatives was the loss of respite for carers that the hospital provided. Rob Ellis, "Heritage and Stigma, Co-producing and Communicating the Histories of Mental Health and Learning Disability," *Medical Humanities* 43, no. 2 (2017): 92–98.
49. Recovery Colleges are a new educational form of intervention based on the reintegration of people with psychiatric disabilities into society that supports self-management through education; for a comprehensive review of this new initiative, see M. Slade, M. Amering, M. Farkas, B. Hamilton, M. O'Hagan, G. Panther, R. Perkins, G. Shepherd, S. Tse, R. Whitley, "Uses and Abuses of Recovery: Implementing Recovery-oriented Practices in Mental Health Systems," *World Psychiatry* 13, no. 1 (2014): 12–20.
50. Acute inpatient units, on the site of district general hospitals, are designed for short-term hospitalisations. Ray Higgins, *Psychiatric Nursing Revisited: The Care Provided for Acute Psychiatric Patients* (London: Whurr, 1999).
51. Helen Killaspy, "From the Asylum to Community Care: Learning from Experience," *British Medical Bulletin* 79, no. 1 (2007): 245–258; Jose Miguel Caldas, Helen Killaspy, Long-term Mental Health Care for People with Severe Mental Disorders, *IMPACT Consortium, European Union* (2011). Url: https://sante.public.lu/fr/publications/l/long-term-mental-health-care-people/long-term-mental-health-care-people.pdf. Accessed 1 January 2019; S. McAndrew, M. Chambers, F. Nolan, B. Thomas and P. Watts, "Measuring the Evidence: Reviewing the Literature of the Measurement of Therapeutic Engagement in Acute Mental Health Inpatient Wards," *International Journal of Mental Health Nursing* 23, no. 3 (2014): 212–220.
52. Rex Haigh, "Acute Wards: Problems and Solutions: Modern Milieux: Therapeutic Community Solutions to Acute Ward Problems," *Psychiatric Bulletin* 26, no. 10 (2002): 380–382; L. Bowers, A. Simpson, J. Alexander, D. Hackney, H. Nijiman, A. Grange and J. Warren, "The Nature and Purpose of Acute Psychiatric Wards: The Tompkins Acute Ward Study," *Journal of mental Health* 14, no. 6 (2005): 625–635.
53. Therapeutic practice has been largely unattainable in acute inpatient settings since the 1980s as a result of rising demands of beds, coupled with the reduction in number of beds; more than half of NHS hospital beds have been cut in 30 years. See Ray Higgins, *Psychiatric Nursing Revisited*; Graham Moon, "Risk and Protection: the Discourse of Confinement in

Contemporary Mental Health Policy," *Health & Place* 6, no. 3 (2000): 239–250; Leo Ewbank, James Thompson, Helen Mckenna, Siva Anandaciva, *NHS Hospital Bed Numbers: Past, Present, Future* (London: The King's Fund, 2017).

54. Helen Gilburt, *Mental Health under Pressure* (London: The King's Fund, 2015); Mark Trewin, *Social Care and the Mental Health Forward View: Ending Out of Area Placements* (Centre for Mental Health, 2017).
55. Goffman, *Asylums*; Robb, *Sans Everything*; Martin, *Hospitals in Trouble.*
56. Gary Winship, "A Meta-recovery Framework: Positioning the 'New Recovery' Movement and Other Recovery Approaches," *Journal of Psychiatric and Mental Health Nursing* 23, no. 1 (2016): 66–73.
57. Goffman, *Asylums*; Andrew Scull, "A Convenient Place to Get Rid of Inconvenient People: the Victorian Lunatic Asylum," *Buildings and Society: Essays on the Social Development of the Built Environment* (1980): 46; Ramon, *Professional Theories and Value Preferences.*
58. Peter Barham, *Closing the Asylum: The Mental Patient in Modern Society* (London: Penguin, 1992). Peter Barham, *Relocating Madness: From the Mental Patient to the Person* (London: Free Association, 1995). Taylor. "The Demise of the Asylum in Late Twentieth-century Britain;" Taylor, *The Last Asylum: A Memoir of Madness in our Times.*

PART III

The Visual and the Material

CHAPTER 11

Tracking Traces of the Art Extraordinary Collection

Cheryl McGeachan

The pink plastic folder lies curiously open on the darkly coloured tabletop. The brightly lit room accentuates the white pages with glimmering ripples of light, drawing to attention the bold black ink of the poetry and drawings that lie within. Lynda edges towards the table that is awash with unusual objects—guitars made of paper and plasticine portraits, to name but a few—and stops to consider the folder. Tracing her fingers along the protective tablecloth, her fingertips stop fractionally before the plastic edges. She nervously peers to her left and catches the eye of a red-haired woman wearing an official-looking badge hanging loosely around her neck, who smiles back in her direction. Without a word being spoken, an invisible line of communication is uttered; Lynda knows that it is okay to let her twitching fingertips touch. She carefully picks up the folder and begins to read.

The folder that catches Lynda's attention is a collection of poems and ink drawings by Marylène Walker, entitled 'Drawing on Lullabies' that was sent to Scottish art therapist Joyce Laing on the 1 February 1999.

C. McGeachan (✉)
School of Geographical & Earth Sciences, University of Glasgow, Glasgow, UK
e-mail: Cheryl.McGeachan@glasgow.ac.uk

R. Ellis et al. (eds.), *Voices in the History of Madness*, Mental Health in Historical Perspective,
https://doi.org/10.1007/978-3-030-69559-0_11

Laing, a collector of art brut since the 1970s, donated a body of work to Glasgow Museums, Scotland, in 2012 for long-term care. The folder is stored in Glasgow Museums Resource Centre (GMRC) and labelled under the banner of the Art Extraordinary Collection. Art Extraordinary refers to visual art forms created by individuals who paint, sculpt or draw due to a compulsion to express an intense personal vision. Most of these individuals have no formal art education or training and often exist on the margins of conventional society, held within the care of various institutions and experiencing mental health difficulties of varying kinds. Connections here can be made to the 'outsider art' tradition and the contentious debates surrounding alternative and raw art.[1] However, whilst the Art Extraordinary collection is clearly indebted to these traditions, Laing was keen to label these pieces differently, choosing what she felt was the more positive term 'art extraordinary' in order to raise up these artists rather than to push them further to the margins. 'Drawings on Lullabies' contains a diverse mix of 80 poems relating, in part, to experiences of mental ill-health, including work entitled 'Schizoid Listening', 'Alone Unborn. (A Schizophrenic Voice)' and 'Born into Pain'.[2] The intricate ink images that align every page showcase, at times, a shifting human form, such as a female face, alongside anamorphic hybridisations of birds, trees and flowers aligning in swirling patterns and seemingly never-ending shapes. Working together these carefully crafted words and images convey an intricate inner landscape of mental ill-health, highlighting the often-unheard experiences of living with mental health difficulties in a deinstitutionalised landscape.

Lynda's happenstance encountering of 'Drawing on Lullabies' was within the context of a small exhibition of Art Extraordinary displayed as part of the annual Scottish Mental Health Arts and Film Festival (SMHAFF) in the Recreational Therapy Department of Leverndale Hospital, a psychiatric institution located on the edges of Glasgow. The hospital's original manifestation was Govan's district asylum opened in 1895, but reconfigured in 1964 as Leverndale and home to one of the only Recreational Therapy Departments still in existence in Scotland. Recent attention to Scotland's histories of asylums and psychiatry shows a diverse set of Scottish approaches to containment and treatment of those seeking mental health care across the centuries.[3] In the recent era of deinstitutionalisation in Scotland, a range of post-asylum spaces have emerged that often fuse together the old and new worlds of mental health care due to their location in old asylum sites. Leverndale Recreational Therapy is one such post-asylum space that whilst placed within the hospital network, and the deep histories of the asylum, demonstrates a community-facing feel that connects those experiencing mental health difficulties with both clinical and community care. In partnership with the Open Museum, a branch of Glasgow Museums that specialises in taking museum objects out into the community, patients and staff from across the hospital had been involved in visits to GMRC to select items for their exhibition. Intent on inspiring curiosity through tours around the museum storerooms, the museum also sought to reveal the hidden and undisplayed inner landscape of its collections. Current research into the Art Extraordinary collection enabled story workshops to take place, bringing to life the unusual objects and the people behind their creation. Alongside other artists such as Adam Christie and Gordon Anderson, Marylène's work captured the visitors' imagination and was selected by the group for display at the Leverndale exhibition.

Lynda was not part of the visiting group that had selected the folder for public display. She was instead one of the many visitors to the Recreational Therapy Department for the annual event. During the evening event, the walls of the department are awash with patient art from the multiple wards around the hospital, filling the space with bright colours and tactile textures. Words written about illness, family, home spaces and belonging hang from the branches of 'memory trees', sentences fluttering in tune to the continuous traffic of human bodies that move between the different spaces of the room. Music from the visiting band cascades into the crevasses of the space, filling ears and hearts with familiar words and rhythms. Art Extraordinary sits within this, positioned carefully on a tabletop that is designed to invite curiosity, intrigue and touch. As the music begins to fade and the last of the visitors deposit their teacups back to the hatch before leaving, Lynda continues to read. Clearly captivated by the work, she wishes to spend more time in Marylène's company. Yet, sensing a change in atmosphere in the room, she looks up for the first time and clasps the folder closed to return it to the empty space on the table. As she delicately places the piece back in its original spot, she speaks aloud for the first time. She explains the profound connection she has to the work and the meaningful nature of the experiences that it expresses. Lynda relays that she is a recently departed resident of Leverndale and conveys her uncertainty over whether she will be able to stay away for long. As she turns to leave, she notes that she has written to Marylène to express her thanks for giving her the strength and inspiration to finish her own poems.

The letter had been carefully slotted into an empty plastic wallet in the front of the folder that now awaits its careful repacking. The folder is then returned back to the museum storeroom.

Lynda, Marylène and Leverndale's intertwining story, adapted from my own field notes during the 'Passionate about Everything' event in October 2015, is used here to introduce the intricate and intriguing connections between people, objects and places, and the multiple voices of mental ill-health that they convey. This work draws upon aspects of 'voice' and experience that can be traced through attention to individual and collective expressions of creativity in relation to mental ill-health by focusing upon the material remnants of these processes.[4] By centring upon the tradition to tell 'small stories' that draw attention to the affective dimensions of how people know and understand their worlds, new 'voices' of encounter, place and practice emerge.[5] Lynda's encountering of 'Drawing on Lullabies' that evening in Leverndale showcases in miniature the important travelling nature of mental health histories as the stories of individuals' experiences move, often unexpectedly, across space and time in material, emotional and embodied form. Research into the histories of 'madness' from an embodied, emotional and biographical perspective has tended to rely heavily on an engagement with shards, gaps and silences in order to gain fragmentary access into these worlds.[6] Yet, arguably, more needs to be known about the variety of *practices* involved in tracing the lives, worlds, voices and experiences of individuals experiencing mental ill-health across time and space that remain difficult to uncover.

This chapter seeks to discuss such practices by highlighting the various ways in which I have sought to track the traces that remain of the lives lived (and died) of the Art Extraordinary Collection. Uncovering the lives of the patient-artists in the collection continues to be exceptionally challenging due to the complex nature of the many worlds they inhabit. Coupled with this, the marginalisation of their stories and journeys through a range of (medical) sites and spaces leaves their experiences largely uncharted and unknown. However, in following the traces that remain of the collection, a variety of spaces emerge which reveal a layered set of histories and geographies of mental ill-health that in turn fuse people, objects and place together in intriguing formations. Using two short case studies from collaborative work undertaken with Glasgow Museums in a gym hall in Barlinnie Prison in Glasgow and an unmarked grave in Sleepyhillock Cemetery in Montrose, alongside Lynda's experiences at Leverndale, this work aims to raise ideas relating to the *practice* of following the trace to uncover lost voices and forgotten stories from the collection. In doing so, this chapter suggests different ways of working beyond the traditional bounded walls of the archive to seek out the voices of 'madness', and instead proposes a turning towards the collisions between archives/collections and the hearts, minds, bodies and landscapes of those bound up with these histories in the making.

Archives, Voices and Traces

Recent methodological innovations in historical examinations of mental health have diversified the nature of archival research into the lives, worlds and experiences of mental ill-health. Attempts to utilise a wide range of sources in varied and creative ways such as asylum photographs (see Rawling, this volume),[7] case notes,[8] patient art,[9] memoirs and interviews,[10] and patient magazines to name but a few,[11] demonstrate a collective desire to seek out the unknown histories of mental health, often from a patient perspective. Since Roy Porter's (1985) pioneering call for mental health histories 'from below',[12] a range of scholars have pushed the archive, in its multiple formations, in order to illuminate the darkened corners of asylum histories, patient/staff encounters and the newly emerging spaces of a deinstitutionalised landscape.[13] This work has developed a stronger account of mental health histories 'from below', teasing out the complex and messy relations between the experiences of mental ill-health and the worldly spaces that individuals, groups and institutions occupy. Yet there is still much more to know about these experiences and encounters. Recent work within the medical humanities has called for increased attention to be given to discussing and debating the historical contexts to communicating mental health, with Rebecca Wynter and Leonard Smith noting that 'history infuses, influences and informs how we discuss and approach mental health and practice mental health care today'.[14] An emphasis on *listening* and *hearing* in the construction and analysis of mental health histories has come to the fore, in line with Brendan Kelly's notion that methodologically 'we just need to listen harder and, perhaps, listen better', developing a new set of work that moves forward into ever-increasing innovative terrains.[15] This has included attention to the amplification of 'patient' voices and experiences that are often drowned out or lost completely to the voices of power, and to the decentring of asylum narratives from different spatial perspectives.[16] As Kelly thoughtfully construes, while patients' voices from the past are unknown, they are certainly not unknowable, and this way of thinking, dispersed throughout the history of psychiatry, medical humanities and asylum geographies, has prompted new methodological ways of conceiving research into the histories of mental ill-health.[17]

These calls for a more amplified, attuned and attentive set of mental health histories to 'voice' chime with recent discussions in historical geography regarding the idea of the trace in (geo-)biographical work.[18] Traces can be described as the vestiges or marks of lives once lived and existence once experienced, scattered across space and time.[19] Miles Ogborn, in his editorial discussing Atlantic geographies, notes that 'attending to the trace involves tracing journeys, interpreting located moments of negotiation and listening for the presence of ghosts'.[20] For Ogborn, a focus on the trace can also bring to the fore moments of movement, negotiation and their residual effects, and therefore 'might follow individual journeys, demonstrating how both intimate and large-scale histories and geographies intersect in wandering paths and personal transformations'.[21] These moments change the perspective on examining certain time–space collisions, opening up avenues for exploring flows of movement and points of intersection at differing times and scales. This attention to the trace as a methodological tool in the (re)construction of forgotten or neglected histories brings to the fore the importance of connecting across objects, people and place in the writing of these histories. It, therefore, turns attention to the ruptures, turning points and disturbances of history that human beings have encountered, processed and infused with meaning, and lived through and died for in certain times and places.[22] An attraction to the trace as a way to consider how the archive and the worlds beyond come together in the making of new histories of mental ill-health, also brings to light the significance of a nuanced exploration of the different ways and means of communicating more diverse and inclusive mental health histories.

This chapter seeks to work at that juncture between creative workings of the trace and the desire to 'listen harder and listen better' in the creation of new histories of mental ill-health. Beginning with a discussion of the gym hall in Barlinnie Prison in Glasgow, this section discusses the various ways in which the excavation of hidden histories of prison reform can reveal unheard experiences of mental ill-health buried deep within the prison system. Turning towards an unmarked grave in Sleepyhillock Cemetery in Montrose in the North of Scotland, this section will draw attention to the (re)writing of mental health histories through layers of time–space collisions. Finally, in returning to discuss the tracing of the Art Extraordinary collection, this piece aims to showcase the importance of continuing to focus on the practice of developing methodological interventions for listening differently in order to excavate new voices of experience in historical mental health research.

Gym Hall, Barlinnie Prison

The siren signalled that the door was ready to be unlocked in Barlinnie Prison, Glasgow, and that the visitors were able to be escorted to the gym hall. A short walk through the quiet courtyard led easily to the unassuming building that is used as a central sports facility for the prison. As the door is pushed open, it is not, however, the standard sports equipment that greets the eager visitor, but instead an array of objects, artworks and display panels relating to prison reform that fills the room. The exhibition entitled 'A Way Out of a Dark Time' is the output of an extensive collaboration between the Open Museum, Scottish Prison Service (SPSS), New College Lanarkshire and the University of Glasgow that sought to uncover the histories of one of Scotland's most controversial experiments in penal reform: The Barlinnie Special Unit (BSU). The BSU opened in 1973 and became renowned for its ground-breaking use of the 'Arts' as a tool of prison reform.[23] The introduction of the Murder (Abolition of Death Penalty) Act in 1965 fundamentally changed the physical and psychological terrains of prisons across the United Kingdom. Prisons in Scotland were now faced with a population of individuals who, with no hope of release, became increasingly unsettled and an upsurge in violent altercations began to take place between prisoners and staff.[24] This unrest triggered a change, and in 1971 the Scottish Home and Health Departmental Working Party recommended that a 'Special Unit' should be set up under the ethos of a 'therapeutic community' whereby prisoners and staff would work together to create mutually beneficial relations in a supportive environment.[25] This unit came to fruition and was set up in Barlinnie, one of Scotland's largest male prisons. Despite the BSU being one of Scotland's longest experiments in penal reform, closing in 1994, it has received minimal public or academic attention, leaving a host of unexamined histories still to be explored. The one-week exhibition in the gym hall at Barlinnie in November 2016, curated by a group of current prisoners, attracted an array of media and public interest intrigued to hear about the unknown inner worlds of the unit.[26] As all the visitors gathered around the room at the launch event to hear the curators' relay their experiences of undertaking this unusual project, people suddenly realised where they were: everyone was standing on the reused site of the BSU and playing a fragmentary part in the continuously overlaid histories of prison reform.

The shuffling noises of paper being cleared away and the hasty removal of half-drunken mugs from the table fills the small teaching space in the education centre of the prison. A protective tablecloth is dutifully laid out, covering the table with a crisp coating of white. As the heavy metal objects are carefully removed from their tissue-laden boxes, the class stands well back at the edges of room, watching with intrigue and bewilderment at the peculiar set of items being arranged in front of them. Among the array of objects brought by the curator of the Open Museum for today's session is a delicate ceramic rose.[27] The rose, made by BSU prisoner Bob Brodie, is part of a collection of BSU objects held in Glasgow Museums as part of the Art Extraordinary collection. Unlike other items in the collection, these works fall outside of the parameters of the Art Extraordinary definition due to their production as part of a wider implementation of art therapy in the BSU by Joyce Laing. Throughout the BSU experiment, Laing encouraged prisoners to paint, sculpt, write and draw in order to express their experiences of confinement in a non-violent way.[28] Laing's wealth of experience working as an art therapist in psychiatric and young offenders institutions across Scotland from the 1950s allowed her to develop different strategies of working in this unique setting that remain to date one of the most significant uses of the arts in Scottish prison history.[29]

Something about the rose captured the class's imagination with speculative stories filling the room regarding the imagined receiver of this romantic symbol. Brodie became a prolific creator of ceramic sculptures in the BSU using the process as an important and valuable expressive outlet for his self-confessed violent nature. When commenting on his art, Brodie notes:

> Some pieces show my desire for things beyond my reach, for things I admire and things I want. On the other hand some pieces will show inner turmoil, frustrations, anger, conflict, despair and hate.[30]

Whilst researching Brodie, in order to uncover stories about the rose, the class were intrigued by the rawness of the experiences his art was conveying, and the intelligibility of these in terms of their own experiences.

The rose, for Brodie, symbolised love that he had both lost and desired for during his confinement but that he had also gained through his use of the arts in the BSU, and it became evident that this was a point of real connection for many in the class. Billy, a key contributor to the project, captures this in a poem he wrote about Brodie for the exhibition:

> Ceramics fired, glazed for long,
> playing his guitar,
> singing his song,
> To release the tension
> He feels so strong.
>
> Bob's art will never wither away,
> It gives him hope for the coming day.[31]

Exploring Brodie's work opened up resonances between experiences of confinement across different times and spaces, and the rose offered a routeway to discussing a commonly ignored or overlooked aspect in the prison setting: love and passion. However, it also enabled the feelings of empowerment, joy and hope that were being felt by many of the current prisoners undertaking the project to come to the fore. In discussing and researching the BSU objects, art was also being created, such as Billy's poem that revealed new voices of possibility for what can be achieved by such a process. In an interview for the project, Laing noted:

> I always saw that art had a much wider ability to invoke people who were under any sort of unhappiness or stress .... If you can involve them in the arts, they will find their own way through.[32]

During their research, the group discovered that the rose had been gifted by Brodie to Laing, a symbolic gesture marking the care felt towards Laing and the arts in the BSU. The rose, and its newly uncovered story, is enthusiastically selected for the exhibition.

The gym hall is a space overwritten by hidden histories. Once home to Scotland's longest experiment in penal reform, it now shows little sign of its previous revolutionary past; the cracks of history painted over by the installation of creaking basketball nets and chipped wooden flooring. In the brightly coloured exhibition guide created by the prisoners, they dedicate a section to discussing mental health in prison. In this section, Mark highlights the loneliness of experiencing mental health difficulties while incarcerated, stating:

> Mental health problems in prison are never easy. Anxiety and stress can bring on panic attacks, even depression and many of these symptoms are extremely difficult to handle. So unless you've been diagnosed previously with regular medication to take, it will be a harrowing and frightening time within the prison environment.[33]

During the research sessions, a number of prisoners discussed the strains that mental ill-health placed on individuals and on the system itself. In 2015, the Scottish Institute reported that Scotland's prison population is made up overwhelmingly of individuals with mental health problems, learning difficulties and dependency problems, placing an enormous strain on limited services and forcing individuals to encounter a fragmented system of care.[34] The significance of the space of prison life and its connections to the experiences of mental ill-health is also relayed in the exhibition guide, with Mark explaining:

> When everything is getting on top of you, the slightest problem can feel so much more extreme. Talking helps, but due to a lack of confidence or being confined to set areas for security reasons, you can feel isolated.[35]

Many of the original prisoners in the BSU, such as Jimmy Boyle, Bob Brodie and Hugh Collins, had experienced many years of solitary confinement in the 'cages system' in Inverness and bore the mental scars of an incarceration system that current prisoners were not a direct part of, but felt in some way connected to.[36] Boyle, labelled in the 1970s as one of Scotland's most violent men, discussed openly in his memoirs the pain of confinement and the effects on his mental health that this entailed.[37] When discussing his first sculpture made in the BSU entitled 'Solitary—Inverness', Boyle reveals the terror of confinement and the mental effects this can have:

> In this sculpture I've tried to portray how it feels to live there [punishment cell in Inverness]; isolation, loneliness and despair. … The most important fact of all is the individual's total helplessness. The bars in this piece are not in perimeter formation, as to my mind the visible bars in any prison are not the ones that count. The bars here are actually entangling the figure. These are the bars that matter.[38]

Through researching this artwork from the BSU, the class were able to trace lines of emotional connection between the then and the now that allowed new conversations about mental health to enter into the classroom.

The nature of the experiences of mental health difficulties voiced by Boyle and other's artwork in the collection allowed channels of connection to emerge that were unexpected and illuminating. Whilst the project was fundamentally about revealing the underexplored histories of prison reform, an important space was created to hear previously unspoken experiences of mental distress, illness and fear. These experiences were uttered, shared and rewritten through the exhibition process, culminating in a new set of voices emerging in the form of exhibition guides, talks, poetry and writings, which shared a variety of experiences of mental ill-health. Through the exhibition and the process of its development, these voices have the ability to leave the prison setting and to be transported to other times, people and places. By successfully uncovering the lost voices of the BSU, some individuals found their own voice and ways of expressing their own histories buried deep within.

An Unmarked Grave, Sleepyhillock Cemetery

Tucked away in the corner of Montrose in the North-East of Scotland lies a cemetery called Sleepyhillock. Rows of carefully planted trees act as protective canopies for the bodies resting beneath. At the outer edge of the plot, the cemetery looks set adrift from the land, the hazy eyes of the town kept at bay, maintaining a healthy distance between the living and the dead. In an unmarked spot lies the remains of patient-artist Adam Christie, laid to rest in a pauper's grave on the 7 May 1950, forty-nine years after his initial admission to the Montrose Asylum. Increased scholarly attention has recently been given to issues of death, dissection and burial in asylum histories, highlighting the significance of considering not just the lives but also the afterlives of patients.[39] A concern for the 'pauper' patient and their erasure in death from wider histories of mental health coincides with an emerging interest in the spaces of asylum cemeteries themselves.[40] Adam shares eternity with a host of once-familiar faces of Montrose Asylum's patients from across the centuries, many of them unknown to Adam during his incarceration, yet their invisibility holds them in common regard. A growing concern for asylum histories is with the unknown patient, the individuals lost to history in life and in death, and increasing attempts are being made to awaken the asylum dead from their restless slumber.[41]

The haunting melody played on a single violin catches in the January air, dancing its way through the now-naked branches of Sleepyhillock. This specially composed piece, entitled 'Slow Air to Adam', written and performed by local music teacher Beth Wylie, demarcates the emotional end to an event held to commemorate Adam Christie's life and death. Gathered together in the cemetery, a small crowd have come from far and wide to say a final farewell to Adam and to watch as a sculpture is revealed that marks his place in the graveyard and into the official history of Montrose Asylum (see Gibbeson and Beattie, this volume, for more on community memory and asylums). Adam was a Shetlander, brought to Montrose Asylum—later known as Sunnyside Hospital—at his family's request in 1901. Adam was thirty-two years of age when he entered Montrose, and previous to this, Adam had become increasingly withdrawn, developing a state of agitation which his family felt left them no alternative but to seek him asylum across the sea to the mainland of Montrose. Once admitted, Adam was diagnosed with 'delusional insanity', with records stating that he consistently contemplated committing suicide, felt persecuted and frequently refused food.[42] The hospital records frequently reported that Adam was always busy with his hands. Whether playing the organ, making fiddles, writing letters home or carving in wood and stone, Adam was clearly compulsive in his artistic creation. At the age of fifty-five, twenty-two years after entering the asylum, Adam developed an obsessive interest in carving stone.[43] With tools of his own making, Adam would collect discarded stones from the hospital grounds and carve them into intricate faces, using glass from a broken bottle to scratch the intricate details slowly into the solid surface. Once complete, Adam would hide these heads around the grounds or gift them to friends in the hospital. It was these heads that revealed Adam's story, long after his bones were buried in the unmarked spot, and which gave voice to Adam's experiences of mental ill-health. For it was also a selection of these heads that turned up in the store room of GMRC as part of Laing's Art Extraordinary collection.

A chance encounter in the 1970s between Laing and the then current psychiatrist in Sunnyside, Dr Kenneth Keddie, began the ongoing journey to bring Adam's memory back to life. Laing had spent a two-week period in 1977 searching psychiatric facilities across Scotland for her version of art brut. She had been inspired by a patient named Antonia Jabloner at an

Aberdeen hospital where she worked as one of the first art therapists in Scotland, during the 1960s, who was compulsive in her art-making. For Laing, Jabloner's work fitted Dubuffet's description of art brut, and inspired by this she wished to seek out as much as she could from different institutions around Scotland. With photographer Jim Waugh in tow, they vowed 'we'd start at the north of Scotland and work out way south. So Craig Dunain was our first call'.[44] Keddie had heard about Laing's expedition and knew that she had searched in gardens, wards, hedges and rubbish bins to find work that had been discarded, lost or overlooked. Keddie, in 1966, had first come across a number of head sculptures in the grounds of the hospital and had set about inquiring their lineage. Nobody at the time seemed to know where they had come from or who would have made them until one day a hospital Steward, James McLennon, who was just about to retire, suddenly recalled the name 'Adam Christie'.[45] The head sculptures, left behind by Adam in life, rescued his voice and allowed some of his experiences at Montrose to be excavated over half a century since his burial in an unmarked grave.

The large stone slab sits proudly in the workshop at the end of Brian's garden. The carving of the facial features have begun, and it is startling how much it already resembles the work of Adam. Brian is anxious to continue carving. The deadline for the commemoration event is looming, and the sculpture is at a particularly delicate stage. One small slip of the chisel, Brian nervously conveys, and the stone will split: the damage is irreparable. The replica stone head is to be laid at the gravesite of Adam, facing both towards the hospital and his beloved Shetland home to which he could never return. Back in Brian's cottage, over coffee, he shares his reflections on the process of making that he is undertaking. He stresses that there is an invisible line of connection between him and Adam that is being forged through the carving process, a stone–metal–flesh dialogue that fuses relations between the past and present.[46] He notes that he tries to imagine how Adam must have felt in the gardens of the asylum as he slowly carved in stone. He speaks of Adam's potential feelings of loneliness and a lost sense of identity to the world he left behind. He mentions that these chime with his own. The art-making process undertaken is doing more than providing salvation for Adam's memory, Brian too feels that it is helping him to rebuild and recuperate from a stressful period of the life he is moving on from. In discussing Adam, the potential to hear Brian's own experiences come to the fore, highlighting the power of following the trace to forge new time–space collisions. As the stone carving is finally revealed to the visitors to Sleepyhillock, the local press ask questions about Adam to the local community. Everyone there knows his name. Everyone can recognise his carvings. Everyone now knows where he is buried.

Conclusions

This chapter has sought to demonstrate some of the *practices* involved in tracing the lives, worlds and voices of individuals experiencing mental ill-health across time and space that remain difficult to uncover. In drawing attention to three specific examples of work undertaken with the Art Extraordinary collection through giving attention to the trace, this chapter has aimed to show the varying ways in which new voices of mental ill-health can emerge from unexpected encounters between people, objects and places. While increased scholarly attention is being given to the role of the museum as a space of exhibiting mental health histories, the examples used here seek to extend these ideas to consider the voices revealed when objects and archives travel beyond their institutional boundaries and collide in interesting ways with hearts, minds and bodies.[47] The fragmented stories shared from different fieldwork encounters illuminate the often-forgotten or overlooked spaces of mental ill-health and highlight their significance for understanding the variety of voices wrapped up in the histories of mental health. The attention given to the partial, the unknown and the remembered in all of the case studies reveals the significance of attending to the trace in the *hearing* and *listening* of other voices of 'madness' for revealing a more diverse and inclusive set of mental health histories.

Ogborn's notion of the trace as a way to uncover hidden journeys, located moments of negotiation and listening for the presence of ghosts comes to the fore in all of the examples used, demonstrating how past and present experiences collide and create new ways of understanding and telling the experiences of mental ill-health. As the 'archival turn' continues to provide a pause for reflection on the practices of 'doing' historical work, an interesting opportunity emerges for a (re)consideration of the ways in which historical mental health research is undertaken and shared.[48] In paying attention to the multiple ways in which objects inspire conversations about mental health care and the places this occupies, a crucial space is generated in which new stories of mental ill-health are revealed that bring to the fore the continuous jostling between the then and the now. In finally returning to Lynda and her chance encounter with the pink plastic folder one evening in Leverndale, it is clear that while the folder now sits quietly on a shelf in the museum storeroom, its ability to provoke further conversation and to communicate different voices of experience is revealed. By illuminating the momentary intersections between Lynda, Marylène and the space of the Recreational Therapy Department, a new set of emotional, embodied and material stories appear that help amplify the voices of the unknown and the unheard. By focusing upon intertwining stories of people, objects and place an opportunity emerges to really hear the voices of human experience that are so incredibly meaningful in creating inclusive mental health histories. The often very different voices of experience that appear in these three small examples begin to highlight the power of paying attention to the small stories of mental ill-health and the humanising qualities that sharing these stories can have across time and space. Through highlighting the different ways in which I have attempted to track the traces of the Art Extraordinary collection, it is clear that voices travel and their presence trickles through history. By drawing attention to the variety of practices undertaken through fieldwork stories, this chapter has shown the importance of continuing to develop innovative methodological approaches for 'listening harder and listening better' in order to continue to excavate new voices of experience in historical mental health research.

Acknowledgements This piece is dedicated to Katie Allan and to the Allan family's fight for better mental health provision in Scottish prisons.

Notes

1. Roger Cardinal, *Outsider Art* (London: Studio Vista, 1972); Colin Rhodes, *Outsider Art: Spontaneous Alternatives* (Thames & Hudson, 2000).
2. Marylène Walker, *Drawing on lullabies* (Art Extraordinary Collection: Glasgow Museums, 1999), A.2012.4.834.
3. Chris Philo and Jonathan Andrews, "Introduction: histories of asylums, insanity and psychiatry in Scotland," *History of Psychiatry* 28 (2017): 3–14.
4. Cheryl McGeachan, "The 'Head Carver': Art Extraordinary and the small spaces of asylum," *History of Psychiatry* 28 (2017): 58–71.
5. Hayden Lorimer, "Telling small stories: spaces of knowledge and the practice of geography," *Transactions of the Institute of British Geographers* 28 (2003): 197–217.

6. Kerry Davis, "'Silent and Censured Travellers'?: Patients' Narratives and Patients' Voices: Perspectives on the History of mental Illness since 1948," *Social History of Medicine* 14 (2001): 267–292.
7. Caroline Bressey, "The city of others: photographs from the City of London asylum archive," *19: Interdisciplinary Studies in the Long Nineteenth Century* 13 (2011).
8. Morag Allan Campbell, "'Noisy, restless and incoherent': puerperal insanity at Dundee Lunatic Asylum," *History of Psychiatry* 28 (2017): 44–57; Hazel Morrison, "Constructing Patient Stories: 'Dynamic' Case Notes and Clinical Encounters at Glasgow's Gartnavel Mental Hospital, 1921–32," *Medical History* 60 (2016): 67–86; Lorelle Barry and Catharine Coleborne, "Insanity and ethnicity in New Zealand: Māori encounters with the Auckland Mental Hospital, 1860–1900," *History of Psychiatry* 22 (2011): 285–301.
9. Cheryl McGeachan, "The 'Head Carver': Art Extraordinary and the small spaces of asylum," *History of Psychiatry* 28 (2017): 58–71; Allan Beveridge, "A Disquieting Feeling of Strangeness?: The Art of the Mentally Ill," *Journal of the Royal Society of Medicine* 94 (2009): 595–599.
10. Gayle Davis, Gayle, *'The Cruel Madness of Love': Sex, Syphilis and Psychiatry in Scotland, 1880–1930* (Amsterdam and New york: Rodopi, 2008).
11. Pauline Prior and Gillean McClelland, "Through the lens of the hospital magazine: Downshire and Holywell psychiatric hospitals in the 1960s and 1970s," *History of Psychiatry* 24 (2013): 399–414.
12. Roy Porter, "The patient's view: doing medical history from below," *Theory and Society* 14 (1985): 175–198.
13. Helen Spandler, *Asylum to action: Paddington day hospital, therapeutic communities and beyond* (London: Jessica Kingsley Publishers, 2006); Mark Gallagher, From mental patient to service user: deinstitutionalisation and the emergence of the Mental Health Service User Movement in Scotland, 1971–2006 (Unpublished PhD Thesis: University of Glasgow, 2017).
14. Rebecca Wynter and Leonard Smith, "Introduction: historical contexts to communicating mental health," *Medical Humanities* 43 (2017): 73–80, 9.
15. Brendan D Kelly, "Searching for the patient's voice in the Irish asylums," *Medical Humanities* 42 (2016): 87–91.
16. Natalie Mullen, '"The Geography of License': Asylum Architecture and Patient Agency in Lancaster's County Asylum, 1840–1915," talk at the Inaugural Congress of the Northern Network for the Medical Humanities. University of Durham: September (2017); Hazel Morrison, Conversing with the Psychiatrist: Patient Narratives within Glasgow's Royal Asylum 1921–1929. *Journal of Literature and Science* 6 (2013): 18–37.
17. Brendan D Kelly, "Searching for the patient's voice in the Irish asylums".

18. Cheryl McGeachan, "Historical Geography II: Traces Remain," *Progress in Human Geography* 42 (2018): 134–362.
19. Charles Nicholl, *Traces Remain: Essays and Explorations* (London: Allen Lane: Penguin Group: 2011).
20. Miles Ogborn, "Editorial: Atlantic geographies," *Social & Cultural Geographies* 6 (2005): 379–385, 383.
21. Ibid., 382.
22. Volker Berghahn and Simone Lässig, eds., *Biography between Structure and Agency: Central European Lives in International Historiography* (Oxford: Berghahn Books, 2008).
23. Christopher Carrell and Joyce Laing, *The Special Unit Barlinnie Prison: Its Evolution through its Arts* (Glasgow: Third Eye Centre, 1982).
24. Scottish Prison Service, *Small Units within the Scottish Prison Service* Occasional Paper No 1/2002 (Edinburgh: Red Howie Associates Ltd, 2002).
25. Scottish Home and Health Department, *Treatment of Certain Male Long Term Prisoners and Potentially Violent Prisoners* (Edinburgh: Departmental Working Party, The Scottish Office, 1971).
26. Jan Patience, "The art that changed the men in Barlinnie," *The Herald* (May 5 January 2017).
27. Bob Brodie, "Rose," (Art Extraordinary Collection. Glasgow Museums. A.2012.4.1121: undated).
28. Christopher Carrell and Joyce Laing, *The Special Unit Barlinnie Prison.*
29. Mike Nellis, "Creative Arts and the Cultural Politics of Penal Reform: the early years of the Barlinnie Special Unit, 1973–1981," *Journal of Scottish Criminal Justice Studies* 20 (2010).
30. Quoted in Christopher Carrell and Joyce Laing, *The Special Unit Barlinnie Prison*, 100.
31. 'A way out of a dark time: Barlinnie Special Unit', Exhibition Guide produced by New College Lanarkshire, Scottish Prison Service and Glasgow Museums (2016).
32. Ibid.
33. Ibid.
34. The Scotland Institute, *Mental Health and Scotland's Prison Population* (Glasgow: The Scottish Institute 2015).
35. 'A way out of a dark time: Barlinnie Special Unit'.
36. James Freeman, "Keys of infamous prison 'cages' are put away for good," *The Herald* (March 1 1994).
37. Jimmy Boyle, *A Sense of Freedom* (London: Pan Books, 1977).
38. Christopher Carrell and Joyce Laing, *The Special Unit Barlinnie Prison*, 65.

39. Jennifer Wallis, *Investigating the Body in the Victorian Asylum: Doctors, Patients and Practices.* (Palgrave-Macmillan, 2017); Jonathan Andrews, "Introduction: Lunacy's last rites," *History of Psychiatry* 23 (2012): 3–5.
40. Chris Philo, "Troubled proximities: asylums and cemeteries in nineteenth-century England," *History of Psychiatry* 23 (2012): 91–103.
41. Nathan Flis and David Wright, 2012. "'A Grave Injustice': The Mental Hospital and Shifting Sites of Memory" in *Exhibiting Madness in Museums*, eds. Catharine Coleborne and Dolly MacKinnon (Routledge: 2012), 101–115.
42. Kenneth Keddie, *The Gentle Shetlander: The Extraordinary Story of an Artist in the Shadows* (P. Harris: 1984).
43. Cheryl McGeachan, "The Head Carver: Art Extraordinary and the small spaces of asylum".
44. Roger Hutchinson, *The Silent Weaver: The Extraordinary Life and Work of Angus MacPhee* (Edinburgh: Birlinn: 2011), 118.
45. Kenneth Keddie, *The Gentle Shetlander.*
46. Cheryl McGeachan, "The 'Head Carver'.
47. Amy Jane Barnes, "Museums and Mental Health," *Museum Worlds: Advances in Research* 2 (2014): 133–167.
48. Kirsty Reid and Fiona Paisley, eds., *Sources and Methods in Histories of Colonialism: Approaching the Imperial Archive.* (Routledge: 2017).

CHAPTER 12

Patient Photographs, Patient Voices: Recovering Patient Experience in the Nineteenth-Century Asylum

Katherine Rawling

Introduction

Do voices always have to be spoken? What do we really *mean* when we imagine the 'patient voice' and how can researchers access these marginalised yet potentially powerful 'voices' from the past? When historians search for patient voices in the archive, they often focus on various versions of direct testimony found in patients' life writing, letters, or written speech. Through these channels, we can move closer to finding the elusive patient voice and access what is truly at the heart of this search—the recovery of various forms of patient experiences, agencies, and subjectivities. This approach involves searching archives for evidence of patients communicating; evidence, perhaps, of resistance and compliance, or, simply, of

K. Rawling (✉)
School of Philosophy, Religion and History of Science, University of Leeds, Leeds, UK
e-mail: k.d.b.rawling@leeds.ac.uk

R. Ellis et al. (eds.), *Voices in the History of Madness*, Mental Health in Historical Perspective,
https://doi.org/10.1007/978-3-030-69559-0_12

everyday patient experiences. Often the purpose behind attempts to recover patient 'voices' is really about a quest for recognition, understanding, and even empathy between historical patients and contemporary readers or researchers. But direct evidence of patient voices is notoriously hard to find in medical archives; patient experiences and subjectivities are usually filtered through practitioners' own narratives in case notes or histories recorded in casebooks, with the result that patients can be depersonalised as scientific subjects, specimens, or data. As Sally Swartz notes, when engaging with historical case notes and documents 'the reader learns a great deal about doctors and their systems of self-representation, and almost nothing of the patients of whom they wrote'.[1] For Swartz, concerned as she is with written records, patients are 'subalterns' and, as such, are 'silenced subject[s] of history'.[2] To address the challenge of apparently 'silent' patient records outlined by Swartz, I, like the other authors in this section, employ an expanded concept of patient 'voice' that includes non-spoken or non-written communication, allowing me to consider the alternative visual archival records that might provide insight into patient experiences. This approach is based on two inter-related propositions. The first is that the search for patient 'voices' is, in essence, the search for patient experiences and patient communication. The second is that communication itself is not exclusively verbal, and that photographic images are themselves used to communicate and conceived of as 'speaking' or as having a 'voice'. By taking these two principles together, I suggest that considering the ways in which photographic images might be used to communicate offers another possible avenue for researchers wanting to uncover the patient 'voice' in asylum records.

Almost since its invention, photography was used in medical and psychiatric practice, in fields as diverse as surgery, infectious disease, and dermatology.[3] As the nineteenth century progressed, and photographic technologies became more efficient and accessible, being photographed became an increasingly common experience for many patients. As a result, there are thousands of photographs of patients pasted into asylum casebooks, appearing consistently in English examples from around the 1880s onwards. They are, however, a relatively untapped source of patient records as, with some notable exceptions, historians have preferred to focus their attention on the written case note rather than the patient photograph.[4] And yet, photography was a widespread practice adopted by institutions as diverse as Newcastle-upon-Tyne City Lunatic Asylum, a borough asylum housing a large pauper population, to Holloway

Sanatorium in Surrey, an exclusive private hospital for the middle and upper classes of the South East of England. These hospitals have been chosen to represent two ends of the institutional spectrum and demonstrate the variety of photographic styles and practices that were used in psychiatric institutions in the last decades of the nineteenth century.

A selection of photographs chosen from the surviving casebooks from these two very different hospitals will be used to consider the possibilities of using the patient photograph as a means of accessing the patient 'voice' in its broadest sense. By paying attention to alternative forms of evidence of patient 'voices', two things happen. Firstly, patient experience can be considered more fully, as something that was verbally *and* visually lived and recorded; many casebooks were both textual and visual documents, meaning the image and text were intended to be read and viewed together. There are instances, however, when the patient's case notes and their photograph sit uneasily alongside each other. In drawing attention to these contradictions between image and text in the examples in this chapter, I suggest that giving the patient photograph full consideration moves us closer to recovering patient voices and experiences that would be lost by simply studying the casebook text alone. Secondly, scrutinising casebook photographs offers the opportunity to see psychiatric photography not simply as something done *to* patients, but something that patients could have an active role in. While not recovering the patient's *spoken* voice, some photographs can hint at forms of patient agency and experience ranging from opposition to compliance with the photographic process that might well be overlooked if the visual record is not taken into account. I argue that rather than being only an administrative method of recording the identity and physical appearance of asylum patients, patient photographs are also evidence of the multiple, and sometimes competing, subjectivities and 'voices' that operated within the institution and its records. The examples reproduced in this chapter, some of which show staff as well as patients, shed light on the highly complex relationships between text and image, practitioner and patient, and photographer and photographed that are active in casebook records.

The 'Voice' of a Photograph

The dynamic and complex relationship between image, text, and language is one that has been noted since the introduction of photographic technologies in the first half of the nineteenth century.[5] In a paper read before the Royal Society in 1856, the asylum alienist and pioneering photographer Dr Hugh Welch Diamond (1809–86) was clear that the photographic image had far greater powers of communication than the written word. He claimed:

> The Photographer, on the other hand, needs in many cases no aid from any language of his own, but prefers rather to *listen*, with the picture before him, to the silent but telling language of nature—It is unnecessary for him to use the vague terms which denote a difference in the degree of mental suffering, as for instance, distress, sorrow, deep sorrow, grief, melancholy, anguish, despair; *the picture speaks for itself* with the most marked pression and indicates the exact point which had been reached in the scale of unhappiness between the first sensation and its utmost height—similarly the modification of fear, and of the more painful passions, anger and rage, jealously and envy (the frequent concomitants of insanity) being shown from the life by the Photographer, arrest the attention of the thoughtful observer more powerfully than any laboured description.[6]

A year later, the photograph's ability to communicate was praised by the writer Lady Elizabeth Eastlake (1809–93) in the *Quarterly Review*:

> What are her [photography's] representations of the bed of the ocean, and the surface of the moon…but facts which are neither the province of art nor of description, but of that *new form of communication between man and man*—neither letter, message, nor picture—which now happily fills up the space between them?[7]

In the same essay, Eastlake referred to the use of the camera in psychiatric institutions (no doubt in response to Diamond's attempts to photograph his patients at Surrey County Asylum in the 1850s), stating, 'What are her studies of the various stages of insanity—pictures of life unsurpassable in pathetic truth—but facts as well as lessons of the deepest physiological interest?'[8] These early articulations of the relationship between photography and communication positioned the camera as an invaluable tool in the fields of medicine and psychiatry.

In contemporary photographic theory, too, photographs, voices, and communication have been intimately connected. Allan Sekula has described photographs as 'utterances' which convey a message, a message which is determined by context. Thus, a photograph is only 'readable' when the reader/viewer is fluent in the language that makes the implicit message in a photograph clear. Sekula claims that when seeing a photograph for the first time, a viewer will not understand it unless she or he is 'literate' in the language that gives the image meaning.[9] He states: 'every photographic image is a sign, above all, of someone's investment in the sending of a message.'[10] In addition, Jennifer Green-Lewis has pointed out that photographs are generally conceived of as being able to 'tell stories' and are, therefore, wholly reliant on 'language'.[11] The storytelling inherent in photographic practices has also been made clear by scholars arguing that the materiality of the photograph (its status as an object, not just an image) is central to understanding its meaning. This enables analysis to go beyond the superficial description of what a photograph might 'show' to consider its use, social biography, and social value.[12] Elizabeth Edward's discussion of the sensory theory of photographs relates directly to the idea of photographs having a 'voice' by claiming that they communicate through their material, haptic, and embodied qualities. She gives the example of family members sitting together to view a family album of old photos of relatives. In this scene, some photographs are touched, some are talked to, many are talked about, and a narrative is formed around them that is generated by the viewers' engagement with the photo-object. The oral dimension of viewing photographs, the literal version of 'telling stories', as well as other sensory experiences like listening, all enable the photograph to communicate. Moreover, Edwards claims that it is through this process that 'photographs become active voices' themselves.[13]

Photographs, therefore, are intimately tied to communication. In the context of Edwards' own research on photography and anthropology, the orality of photographs can help in the histories of 'fracture and dispossession', particularly in the colonial context or in the histories of indigenous peoples.[14] I extend this to suggest that photographs are also useful for recovering the histories and experiences of other dispossessed and marginalised groups, in this case, psychiatric patients. When doctors discussed and exchanged photos of their patients with their colleagues, orality and communication were embedded and embodied in practice.[15] Just as relatives might huddle around an old album, handling the photographs as they talk, when doctors swapped and discussed patient photographs as illustrative examples of symptoms or diagnoses, the same principles were at work. In both cases, 'the spoken and the seen cease to be separate modalities; instead they are bound together in and through the human body'.[16]

Examining the photographic record of asylums is not without precedent, and both historical and contemporary photographs have been used to access the apparently closed worlds of mental ill-health and its institutions. The end of large-scale institutional care in Britain and Europe beginning in the 1960s and gaining pace from the 1980s provided opportunities for photographers to enter once-grand nineteenth-century hospitals to photograph decaying infrastructure and empty corridors or wards. The potential power of documentary photography, usually in dramatic monochrome, was well suited to this task as photographs captured these vast, yet silent, spaces in stark realism.[17] Such images were designed to elicit an emotional reaction from viewers, to 'speak' to them of the inhumanity and ultimate failure of institutional therapy. Interestingly, this form of documentary or reportage photography was sometimes the first stage in the afterlife of institutions that may then be demolished or redeveloped, as discussed in Gibbeson and Beatties' chapter in this collection.

In addition, a body of recent work has begun to use patient casebook photographs to explore the role of photography in visualising the insane patient and in the genre of medical portraiture more generally.[18] Moreover, there is growing appreciation of the complexity and fluidity of patient photographs.[19] Rory du Plessis encourages historians to view casebook images, not simply as clinical data, but as representations of individuals, while Caroline Bressey shows how the photographic archive can be used to uncover the experiences of marginalised groups, namely people of colour, in asylums.[20] What this work has in common is the desire to pay attention to the extensive non-textual record of mental ill-health and its institutions, and to use the visual to access patient experiences and subjectivities.

Both evocative documentary-style photography of buildings in decay and historical casebook patient photographs can elicit similar emotional and personal reactions in the viewer. Barbara Brookes claims that coming face to face with a casebook photograph reminds viewers of the 'suffering of individuals' and restores 'humanity' to long-forgotten patients. She continues, '[A]t times the thin biographies in the case notes, varying according to the physical ailments and troublesomeness of the patients, are brought to life by a photograph'.[21] For Brookes, patient photographs clearly have the potential to communicate, to give voice to the silent, by enabling an empathetic connection between past and present that 'the written text rarely can', a process similar to that described by Cheryl McGeachan in this volume.[22] Brookes implies that it is the image, and only the image, that creates this connection. This is problematic on two levels. Firstly, stating that it is only the photograph that can establish a connection between long-gone and present-day people diminishes the potential impact words can have on the emotions or reactions of readers. Secondly, by concentrating attention purely on the photograph, it is extracted from its original context. This means that the intended relationship between the words and image that was so integral to the casebook as a clinical document is obscured. Rather, I wish to emphasise here that case notes and case photographs were part of the same whole. That said, the nature of the relationship between image and text can be highly ambiguous, particularly when the two elements of the document do not appear to match. Here I discuss examples of such cases in an effort to detect the possible traces of competing 'voices' that are at work in patient records.

A Picture Tells a Thousand Words?

William[23] was admitted to the Newcastle-upon-Tyne City Lunatic Asylum on 29 November 1905. He was a 15-year-old labourer, admitted suffering from mania associated with a 'Congenital Mental Defect', a term used in the period to distinguish between those conditions thought to be present in the patient since birth and those that were acquired later.[24] His medical certificate noted that he had a 'strange look', and notes on his present mental state describe him as 'very miserable and frightened and is continually crying'.[25] William's photograph is placed directly next to these notes and is in a standard format for this particular institution—a close-up head shot, the form and style of which might be recognisable to present-day viewers as similar to a standard identity photo, like a modern passport photograph. The photographic print is cut down to size to fit neatly into the margin space of the page and shows a teenage boy, facing into the camera with a calm expression, the slightest trace of a smile visible on his lips (Figs. 12.1 and 12.2).

The first page of a patient's case history was standardised to contain vital information like age, marital status, religion, and condition on admission. From around 1895, the patient photograph became part of this standardised casebook information at Newcastle with each patient being photographed in the same way (seated, in front of a plain background), with the resulting photograph then being placed next to the admission notes.[26] In other cases like those of Margaret admitted in July 1896,[27] Matilda admitted in June 1900,[28] Mary admitted in June 1903,[29] and

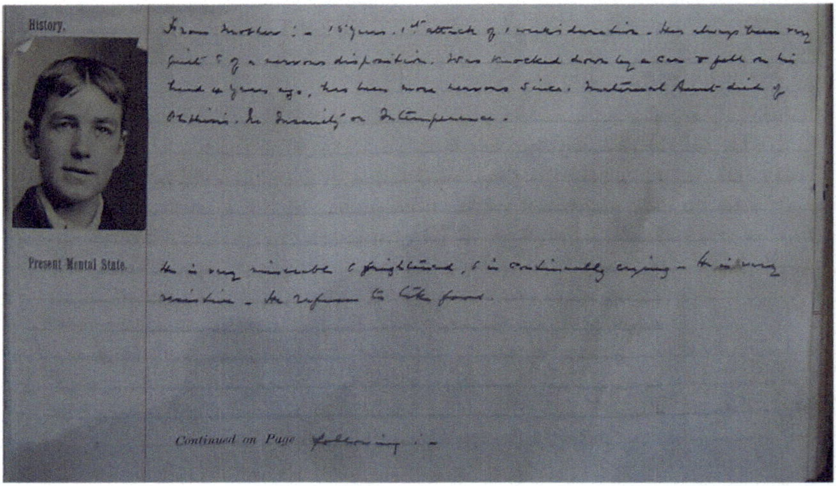

Fig. 12.1 Photographer unknown, William, admitted 29/11/1905. Newcastle-upon-Tyne City Lunatic Asylum Casebook, males, TWAS HO/SN/13/14. 280. Permission to reproduce from Tyne and Wear Archives and Museums

Louisa admitted in August 1904,[30] the description of the patient recorded in the case notes does not match the photograph displayed in the casebook. These patients are described in the written notes as 'frequently crying' and 'melancholic,'[31] 'very much afraid of something,'[32] 'wild and excited,'[33] or 'dazed [and] vacant,'[34] states that are not in evidence in the portraits which show patients with placid or smiling expressions (Figs. 12.3, 12.4, 12.5, and 12.6). This is in marked contrast to earlier psychiatric photography in which photographs were taken as an explicit illustration of the patient's mental state. In the late 1850s, Diamond's portraits of his patients at Surrey were published in a series in *The Medical Times and Gazette*, alongside Dr John Conolly's case studies, with the lithographs from photographs acting as direct illustration of the case histories. Conolly spent much time in his text describing the patients' features and appearance, encouraging the reader to view the 'admirable' and 'faithful' portraits in conjunction with his narrative.[35] In the Newcastle patient notes, there is no such immediate imperative for the reader/viewer to analyse the image provided, or indeed support the text with an illustrative image.

Similar disparities occur in the casebooks from the private Holloway Sanatorium produced in the same period. Photographs of Constance, a

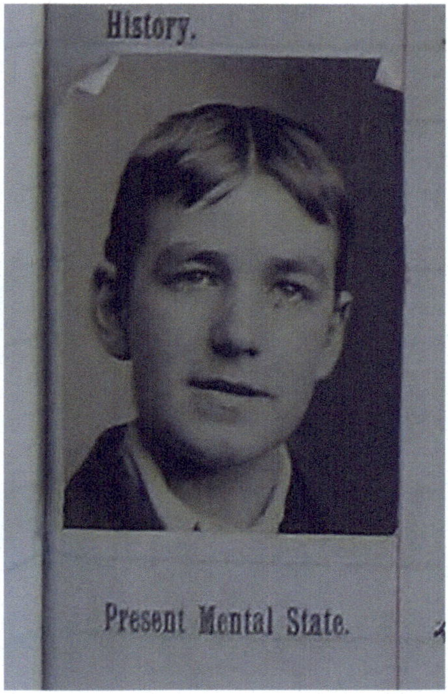

Fig. 12.2 Detail of Figure 12.1. Permission to reproduce from Tyne and Wear Archives and Museums

patient on two separate occasions at the Sanatorium, appear in the female casebooks for the period 1889–91. On her first admission aged 19 in May 1889, the photographs pasted into the ledger alongside her case notes seem entirely consistent with her condition. She is described as acutely maniacal and never still, throwing her arms and legs about and with a habit of sticking out her tongue instead of answering the Medical Officer's questions.[36] The three photographs accompanying these notes suggest a high degree of animation and movement on her part. In the first, a slim photographic object fitted neatly into the page margin, she is shown with female attendants flanking her on either side (Fig. 12.12). In the second and third shots, she is pictured close-up, apparently in a state of high agitation, her mouth open to suggest a scream, shout, or exclamation of some sort (Fig. 12.7). The occasional and rather superficial references in the notes to these photographs ('The annexed photos were taken today') demonstrate the ways in which doctors might use patient photos to add detail or flesh out the narrative; the implication being that the images are

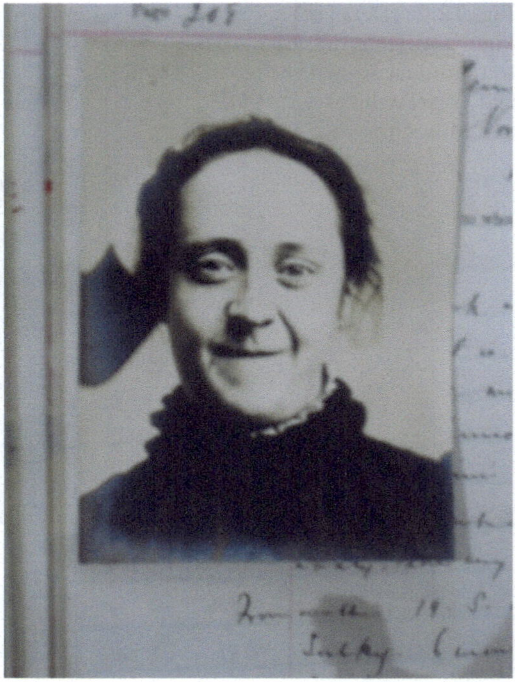

Fig. 12.3 Photographer unknown, Margaret, admitted 29/11/1905. Newcastle-upon-Tyne City Lunatic Asylum Casebook, females, TWAS HO/SN/13/34. 475. Permission to reproduce from Tyne and Wear Archives and Museums

included to provide additional visual evidence or information to complement the case notes.[37] The photographs of Constance taken during her first admission are arresting, evocative, and even alarming. However, the fourth photograph which accompanies the notes for her second admission 14 months later is, considering the immediate material context of the image, possibly even more striking. Constance was admitted for the second time in April 1891, again suffering from acute mania, characterised by excitement, restlessness, noisiness, and general incoherence. This time, her photograph, placed alongside notes that describe her as 'throwing her arms about, laughing, shouting, whistling and talking incoherently' show a lady of calm serenity, her neat dress, smooth hair, and conventional pose all suggesting modesty, order, and respectability (Fig. 12.8).[38]

In all these cases, there would have been some time lapse between the initial clinical assessment and photographs being taken, and, of course, expressions, moods, and conditions change. There is no reason that someone suffering from mental ill-health should look a certain way all or,

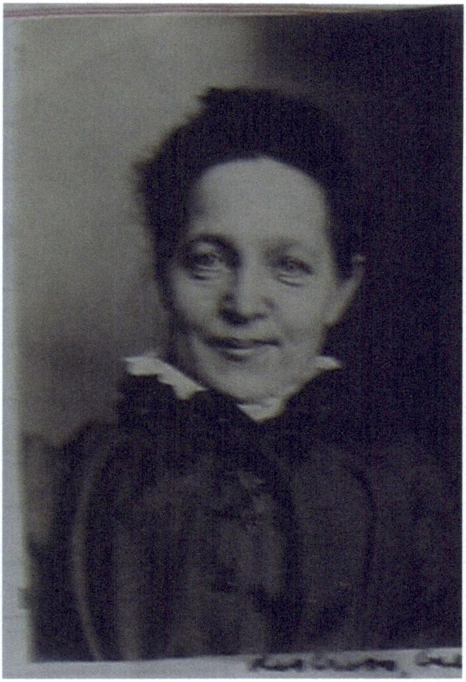

Fig. 12.4 Photographer unknown, Matilda, admitted 1/6/1900. Newcastle-upon-Tyne City Lunatic Asylum Casebook, females, TWAS HO/SN/13/36. 322. Permission to reproduce from Tyne and Wear Archives and Museums

indeed, any of the time. Nonetheless, the discrepancies between the Medical Officers' description of the patient and the (re)presentation of the patient in the photograph raises certain questions, particularly if (as it is commonly assumed) that photographs in this context served purely as illustration or evidence. Why do the photos and description not match? Is it possible that these patients recover themselves sufficiently for their portraits? Were the conventions of how one should sit for one's photograph so ingrained by the last decades of the nineteenth century that posing in such a way became almost second nature? The influence of photographic convention on pose, style, and arrangement is in evidence in many medical photographs in which patients are pictured against decorative backdrops, leaning against columns or chairs, or recreating the recognisable three-quarter angled pose. But despite the conventions of studio photography being evident in some medical photos, there were no standard procedures dictating how institutions should practise photography, if at all. Doctors were still undecided as to whether photography was of use in their work,

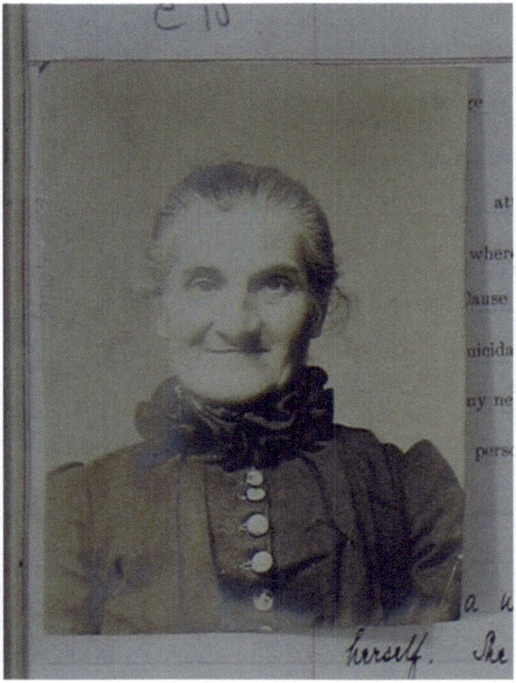

Fig. 12.5 Photographer unknown, Mary, admitted 17/6/1903. Newcastle-upon-Tyne City Lunatic Asylum Casebook, females, TWAS HO/SN/13/38. 115. Permission to reproduce from Tyne and Wear Archives and Museums

and the archives of patient photographs that remain suggest that practices were experimental, fluid, and often improvised.[39] In another example, despite describing Rose, a patient at Holloway Sanatorium in the late 1880s, as 'excitable', 'objectionable', 'exuberant' and 'annoying' in her case notes, the medical officers chose for the casebook a portrait of her leaning on the newel post at the foot of a substantial flight of stone steps in the Sanatorium grounds. Her feet are crossed at the ankles, her hands clasped in the conventional style of numerous professional and amateur portraits of the time.[40] Her pose and demeanour suggest ease and comfort, an assured familiarity with how one should present oneself for a photo (Figs. 12.9 and 12.10).

The surviving archives of numerous asylums indicate that photographs formed a part of the patient record. Different institutions had different approaches to photography; while all patients at Newcastle were photographed as part of standard procedure, photography at Holloway Sanatorium was more erratic and irregular. Nevertheless, photography

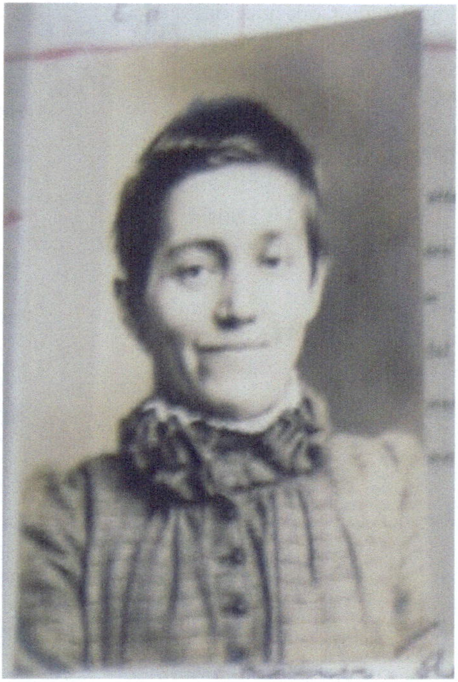

Fig. 12.6 Photographer unknown, Louisa, admitted 15/8/1904. Newcastle-upon-Tyne City Lunatic Asylum Casebook, females, TWAS HO/SN/13/38. 442. Permission to reproduce from Tyne and Wear Archives and Museums

and photographs were deemed important and useful at both institutions. However, it seems that in some cases it was not considered necessary for the two types of evidence to match or for the image to support the statements in the notes. When considering the materiality of these image-objects, the placement of the photograph directly next to the case note text has a jarring effect on the reader/viewer; when one is confronted by the text saying one thing and an image suggesting another, the usual assumed function of photographs as illustration, or as supporting evidence of the patient's condition, is disrupted.

No such disruption exists in other records that contain both patient photographs and text. In published sources like medical textbooks and journal articles, whilst images appear less frequently, they serve a more clear-cut purpose. In standard textbooks of the day like Savage and Goodalls' *Insanity and Allied Neuroses* (four editions 1884–1907) or W.H.B. Stoddart's *Mind and Its Disorders* (five editions 1908–26), photographic plates are used to illustrate explicit examples, with the reader being

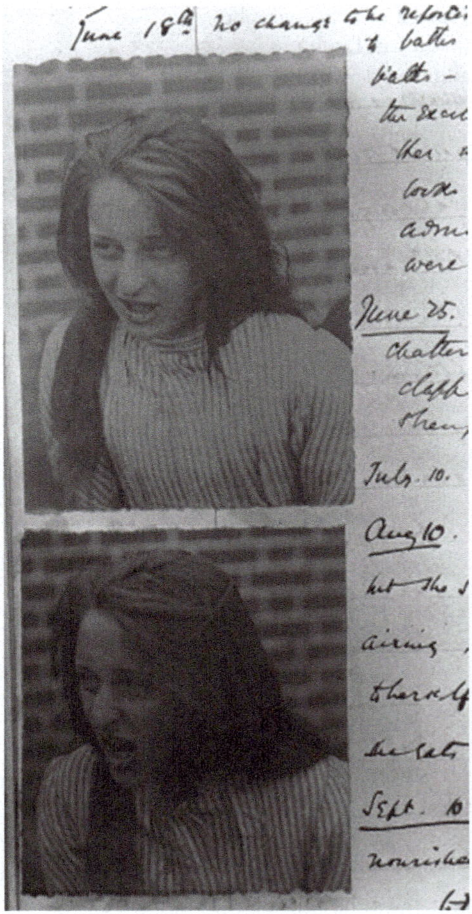

Fig. 12.7 Constance on first admission, Holloway Sanatorium Casebook No.2, females (certified patients admitted January-September 1889), WMS 5157/5157. 193. Credit: Wellcome Collection

instructed in how to 'read' the images correctly through the use of captions or direction in the main text.[41] This cannot be said for the casebooks in which medical officers rarely make any direct reference to photographs, or even acknowledge their presence on the page. The standardised and regular photographing of patients at Newcastle suggests that it was an important activity, even an integral part of clinical and administrative practice, but, at the same time, not a practice that required comment and not one in which any disjunction between image and text was deemed problematic. The relationship between photographs and case notes, then, is an

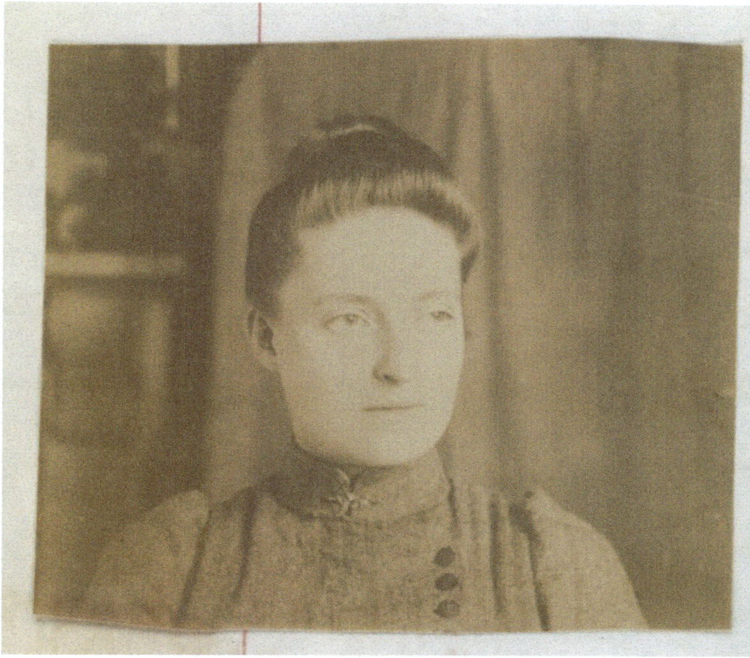

Fig. 12.8 Constance on second admission, Holloway Sanatorium Casebook No. 4, females (certified patients admitted July 1890-June 1891), WMS 5157/5158: 249. Credit: Wellcome Collection

ambiguous and disorientating one, especially in the context of photography's assumed (though highly problematic) evidential or factual status.

Medical case notes are, of course, mediated; they are versions of patient experience filtered through, interpreted, and presented by the doctor. However, it is in cases like those above that we can begin to consider other factors apart from the medical officer's voice in these official records. When text and photograph seem mismatched, contradictory even, patients might begin to compete with the dominance of the doctor's narrative and something apart from the doctor's voice emerges—some form of subjectivity on the patient's part that makes them sit for a photograph in a particular way. Such cases open up the possibility of multiple voices and subjectivities within the documents, in the form of not just certifying doctors, family and friends, recording medical officers, and the patients

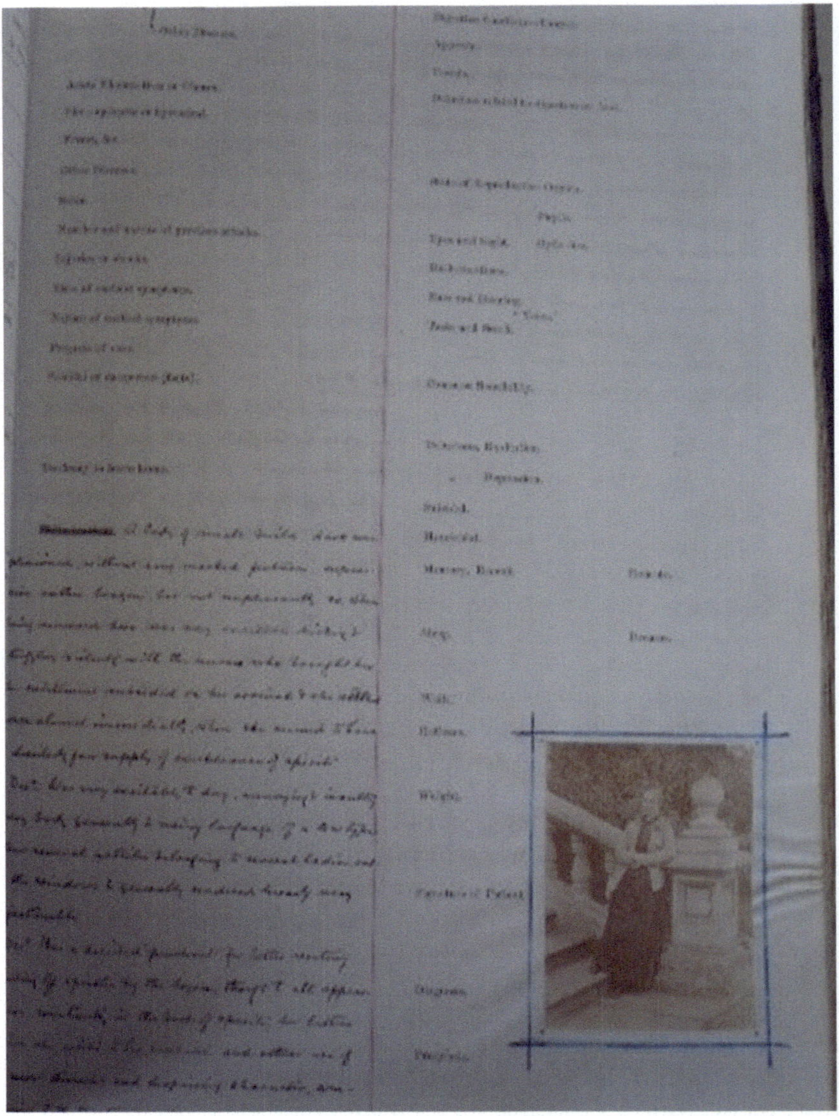

Fig. 12.9 Photographer unknown, admission page for Rose, Holloway Sanatorium Casebook (certified patients admitted Jun 1885-Jan 1889) Surrey History Centre 3473/3/1.94. Reproduced by permission of Surrey History Centre

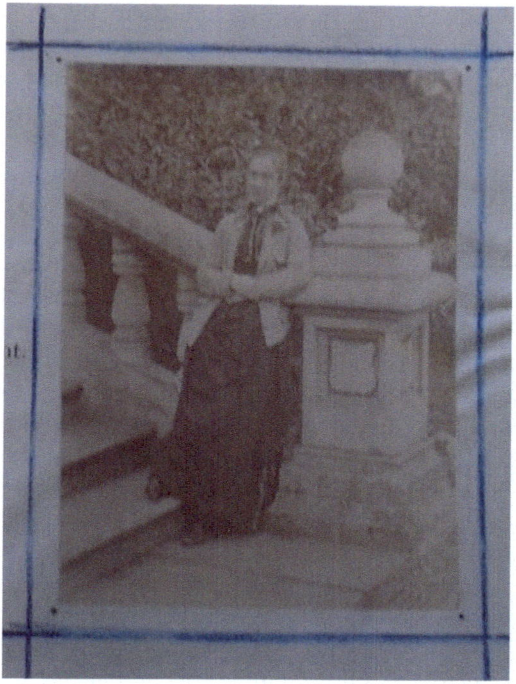

Fig. 12.10 Detail of Figure 12.9. Reproduced by permission of Surrey History Centre

themselves (sometimes direct testimony in quotation marks, sometimes paraphrased by others), but also the patient image. These examples are a reminder of the complex relationship between the two types of evidence presented in official patient records.

Multiple Voices

For Brookes, viewing patient images 'provides one vivid way into their lives'.[42] If patient photographs can help present-day viewers access the past by offering traces of people's experiences of mental ill-health and institutional life, those casebook photos that show staff, as well as patients, are a direct reminder of one aspect of patient experience—the practitioner–patient encounter. The inclusion of staff in patient photographs is a visual reminder of relationships within the asylum, and of the potential connections made between staff and patients. The asylum was a place of human interaction, dialogue, and communication. In the instances in which staff do appear in the photograph, their role is often highly ambiguous. Staff might feature in patient photographs by way of a comforting or restraining hand, holding the patient in their chair for the duration of the exposure or holding up the patient who is having trouble standing. Sometimes it can be hard to determine whether we are seeing images of resistance and restraint or assistance and practical physical (or, indeed, emotional) support. Take, for example, the photo of Agnes, a patient admitted in December 1890 to Holloway Sanatorium (Fig. 12.11).[43] The rather large photographic print appears on her admission pages next to her physical condition on admission notes.[44] Two female attendants appear in the image with her—a relatively rare glimpse of staff in these documents. But are they holding her up or holding her back? Keeping her still for what reason—because she cannot physically stand up or will not? On the same point, do the attendants who are visible either side of Constance in her first casebook photograph (Fig. 12.12) help her to stand, or, hold her still because she will not do as she is instructed? Does the nurse that Frances clings to offer this close contact with her patient, or resist it by stepping back from her (Fig. 12.13)?

Any answers to these questions will inevitably be informed by individual and subjective views of the institution; after all, our selves are always present in how we view, read, or interpret the past. It is a well-established principle of photographic theory that, as Susan Sontag notes, 'a photograph changes according to the context in which it is seen'.[45] For Swartz, this might be an example of the way patient experiences are 'appropriated' both by the historical discourses of psychiatry, asylum management, and clinical practice and by historians or other researchers who read, view, and interpret the case note material. But that said, while these examples seem to offer up more questions than answers, in other examples it is easier to explain the presence of staff within the frame. The Newcastle casebooks contain occasional photographs of patients in which they are being held by the head by an attendant, and the hands placed on the elderly Thomas' shoulders while a patient at the Sanatorium are clearly there to prevent him rising out of his chair and spoiling the photo (Figs. 12.14 and 12.15). Such images can make uncomfortable viewing, especially if one takes Brookes' point that, not only do we view these images in the full knowledge that, at the time, mental illness led to incarceration, but that coming 'face-to-face' with a photograph restores 'humanity' to a patient and 'reminds us of our own mortality'.[46] While Brookes goes too far in implying that written case notes cannot have the same effect, what the patient

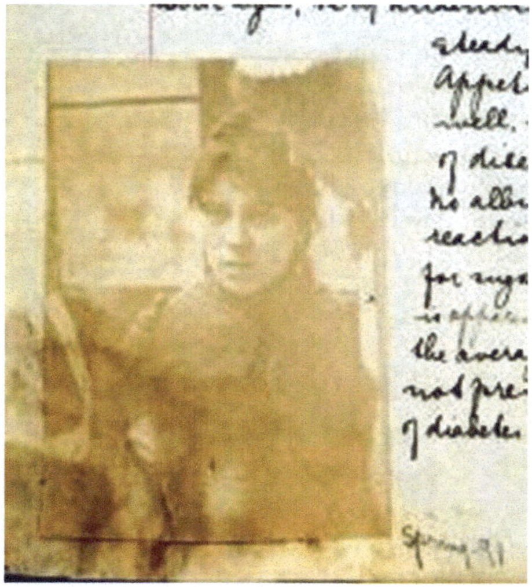

Fig. 12.11 Photographer unknown, Agnes and attendants (1891), Holloway Sanatorium Casebook No.4, females (certified patients admitted July 1890-June 1891), WMS 5157/5158. 143. Credit: Wellcome Collection

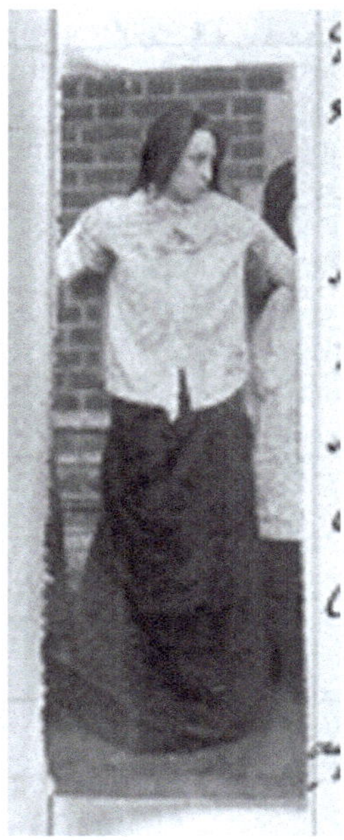

Fig. 12.12 Photographer unknown, Constance and attendants, Holloway Sanatorium Casebook No.2, females (certified patients admitted January - September 1889), WMS 5157/5157. 192. Credit: Wellcome Collection

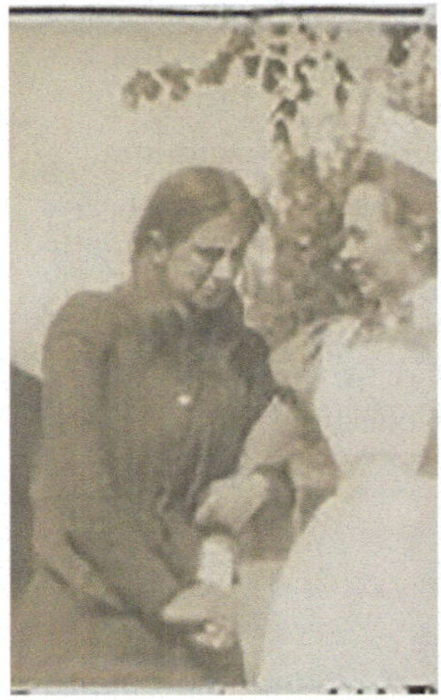

Fig. 12.13 Photographer unknown, Frances and attendant, Holloway Sanatorium Casebook No.11, females (certified patients admitted May 1898-May 1899), WMS 5157/5159. 17. Credit: Wellcome Collection

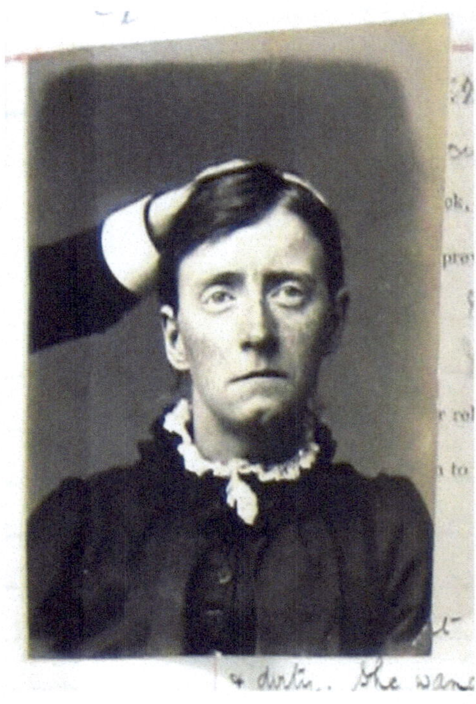

Fig. 12.14 Photographer unknown, Ellen, admitted 3/6/1904. Newcastle-upon-Tyne City Lunatic Asylum Casebook, females, TWAS HO.SN/13/38. 382. Permission to reproduce from Tyne and Wear Archives and Museums

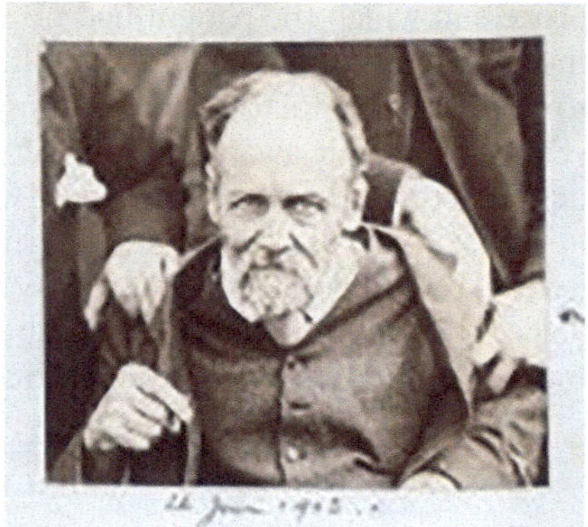

Fig. 12.15 Photographer unknown, Thomas, June 1903. Holloway Sanatorium Casebook No.11, males. WMS 5157/8160. 338. Credit: Wellcome Collection

images certainly *do* add is another striking layer of information and context to the search for patient voices that cannot be accessed through textual references alone.

Patient photographs can suggest both resistance and complicity, both of which, as I argue elsewhere, are reliant on subject agency.[47] In photographs in which the patient attempts to look away *and* in examples in which they arrange themselves as if for a professional studio portrait, they are responding to the circumstances they find themselves in.[48] Both types of image, then, are evidence of their experience. Photography can offer an opportunity to present a particular identity, one that might be aspirational, validating, or fantasised. It is well known that professional photographers gave their clients props, costumes, and backdrops to help them construct an imagined identity which was then captured on camera.[49] The photograph of a working-class client posing with the borrowed trappings of someone better off might be relatively straightforward to analyse; patient photographs are more complex, however. It is hard to know for certain what dynamics of power were operating in any given photography session—who was directing the shot? What instructions were given? Were these followed or ignored? The shifting dialogue between photographer and sitter is further complicated by the influence of the doctor–patient relationship, which assigned to the doctor who also took photographs a double dose of authority over their patient–sitter. We might assume that power was distributed unevenly in this encounter, but the precise attribution of power to those present (as is arguably the case in any photograph) is much harder to gauge. Again, we might speculate that a photographic process in which the patient had no say would be entirely in keeping with their status as a patient in in an asylum, and there is little extant evidence to suggest that doctors sought consent from their patient subjects. And yet, the apparent awareness of how one should be photographed or the desire to resist this process in some way is a tangible force in some patient images.[50] What is clear is that the uncertainty of patient photographs is itself a reminder of the complexity of patient records and the multiple voices that operate within them; their trickiness is a characteristic of the fractured and uneven record of patient experience in the past.

Conclusion

Photography was introduced into medical practice because of its apparent ability to capture 'faithful' images of patients and their symptoms. Seemingly devoid of the artist's interference, the 'facts', as Lady Eastlake called them, offered the possibility of a 'new form of communication between man and man'.[51] In practice though, the meaning of patient photographs was much more ambiguous, especially in cases in which the image and text contradicted each other; in these instances, the evidential or factual function of the patient image is called into question. The smiling patient who is described as crying in the notes should alert us to competing, or, at least, *alternative*, subjectivities and voices that might be present in the documents. Moreover, photographs in which staff are pictured also can act as a prompt to consider the asylum as a place of human interaction.

Recovering patient experience should no doubt be a priority, not only because it continues the now well-established call for a history 'from below', but because it furthers our understanding of the past by including many standpoints and experiences. It is important to note that the examples discussed in this chapter span a range of cases in terms of gender, age, social class, diagnosis, and symptoms.[52] Both Edwards' sensory theory and Brookes' description of the powers of emotional connection inherent to historical photographs can be used to think about the notion of the patient voice and patient experience within psychiatric institutions. Considering the patient photograph pasted on to a patient record, as well as the notes, not only appreciates the archive in full, but adds another voice to the multiple traces of voices that are active at any one time in the documents. Despite the complexity, it is this layering of voices that helps the historian and present-day viewer/reader access past patient experiences. In examining the photographic record of psychiatric medicine, we are reminded that we need not look to written testimony only in the search for patient voices, if, as Diamond suggested, we 'listen' to the voice through the photograph and let the picture 'speak'.[53]

Acknowledgements I would like to thank Tyne and Wear Archives, Surrey History Centre and the Wellcome Collection for their kind permission to reproduce images from their collections. Regrettably, I could not ask permission from the patients themselves.

Notes

1. Sally Swartz, "Can the Clinical Subject Speak? Some Thoughts on Subaltern Psychology," *Theory and Psychology* 15 (2005): 505-525, 507.
2. Ibid. Swartz is, of course, referencing here Gayatri Spivak, "Can the Subaltern Speak?" in *Colonial Discourse and Post-Colonial Theory*, eds. P. Williams and L. Chrisman (New York: Harvester Wheatsheaf, 1993), 66-111.
3. Daniel Fox and Christopher Lawrence provide a general overview of the varied applications of photography to medicine from the 1840s; see Daniel M. Fox and Christopher Lawrence, *Photographing Medicine: Images and Power in Britain and America since 1840* (New York and London: Greenwood Press, 1988).
4. Notable recent exceptions to this are Rory du Plessis, "Beyond a Clinical Narrative: Casebook Photographs from the Grahamstown Lunatic Asylum, c. 1890s," *Critical Arts* 29 (2015): 88-103; Katherine D.B. Rawling "'The Annexed Photos Were Taken today': Photographing Patients in the Late-Nineteenth-century Asylum," *Social History of Medicine* (2019) https://doi.org/10.1093/shm/hkz060; Jennifer Wallis, *Investigating the Body in the Victorian Asylum: Doctors, Patients, and Practices*, (Basingstoke: Palgrave MacMillan, 2017).
5. The generally accepted date of the 'invention' of photography is 1839 when Daguerre announced his photographic process in France. However, the concept of, and the desire to photograph, predates this by many years. Most general histories of photography discuss its origins and 'invention'. See for example John Falconer and Louise Hide, *Points of View: Capturing the Nineteenth Century in Photographs*, (London: The British Library, 2009); Mary Warner Marien, *Photography: A Cultural History* (London: Laurence King, 2006); Ian Jeffrey, *Photography: A Concise History* (London: Thames and Hudson, 1981).
6. Hugh W. Diamond, 1856, "On the Application of Photography to the Physiognomic and Mental Phenomena of Insanity" (1856) reprinted in

Sander L. Gilman, *The Face of Madness: Hugh W. Diamond and the Origins of Psychiatric Photography* (New York: Brunner/Mazel, 1976), 19-24, 19-20. Emphasis added.

7. Lady Elizabeth Eastlake, "Photography" *The Quarterly Review* 101 (1857): 442-468, 465. Emphasis added. Her remarks were made regarding the question of whether photography could be regarded as 'Art'. She argued that the camera's ability to record 'fact' made it a wholly different enterprise to Art and a comparison between the two was futile.
8. Ibid.
9. Allan Sekula, "On the Invention of Photographic Meaning" in *Thinking Photography*, ed. V. Burgin (London: MacMillan, 1982), 84-109, 85-86.
10. Ibid. 87.
11. Jennifer Green-Lewis, *Framing the Victorians: Photography and the Culture of Realism*. (Ithaca: Cornell University Press, 1996), 20-21.
12. Elizabeth Edwards, "Thinking Photography Beyond the Visual," in *Photography: Theoretical Snapshots*, eds. J.J. Long, A. Noble and E. Welch (London and New York: Routledge, 2009), 31-48, 37-43.
13. Ibid. 42.
14. Ibid. 41.
15. I discuss evidence of this practice in Katherine D. B. Rawling, "'She Sits All Day in the Attitude Depicted in the Photo': Photography and the Psychiatric Patient in the Late-nineteenth Century," *Medical Humanities* 43 (2017): 99-110, DOI: 10.1136/medhum-2016-011092: 104.
16. Edwards, *Thinking Photography*, 39.
17. For an example of photography in an Italian institution, see John Foot, "Photography and Radical Psychiatry in Italy in the 1960s. The Case of the Photobook *Morire di Classe* (1969)," *History of Psychiatry* 26 (2015): 19-35. For a discussion of the 'repurposing' of asylum photography and the use of psychiatric images by the creative arts, see Barbara Brookes, "Pictures of People, Pictures of
Places: Photography and the Asylum," in *Exhibiting Madness in Museums: Remembering Psychiatry through Collections and Display*, eds. C. Coleborne and D. Mackinnon, (New York: Routledge 2011), 30-47, 31, 38-44.
18. Katherine D.B. Rawling, *Visualising Mental Illness: Gender, Medicine and Visual Media, c.1850-1910* (Ph.D. Thesis, University of London, 2011) and Rawling, "She Sits All Day"; Susan Sidlauskas, "Inventing the Medical Portrait: Photography at the 'Benevolent Asylum' of Holloway, c.1885-1889," *Medical Humanities* 39 (2013): 29-37. DOI:10.1136/medhum-2012-010280.
19. Rawling, "The Annexed Photos".

20. du Plessis, "Beyond a Clinical Narrative"; Caroline Bressey, "The City of Others: Photographs From the City of London Asylum Archive," *19: Interdisciplinary Studies in the Long Nineteenth Century* 13 (2011). DOI: https://doi.org/10.16995/ntn.625.
21. Brookes, "Pictures of People," 34.
22. Ibid. 36.
23. The decision to anonymise patient names can be a contentious one; in a collection that seeks to recover the 'voice' of silenced people, anonymising those very people can be construed as another marginalising act, as well as being counterintuitive when their images are reproduced on the pages. However, anonymisation is a standard condition of archival use and one that I am bound by here. For discussion of some of the ethical issues around patient images and names, see Wallis. *Investigating the Body*, 32-34 and Tania Woloshyn, *Soaking up the Rays: Light Therapy and Visual Culture in Britain, c.1890-1940* (Manchester: Manchester University Press, 2017), 34-37.
24. This term is also linked discursively to other historically contingent diagnostic categories like 'feeblemindedness', 'idiocy', and 'imbecility'. For more on these categories, see Anne Digby and David Wright, eds. *From Idiocy to Mental Deficiency: Historical Perspectives on People with Learning Disabilities* (London: Routledge, 1996); Mark Jackson, *The Borderland of Imbecility: Medicine, Society and the Fabrication of the Feeble Mind in Late Victorian and Edwardian England* (Manchester: Manchester University Press, 2000); Patrick McDonagh, *Idiocy: A Cultural History* (Liverpool: Liverpool University Press, 2008); Rebecca Wynter, "Pictures of Peter Pan: Institutions, Local Definitions of 'Mental Deficiency', and the Filtering of Children in Early Twentieth-century England," *Family and Community History* 18 (2015): 122-138.
25. Notes for William, Newcastle-upon-Tyne City Lunatic Asylum, Casebook Males, Tyne and Wear Archives Service (hereafter TWAS) HO. SN/13/14. 280.
26. This is a good deal later than other institutions. Dr Diamond and the professional photographer Henry Hering were photographing patients at Surrey and Bethlem, respectively, in the 1850s. Doctors at the West Riding Pauper Lunatic Asylum, Wakefield began compiling an album of patient photographs from the 1870s. For a discussion of this album, see Wallis. *Investigating the Body*, 21-59.
27. Notes for Margaret, Female Casebook, TWAS HO.SN/13/34, 475.
28. Notes for Matilda, Female Casebook, TWAS HO.SN/13/36, 322.
29. Notes for Mary, Female Casebook, TWAS HO.SN/13/38, 115.
30. Notes for Louisa, Female Casebook, TWAS HO.SN/13/38, 442.
31. Notes for Matilda, Female Casebook, TWAS HO.SN/13/36, 322.

32. Notes for Margaret, Female Casebook, TWAS HO.SN/13/34, 475.
33. Notes for Mary, Female Casebook, TWAS HO.SN/13/38, 115.
34. Notes for Louisa, Female Casebook, TWAS HO.SN/13/38, 442.
35. John Conolly, "Case Studies from the Physiognomy of Insanity" *The Medical Times and Gazette* (1858-59) reprinted in Gilman, *Face of Madness*, 27-72.
36. Notes for Constance, Holloway Sanatorium Casebook No. 2, Females (Certified patients admitted January-September 1889) Wellcome Manuscript (Hereafter WMS) 5157/5157, 192.
37. Ibid. 193.
38. Notes for Constance, Holloway Sanatorium Casebook No. 4, Females (Certified patients admitted July 1890-June 1891) WMS 5157/5158, 249.
39. No author, "The Photographing of Insane Patients: Notes From a Meeting of the Northern and Midland Division of the Medico-Psychological Association," *Journal of Mental Science* 48 (1902): 202-204.
40. Notes for Rose, Holloway Sanatorium Casebook Females (Admitted June 1885-Jan 1889) Surrey History Centre 3473/3/1, 94.
41. George H. Savage with Edwin Goodall, *Insanity and Allied Neuroses: A Practical and Clinical Manual* (London: Cassell & Co., 1884); W.H.B. Stoddart, *Mind and Its Disorders: A Text Book for Students and Practitioners* (London: H.K. Lewis, 1908). Textbook images are discussed further in Rawling, "She Sits All Day", 102-106.
42. Brookes, "Pictures of People," 33.
43. Notes for Agnes S., Holloway Sanatorium Casebook No. 4, Females (Certified patients admitted July 1890-June 1891) WMS5157/5158, 143-46, 169-70, 198, 226.
44. Ibid. 143. The photograph measures 7.8 x10.5 cm.
45. Susan Sontag, "The Heroism of Vision," in *On Photography* (London: Penguin, 1977), 85-112, 106.
46. Brookes, "Pictures of People," 36.
47. Rawling, "She Sits All Day," 107-108; Rawling, "The Annexed Photos".
48. Ibid. See also Rawling, *Visualising Mental Illness.*
49. Audrey Linkman, *The Victorians: Photographic Portraits* (London and New York: Tauris Parke, 1993). I expand on the influence of photographic convention on casebook photographs in Rawling, "'She Sits All Day,'" 106-108.
50. See Rawling, "She Sits All Day," 106-109, for a fuller discussion of the patients' role in casebook photography.
51. Eastlake "Photography," 465.
52. Roy Porter, "The Patient's View: Doing Medical History From Below," *Theory and Society* 14 (1985): 175-198.
53. Diamond, "On the Application," 19.

CHAPTER 13

A Boundary Between Two Worlds? Community Perceptions of Former Asylums in Lancashire, England

Carolyn Gibbeson and Katie Beattie

Introduction

Historians and geographers have explored the voices of those patients who lived within former asylums,[1] and these studies have helped to illuminate many previously forgotten voices (as Rawlings argues in this volume) and the wider histories of asylums. Existing literature describes former asylums as both places of fear and complicated places comprising multiple possible narratives. Much of this literature focuses on their history,[2] the move to community care and wider healthcare issues,[3] patient histories[4] and former staff voices.[5] Since the mass closure of asylum sites in the late 1990s and early 2000s, many of these large sites have now been converted into residential uses. The redevelopment of historic buildings is often contentious,[6] and there is little literature that explores how the emotions, attachments, different meanings and values that people place on these sites

C. Gibbeson (✉) • K. Beattie
Sheffield Hallam University, Sheffield, UK
e-mail: c.gibbeson@shu.ac.uk

R. Ellis et al. (eds.), *Voices in the History of Madness*, Mental Health in Historical Perspective,
https://doi.org/10.1007/978-3-030-69559-0_13

affects the decisions taken in respect of their management and reuse. What is missing from existing studies is the study of the buildings themselves and the community memories associated with them.

As the voices of those who could relate their stories about life in these institutions begin to disappear through time, new voices and stories of these places are emerging (see McGeachan in this volume). It is important to hear the voices of former patients and staff but the voices of people living near the institutions are also part of the story. Little has been written about those who lived outside the asylum walls in the surrounding communities,[7] and their experiences of watching their local asylum during its closure, subsequent decline and demolition or reuse is missing from these narratives. Therefore, in this chapter, we focus on voices from the communities 'outside the asylum walls'[8] from those who live around the sites, who likely knew them when they were functioning mental hospitals and who still see them now as converted, residential housing. This chapter will briefly discuss how former asylums came to be seen as places of fear before detailing the methodology used in the two studies from which the data in this chapter is drawn. It will then give a history of the two asylums investigated, Lancaster Moor and Whittingham hospitals, before examining the data from the two studies in detail through the themes that emerged from the data: memory and legacy and former asylums as heritage. In this chapter, 'heritage' is seen as a building, place or site that people value and as having a degree of significance that requires additional consideration in planning decisions.[9]

An Image of Fear and Isolation

Asylums are often depicted as places of fear with 'tainted reputations',[10] and were once viewed as the most feared places in Western society.[11] The buildings themselves have becomes symbols of the fear of madness.[12] The semantic connotations of the word asylum are predominantly negative and add to the prevailing narrative as somewhere wholly undesirable, particularly when contrasted to the term 'mental hospital' which implies a more caring outlook. Landscapes and places, like people, can retain a sense of guilt[13]; places become 'mnemonic containers'[14]—places that stimulate memories of events that took place in that particular building. Richardson[15] has argued that 'people alive at the time of the New Poor Law [1834] feared what was to be done to them in hospitals and workhouses', and this included the large county asylums that are at the heart of this chapter.

The idea of the asylum as a prison and a place of incarceration has been present in patient accounts since the early days of the asylum,[16] although it should be noted that these accounts were written as arguments for reform and were therefore likely to present a particularly negative view of these institutions. These narratives for reform continued throughout the history of asylums.[17] These sites were, however, part of their local communities and drew their staff from the surrounding area. The idea of the asylum as being isolated or separated from the rest of the world has been challenged by Bartlett and Wright,[18] who argue that the relationship between the institutions and the community was more complicated than is often presented. The traditional view of asylums as solely places of fear is being dismantled[19] but the voices of local communities offer an opportunity to analyse this further.

Methodology

The two research projects[20] on whose data this chapter is based were conducted during the redevelopment phase of two hospital sites. Surveys were carried out by the two authors with residents of Lancaster and the Whittingham area, and they explored residents' views of the two developments, their attitudes towards the sites prior to and during redevelopment. The two sites of Lancaster Moor and Whittingham were chosen because both sites at the time of the studies were in the process of being redeveloped. There were other sites both in the North West of England and elsewhere in the country but many of these had already been either redeveloped or demolished.

In total 80 residents were surveyed in Lancaster and 36 in the Whittingham area, providing a total of 116 completed questionnaires. The questions were designed to examine whether the local communities had a desire to protect these former asylums as historic buildings and how they interpreted these sites. These surveys were carried out in person by the two authors. Both samples were carried out using convenience sampling; members of the public who passed the researchers were asked if they wished to participate or were given the questionnaires by the researcher at local parish meetings (in the case of Whittingham study). Both authors asked the respondents for their local knowledge of the hospitals and the redevelopments as well as asking what they felt should happen to these former institutions, their views on the conversion to residential use and whether the history of these former sites should be acknowledged in the redevelopments.

The questionnaire results were both quantitative and qualitative, with qualitative data forming the large majority of data gathered. The process of analysis of that qualitative data followed Boyatzis'[21] approach to thematic analysis by identifying recurring themes within the data. A predominantly inductive process was adopted as the insights gained through the data led the themes used to draw conclusions and insights. The data itself therefore directed the thematic analysis from all the response by seeking out common themes that reoccurred within the data as well as looking for any exceptions. This was done within each research site and then compared. This data therefore provides us with the voices of those who now live around the sites, whether in the Whittingham area or the small city of Lancaster. These voices are important in the history of the former asylum sites as they provide the next chapter in their story; these sites are where the local communities, or their families, lived, worked and spent large parts of their lives, or whose families who worked in, and lived near, the hospitals.

Lancaster Moor and Whittingham Hospitals: A Brief History

Lancaster Moor, or the first Lancashire County Lunatic Asylum, was one of the early county asylums to be built following the 1808 County Asylums Act, which created the principle of public mental asylums in each county in Britain. The typically Georgian building, designed by T. Standen, opened in July 1816, its design having been based on a Georgian country house.[22] Originally the Lancaster County Lunatic Asylum, Lancaster Moor Hospital was located on the outskirts of Lancaster. As would become a feature of asylums, the Lancashire County Asylum soon became full, and, so, a further wing was added in 1824 creating the small village-like features of most asylums. The asylum had its own farm, allotments, bakeries, workshops and a laundry.[23] The asylum population continued to expand, and in 1879 an additional wing, which would become known as 'the Annexe', was opened. This wing, unlike its earlier counterpart, was built in the neo-Gothic style and was located on the opposite side of the road to the Georgian wing, standing on the top of the hill and now visible from the M6 motorway. Additional buildings were added throughout the period up to the Great War when the hospital accommodated some wartime patients.[24] Although it was during the 1950s that the possibility of the closure of asylums was first discussed,[25] it was not until the 1980s that the closure process began in force.[26] Lancaster Moor's original wing closed in 1991 and the Annexe in 1999. By the end of its working life, additional hospital services such as an ear and eye clinic had been added. Following the closure of the two sides of the hospital in the 1990s, the buildings then remained empty until 2002, when the Georgian original building was converted into housing and renamed Standen Park. The Annexe remained empty until 2013, when conversion of this building to housing commenced with the addition of new build housing on the site.

Whittingham Hospital was the fourth Lancashire County Asylum located near the village of Goosnargh. As with Lancaster Moor, the asylum was a small, seemingly self-contained village with stores, kitchens, recreational hall, brewery, a church and mortuary.[27] The asylum opened in 1873 to alleviate pressure on the existing three Lancashire County Asylums of Lancaster Moor, Rainhill and Prestwich.[28] As with most asylums, and like Lancaster Moor, Whittingham was expanded through the years and even had its own post office and railway.[29] Whittingham took in military patients during the Great War and building on the site continued well into the 1930s. By the time the hospital was incorporated into the National Health Service in 1948, it was the largest asylum in the UK. During the 1960s, allegations of abuse and neglect were made against the hospital and were brought to the attention of the public by a student nurse which resulted in an inquiry into the behaviour of staff, treatment and poor conditions. A television documentary was made in 1980 examining patient facilities, treatment and the future of the hospital.[30] Whittingham closed in 1995. The site remained unused, gradually deteriorating and subject to several planning applications for housing use that came to nothing. However, in 2016 permission for the demolition of the hospital buildings and the construction of 650 dwellings was granted.

Memory and Legacy

Even though it was nearly 20 years since the sites had closed, they were still well known within the surrounding area for their former use; they appeared not to be hidden or secret or unknown to the local community. The history and former use of the two sites was well known within their local community with 94% of those surveyed knowing the history of the sites. Within the questionnaire, respondents were asked to describe the former use of these two sites. In both cases, the survey did not provide descriptions or tick boxes for people to use, the terminology adopted was proffered by the residents themselves. In Lancaster, 28% of residents described the site as 'a mental hospital' with 45% residents describing it as an 'asylum'. Similarly, for Whittingham, 32% described the history of hospital as a 'mental hospital' and 35% described it as an 'asylum'. The majority of questionnaire respondents were over 40 years old in both studies, due to the fact that the questionnaires and meetings were carried out on weekdays during work hours; therefore, it is difficult to definitely say whether there was a demographic breakdown of the different terminology used to describe these former institutions. However, across all the age ranges (including those in the 21–30 and 31–40 age brackets) the word 'asylum' was used, and was not limited to the older generations.

Despite it being nearly 100 years since the two hospitals changed their names from 'Asylum', the term was still be used by residents, and the use of language is important as it helps to emphasise dominant narratives and stories about these places. It is difficult to conclude the reasons behind the retention of the older terms in the two communities. However, the name change of asylums to mental hospitals precipitated by the 1930 Mental Treatment Act was in response to a desire to change the terminology associated with mental illness. The words 'pauper', 'lunatic' and 'asylum' were all changed as attitudes towards mental illness had changed since the early Lunacy Acts.[31] It should be noted however that a change in legislation does not in itself change attitudes or people's responses to institutions, and this can be seen through the data in this study.

Kenny[32] has argued that memory needs a place or a context and is transmitted through generations in the stories told. Trigg[33] argued that the identity of a place is marked by the events that are constitutive of its identity. As asylums drew their staff from the surrounding population, stories from these staff members are likely to be transmitted down the generations of those living in the Lancaster or Whittingham areas, particularly where the residents of the questionnaires were older and were therefore likely to have lived in the area a long time. This is, however, one possibility as these institutions have particular connotations that have persisted over time,[34] with the stigmatised images are often portrayed in the media and films, reinforcing our views of them. Smith[35] has argued that there was no barrier or boundary between the asylum and the surrounding communities as Gittins[36] suggested. From the data in these studies, both the

Lancaster and Whittingham communities were closely linked with the former asylums. The survey respondents knew these sites and their histories, and this data supports the view that local communities and the local asylum were more intertwined than the image of the asylum as a boundary between those inside and outside would suggest[37]; as Smith[38] showed, admissions to the asylum often came from the family as well as from the nursing staff, and asylums were used as a place of both long-term care and short-term respite.

Retaining the memory of these two former asylums was a recurring narrative that appeared from within the qualitative responses to the surveys. In Lancaster, 86% of those who responded felt that the history of Lancaster Moor should be remembered as opposed to 53% in Whittingham for Whittingham Hospital. The lower percentage from the Whittingham area residents could be attributable to the fact that the hospital suffered from high-profile scandals about the treatment and conditions of the patients during the 1960s and 1970s.[39] It is not possible to be certain of this as the scandals were not mentioned directly within the responses, but the history was seen by some respondents as 'not an easy history but [one] we should remember'. A sense of obligation was felt towards the sites and its previous residents; even when it was seen by some respondents as 'challenging', these places were seen as being part of the social history of the local community. Some residents felt that whilst parts of the history were difficult and hard to deal with, they felt that 'history is where we come from, lessons should be learnt'. Whilst they would be considered as what Pendlebury et al.[40] describe as 'uncomfortable heritage', this was not seen as a barrier to them being remembered.

Some respondents raised the issue of incarceration specifically. It was felt that 'people suffered in there' and that 'lots of lives passed through there, people didn't deserve to be in there'. Responses were as follows:

> 'The wards were too large, people became institutionalised, there was no privacy.'
> 'Victorian ethic regarding mental health—harsh treatment'.
> 'The treatment and solitary confinement'.

And some residents highlighted the incarceration of those who were considered to be in the hospitals in error:

> 'Times have changed, there were many patients who were in there who would not be today.'
> 'People were put in there for no proper purpose.'
> 'Ladies were in there because they had children out of wedlock.'

Whilst the incarceration of patients who should not have been held within these hospitals is often a narrative associated with former asylum sites,[41] and one which early anti-asylum narratives by former patients highlighted,[42] this again presents a one-sided view of asylums. Walton[43] argued that these controversies did exist and were embarrassing for the early psychiatrists but communities often did their own 'casting out' of their mad relatives or citizens to cellars, almshouses or locked rooms. However, this picture is a complicated one as people did not choose to be put in asylums and the community around them were involved in their histories right from the start, whether as patients, as staff or in occupations that worked with or in the hospitals.

For one resident, the past history of the site proved to be too problematic, and they felt that the site 'should be knocked down' due to its difficult reputation. Another remarked that we 'possibly don't want to remember—development is a new lease of life'. Redevelopment here is being viewed as a way of removing or cleansing the former history from the site, something that has been used specifically for asylums, notably in Canada.[44] The past history was seen as being too uncomfortable to remember; therefore, the reputation or stigma should be removed completely. This removal or cleansing often happens where notorious murders or kidnappings have taken place and where the local authorities have decided to demolish the building to expunge the memory from that place.[45] The idea from the quote that the public 'doesn't want to remember' could be meant in respect of the history being too difficult or for the fact that it is a history that is felt should be deliberately forgotten. One respondent offered a cautionary approach to remembering the history of the site in that we should 'remember but not celebrate'. The history was important but again an element of unease was present. Moons et al.[46] and Pendlebury et al.[47] have both argued that there is selective remembrance, particularly in the cases of former asylums and other 'uncomfortable' heritage sites, but they both attribute this to the developers of these sites. This quote would suggest that it is not only those redeveloping the sites that engage in this filtering of history; what is chosen to be kept and what is chosen to be removed, whether that is the physical building or the historical and symbolic associations with that building, is not simply the work of one party involved in the process of finding new uses. Within the quotes above there is a hint of the challenge or difficulty with these sites, their 'stigma',[48] but residents also reflected on the history more generally and not always in a negative way.

Despite the examples above, the majority of the residents surveyed felt positively towards Lancaster Moor and Whittingham. One resident even responded that they felt the former asylum site was a 'national treasure'. This response views asylums in a more preservation-orientated way, seeing it as something architecturally or aesthetically important. This re-appreciation as heritage or for aesthetic qualities has been suggested by Franklin[49] as one way that the stigma of the past history can be removed or reinvented for asylums to enable their reuse. In focusing on the aesthetics and historic nature of former asylums, this has enabled the more negative connotations to become less apparent, as Franklin[50] suggested, or perhaps it is because more time has passed since the events within them occurred; as Moses[51] indicated, a 'temporal or social-cultural distance of context communities from the traumatic histories of a site allows for greater creativity in the interpretation and commemoration of those histories'. Former asylums were not places of purely negative events like the 'guilty houses' that Sniekers and Reijnders[52] discuss, some are listed and are therefore retained, whereas others are not and are demolished. Equally, some are seen as being aesthetically pleasing, whereas others are not, and are therefore retained, and the cost of redeveloping[53] also plays a part in this uneven process of demolition[54] (as in the case of Whittingham) or reuse (at Lancaster Moor) of former asylum sites.

Those who felt positively towards the sites saw them as places of safety for patients, arguing that 'it provided a safe place' or a 'safe haven' and a 'potential sanctuary from the outside world' (See also the Calabria et al. chapter in this volume). These responses echo the original intentions of asylums, that of a place of safety and treatment for patients where early doctors believed asylums were 'to be a home, where the patient was to be known and treated like an individual, where his [sic] mind was to be constantly stimulated and encouraged to return to its normal state'.[55] Scull[56] has argued that these new asylums and the facilities and buildings themselves were designed as part of the curative regime. Similarly, the author and academic, Barbara Taylor,[57] who herself spent time in Friern Hospital (originally the Second Middlesex County Asylum, England), has described that hospital as a sanctuary or safe place when she needed one most. One resident highlighted physical characteristics of the site stating 'the environment for sick people was wonderful and the grounds were beautiful', echoing Scull's[58] view above that the site itself helped to provide the cure. Unfortunately, it is not possible to ascertain whether this individual had any personal connections with the site, but it is, nevertheless, an important challenge the dominant narratives of these places.

From the discussion of residents' views, above, it can be seen that there were both positive and negative opinions in respect of the two sites, although the responses were predominantly positive ones, which in itself is counter-intuitive as the data shows that they are also still being referred to as 'asylums'. As Harrison[59] has argued, the meanings and value of places are socially constructed and not intrinsic to an object resulting in a multiplicity of views, meanings and opinions on a particular place. It could be argued that this is the case for any historic or heritage site, that is, places do not have fixed meanings,[60] and those meanings can and do change even if any heritage designation remains.[61] Given that the 'meaning of artefacts is culturally constituted',[62] perceptions of former asylum sites are clouded by the meanings of asylums culturally, as well as people's personal experience and emotional reactions to them.[63]

Former Asylums as Heritage

One of the residents in the Whittingham area highlighted that the former asylums had been 'a huge employer [and] had character and a sense of community'. Asylums were both communities in themselves and were a large part of their local community.[64] Their closure therefore not only affected the patients but also the staff who often came from that surrounding local community. The closure of these institutions was a major shock and caused anxiety for both patients and staff.[65] This period of emptiness was highlighted by the voices of the community surveyed as one of the issues in how the two sites were perceived today and which influenced their preservation. The majority of residents in Lancaster felt that it was good that the building was being reused. Responses such as 'fabulous it was being reused' and 'better it was used than left empty' echoed the sentiments of 52 out of 80 of those who participated. Only one respondent in Lancaster felt that building should have been knocked down because of its reputation and history.

There was little concern from local residents that the building was being reused; its former history and any negative connotations that have been suggested to be a hindrance to the redevelopment of former asylums[66] did not prevent this. From the surveys, none of the objections or concerns relating to the new developments at both sites were connected to the former history of the sites, the concerns and objections related to the specifics of each development:

> 'Don't like new development'
> 'Good to reuse but poor dev[elopment]—not paid attention to architecture'
> 'Glad it's being redeveloped but not sure about use'
> 'Disgusting—better use could be found'
> 'Shame it's another new housing dev[elopment]'
> 'Need new houses but it's the wrong use'
> 'Use good but it's the wrong use'

Whilst there was disagreement about what the use should be, almost every person surveyed felt that the building should be reused, and the local residents were concerned about the condition of the buildings even though they had lain empty:

> 'Better than [the] state it was in'
> 'Shame for it to stand empty'
> 'Better it [is] used than being left empty'
> 'Better than it going derelict'
> 'Redundant building—good use'
> 'Making a nice job, better than [it] falling to bits'
> 'No point in empty buildings, happy with it'
> 'As long as they preserve it, better than being empty'

Vacant buildings are themselves argued to possess a stigma and have been seen as being problematic both economically and visually.[67] They are often also seen as a source of crime.[68] Urban decay is itself seen as a stigma,[69] and the condition of the sites prior to redevelopment made many of the residents concerned as seen in the quotes, above.

Lynch[70] argued that we fear waste and loss and that we believe things should be clean and permanent; therefore; seeing buildings in a derelict state causes unease as 'buildings, although inanimate, are often assumed to have "life". Death, destruction and deterioration represent the anxiety-inducing flip side to a range of enduring and sometimes contradictory assumptions about built architecture's defining attributes: its material durability, its creative genesis, its productive utility, its aesthetic value'.[71] The suggestion by Lynch[72] and Cairns and Jacobs[73] was that these decaying or ruined buildings make us uneasy and remind us of the past in uncomfortable ways, and, therefore, we dislike these forms of buildings and the state they are in. The process of decay may also have been an influencing factor here, as old ruins are considered 'safe' as they are from the deep past.[74] The reuse of a building, rather than its demolition (as in the case of Whittingham), leaves a physical reminder of the place that would not exist if the building were demolished. As Stromberg[75] has argued, reuse that prevents demolition is in itself a form of preservation and therefore a physical cue to think about the past history of a place and to ask questions about that history that might otherwise be forgotten. Without a building to act as a tie to that memory or a reminder of that past, it can be suggested that the history of these places are more likely to be forgotten, rather than where a redeveloped building remains, acting as a prompt for questions about its history, as explored in this volume.

There is often strong opposition to the change, reuse or redevelopment of historic buildings[76] and a feeling of ownership even where there is no legal basis for one.[77] The heritage sector itself has been subjected to recent criticism that heritage is decided upon by 'experts' or a small elite group of people who control the idea of what heritage constitutes.[78] The heritage sector sees objects as intrinsically valuable,[79] although Harrison[80] has argued that overtime some buildings will become irrelevant and therefore should no longer be considered as heritage. Harrison[81] has also suggested that once something is considered 'heritage', then this status is never questioned. Smith[82] has criticised the control of what is deemed 'heritage' or valuable within the heritage sector as well as argued that heritage seeks a reification of elite values, with buildings such as factories, industrial, asylums and prisons having no social obligation felt towards those that require remembrance.[83]

Alongside this, dereliction and ruin have been seen as a sign of failure[84], because the building had not yet been made lucrative through its potential reuse, but it also posed a problem for the heritage industry which seeks to 'arrest decay' and fix a building within a specific period.[85] Former asylums pose challenges in communicating and remembering their history. As Edensor[86] argues in the case of former industrial sites, former asylums do not provide easy histories with which to create one particular story and therefore are challenging to promote their remembrance to a wider audience as it is possible to do with other heritage sites and buildings. However, as Bangstad[87] has suggested, heritage, in actually seeking to remember our past, in fact enables 'prescribed forgetting'. Particularly in the case of difficult histories however, he suggests that heritage and the remembrance of the past have a social obligation to remember those who have had a less prominent role in the history books.[88] This correlates with the desire of the majority of local residents who felt that, while difficult and potentially challenging, these former asylum sites ought to be remembered as part of their local, but also it could be argued national, social history.

Conclusions

This chapter sought to explore the voices of those 'outside' the walls of two former asylum sites and to investigate how these local communities viewed the former asylum sites. It examined the question of whether there is a boundary that exists between community and asylum, as Gittins[89] argued, or whether the relationship between asylums and the local community was more intertwined, flexible and fluid.[90] From the two sites of Lancaster Moor and Whittingham hospitals discussed in this chapter, the voices of local residents and the communities surrounding the two sites demonstrate that the relationship is complicated even 20 years or more since the closure of the sites. Those surveyed in Lancaster acknowledged the difficult and challenging nature of the site and their past; however, the majority felt that despite this, it was an important site of social and local history that should be remembered, although there was no agreement or common feeling of how this ought to happen. The local community around Whittingham, by contrast, were much more reticent towards the hospital and its past history with fewer people believing that the history of the site ought to be remembered.

Former asylum sites have been seen as liminal sites: Moons et al.[91] argued that they are liminal 'not only in the sense of being at the edge of a city [...] but to the extent that the shadow of their former use must either be embraced, transformed or suppressed' through their reuse. This shadow of their former use appears in the cases of Whittingham and Lancaster Moor; however, it is not straightforward and clearly defined. As Bynum et al.[92] argued, 'historical circumstances are often flexible enough to accommodate, without snapping, a variety of interpretive glosses', and this is certainly the case with the two former asylums examined in this chapter. Only a minority of responses demonstrated a negative response to these sites, responses that would fit with the view that the history needed to be removed from the sites to enable their reuse[93], and that it would cleanse the site of their past in some way. The majority of the responses reinforced the interconnected relationship between community and asylum[94] and presented an image of a community that was still connected to these sites, as they always had been.

Both sites were still seen as being part of their local community. There was not, and did not appear to have ever been, the perceived barrier or boundary between them and the 'outside' community, as Gittins[95] suggested. They were sites of local employment, of providing job opportunities for those within the local communities[96] and of sites where the local community had been involved in or lived alongside since their construction.[97] The data from the studies discussed in this chapter demonstrates how this connection persists even though the sites have now closed and been converted as residents seek to remember their histories. The narratives of local residents therefore give additional weight to the view that 'the characterisation of mental asylums as isolated and segregated from the local community has been dismantled gradually'.[98] These sites have become and are still embedded in the psyche of the local communities surrounding them. The local communities around Whittingham and Lancaster Moor Hospitals are creating and have created their own narratives of their personal pasts and the pasts of these asylum sites based on their experiences of them over time. These include the periods when they were functioning hospitals as well as following their closure and their increasingly derelict states prior to redevelopment. The whole life period of these sites is important when considering the narratives that surround them and shape how they are seen today. These narratives are an important part of the history of these sites and help to challenge the image of them as purely fearful places. In a wider context, the voices and perceptions of existing residents in the communities around these now-closed institutions are important in the discussions about remembering these sites and who is responsible for doing this, as these communities have always been involved in these sites.

Notes

1. For example, see Beveridge, Allan (1998) Life in the Asylum: patients' letters from Morningside 1873–1908, History of Psychiatry, 9, 431–469; Bressey, Caroline (2011) The City of Others: Photographs from the City of London Asylum Archive, Interdisciplinary Studies in the Long Nineteenth Century, 13, 1–15.

2. For example, see Scull, Andrew (1979) Museums of Madness: The social organisation of insanity in 19th century England, London, Penguin Books; Scull, Andrew (2006) The Insanity of Place/ The Place of Insanity: Essays on the history of psychiatry, London, Routledge; Philo, Chris (2004) A geographical History of Institutional Provision for the Insane from Medieval Times to the 1860s in England and Wales, The Space Reserved for Insanity, Lewiston, The Edwin Mellen Press.
3. For example, see Korman, Nancy and Glennester, Howard (1990) Hospital closure, Milton Keynes, Open University Press Kucik (2004); Barham, Peter (1992) Closing the Asylum: The mental patient in Modern Society, London, Penguin; Paulson, George (2012) Closing the asylums: Cause and consequences of the Deinstitutionalisation Movement, Jefferson, McFarland & Company.
4. For example, see Beveridge, Allan (1998) Life in the Asylum: Patients' letters from Morningside 1873–1908, History of Psychiatry, 9, 431–469; Bressey, Caroline (2011) The City of Others: Photographs from the City of London Asylum Archive, Interdisciplinary Studies in the Long Nineteenth Century, 13, 1–15.
5. See Parr, Hester, Philo, Chris, Burns, Nicola (2003) "That Awful Place was home" Reflections on the Contested Meanings of Craig Dunain Asylum, Scottish Geographical Journal, 119 (4), 341–360; Baur, Nicole (2011) On Site. Oral Testimonies in Mental Health History, Social History of Medicine, 24 (2), 484–487; Finnane, Mark (2009) Opening up and Closing down: Notes on the End of an Asylum, Health and History, 11 (1), 9–24.
6. Kalman, Harold D (2014) Heritage Planning, Principles and Process, London, Routledge; Gibbeson, Carolyn (2018) Not always nice: The effect of a whole life perspective on heritage and redevelopment, Journal of Urban Regeneration and Renewal 12 (1), 32–42.
7. Bartlett, Peter, Wright, David, (1999) Outside the Walls of the Asylum, the history of care in the community 1750–2000, London, The Athalone Press.
8. Gittins, Diane (1998) Madness in its place: Narratives of Severalls Hospital 1913–1997, London, Routledge.
9. Ministry of Housing, Communities and Local Government (2019) National Planning Policy Framework, available at: https://www.gov.uk/government/publications/national-planning-policy-framework%2D%2D2; Management of the Historic Environment, London, English Heritage.
10. Moons, Graham, Kearns, Robert and Joseph, Alun (2015) The Afterlives of the Psychiatric Asylum. Recycling concepts, sites and memories, Farnham, Ashgate.

11. Gittins, Diane (1998) Madness in its place: Narratives of Severalls Hospital 1913–1997, London, Routledge.
12. Mellett, David J (1982) The Prerogative of Asylumdom. Social, Cultural and Administrative Aspects of the Institutional Treatment of the Insane in Nineteenth Century Britain, New York, Garland Publication Inc.
13. Sneikers, Maloe and Reijnders, Stijn (2011) An ethnography of guilty houses in Belgium, Intellect Limited: Northern Lights, 9: 27–44.
14. Morton, Christopher (2007) Remembering the house: Memory and materiality in Northern Botswana, Journal of Material Culture, 12 (2), 157–179.
15. Richardson, Ruth (1987) Death, Dissection and the Destitute, London, Routledge & Kegan Paul.
16. Lowe, Louisa (1883) The Bastilles of England or the lunacy laws at work, London, Crookenden and Co; Hamilcar, Marcia (1910) Legally Dead, London, John Ouseley Ltd; Grant-Smith, Rachel (1922) The Experiences of an asylum patient, London, George Allen and Unwin Ltd.
17. Busfield, Joan (1986) Managing Madness, Changing Ideas and Practice, London, Unwin Hyman; Korman, Nancy and Glennester, Howard (1990) Hospital closure, Milton Keynes, Open University Press; Kucik, Lisa M (2004) Restoring Life: The adaptive reuse of a Sanatorium, thesis submitted for Master of Architecture, University of Cincinnati.
18. Bartlett, Peter, Wright, David, (1999) Outside the Walls of the Asylum, the history of care in the community 1750–2000, London, The Athalone Press.
19. Mooney, Graham, Reinarz, Jonathan (2009) Permeable Walls: Historical Perspectives on Hospital and Asylum Visiting, Amsterdam, Rodopi.
20. Gibbeson, Carolyn (2018) After the Asylum: Place, value and heritage in the redevelopment of historic former asylums, PhD thesis Newcastle University; Beattie, Katie (2017) An Investigation into the Re-development of Historic Sites Case Study—Whittingham Mental Hospital, Undergraduate Dissertation, Sheffield Hallam University.
21. Boyatzis, Richard, E (1998) Transforming Qualitative Information, London, Sage Publications.
22. Williamson Peter (2002) 'From confinement to community: The story of 'The Moor', Lancaster's County Lunatic Asylum', in Wilson, S (2002) (ed) Aspects of Lancaster, Discovering Local History, Barnsley, Wharncliffe Books.
23. Williamson Peter (2002) 'From confinement to community: The story of 'The Moor', Lancaster's County Lunatic Asylum', in Wilson, S (2002) (ed) Aspects of Lancaster, Discovering Local History, Barnsley, Wharncliffe Books.
24. Williamson Peter (2002) 'From confinement to community: The story of 'The Moor', Lancaster's County Lunatic Asylum', in Wilson, S (2002)

(ed) Aspects of Lancaster, Discovering Local History, Barnsley, Wharncliffe Books.

25. Wing, John K (1991) "Vision and Reality" in Hall P, and Brockington, I F (1991) (eds) The Closure of Mental Hospitals, London, Gaskell.
26. Wing, John K (1991) "Vision and Reality" in Hall P, and Brockington, I F (1991) (eds) The Closure of Mental Hospitals, London, Gaskell; Korman, Nancy and Glennester, Howard (1990) Hospital closure, Milton Keynes, Open University Press; Kucik, Lisa M (2004) Restoring Life: the adaptive reuse of a Sanatorium, thesis submitted for Master of Architecture, University of Cincinnati.
27. Brandon, Ed (no date), History of Lancaster Moor Hospital and Whittingham Asylum from www.countyasylums.co.uk.
28. Knapman, P., & Ashton, Ken. (2017). Whittingham Hospital 'Asylum' retrieved from http://whittinghamhospital.co.uk.
29. Brandon, Ed (no date), History of Lancaster Moor Hospital and Whittingham Asylum from www.countyasylums.co.uk.
30. Brandon, Ed (no date), History of Lancaster Moor Hospital and Whittingham Asylum from www.countyasylums.co.uk.
31. British Medical Journal (1930), The Mental Treatment Act, The British Medical Journal, 2, 978.
32. Kenny, Michael. G. (1999) A Place for Memory: The Interface between Individual and Collective History, Comparative Studies in Society and History, 4 (3), 420–437.
33. Trigg, Dylan (2009) The place of trauma: memory hauntings and the temporality of ruins, Memory Studies, 2 (1), 87–101.
34. Moons, Graham, Kearns, Robert and Joseph, Alun (2015) The Afterlives of the Psychiatric Asylum. Recycling concepts, sites and memories, Farnham, Ashgate.
35. Smith, Cathy (2006) Family, community and the Victorian asylum: A case study of the Northampton General Lunatic Asylum and its pauper lunatics, Family and Community History, 9 (2), 109–124.
36. Gittins, Diane (1998) Madness in its place: Narratives of Severalls Hospital 1913–1997, London, Routledge.
37. Bartlett, Peter, Wright, David, (1999) Outside the Walls of the Asylum, the history of care in the community 1750–2000, London, The Athalone Press; Walton, 1989; Gittins, Diane (1998) Madness in its place: Narratives of Severalls Hospital 1913–1997, London, Routledge.
38. Smith, Cathy (2006) Family, community and the Victorian asylum: A case study of the Northampton General Lunatic Asylum and its pauper lunatics, Family and Community History, 9 (2), 109–124.
39. Brandon, Ed (no date), History of Lancaster Moor Hospital and Whittingham Asylum from www.countyasylums.co.uk.

40. Pendlebury, John, Wang, Yi-Wen, Law, Andrew, (2018) Re-using 'uncomfortable heritage': The case of the 1933 building Shanghai, International Journal of Heritage Studies, 24 (3), 211–229.
41. Wise, Sarah (2012) Inconvenient People, Lunacy, Liberty and Mad-Doctors in Victorian England, London, Bodley Head.
42. Lowe, Louisa (1883) The Bastilles of England or the lunacy laws at work, London, Crookenden and Co; Hamilcar, Marcia (1910) Legally Dead, London, John Ouseley Ltd; Grant-Smith, Rachel (1922) The Experiences of an asylum patient, London, George Allen and Unwin Ltd.
43. Walton, John K. (1989), 'Casting Out and Bringing Back in Victorian England: Pauper Lunatics, 1840–70', in Bynum, William F., Porter, Roy and Shepherd, Michael. (eds), The Anatomy of Madness: Essays in the History of Psychiatry London, Routledge.
44. See Flis, Nathan, Wright, David (2011) "A Grave Injustice' The mental hospital and shifting sites of memory' in Coleborne, Catharine, MacKinnon, Dolly (2011) Exhibiting Madness in Museums: Remembering Psychiatry Through Collection and Display, London, Routledge.
45. Moses, Sarah (2015) Stigmatized space: Negative Heritage in Historic Preservation, thesis submitted for Graduate Program in Historic Preservation, University of Pennsylvania; Sneikers, Maloe and Reijnders, Stijn (2011) An ethnography of guilty houses in Belgium, Intellect Limited: Northern Lights, 9: 27–44.
46. Moons, Graham, Kearns, Robert and Joseph, Alun (2015) The Afterlives of the Psychiatric Asylum. Recycling concepts, sites and memories, Farnham, Ashgate.
47. Pendlebury, John, Wang, Yi-Wen, Law, Andrew, (2018) Re-using 'uncomfortable heritage': The case of the 1933 building Shanghai, International Journal of Heritage Studies, 24 (3), 211–229.
48. Moons, Graham, Kearns, Robert and Joseph, Alun (2015) The Afterlives of the Psychiatric Asylum. Recycling concepts, sites and memories, Farnham, Ashgate; Franklin, Bridget (2002) Hospital-Heritage-Home: Reconstructing the Nineteenth Century Lunatic Asylum, Housing, Theory and Society, 19 (3), 170–184.
49. Franklin, Bridget (2002) Hospital-Heritage-Home: Reconstructing the Nineteenth Century Lunatic Asylum, Housing, Theory and Society, 19 (3), 170–184.
50. Franklin, Bridget (2002) Hospital-Heritage-Home: Reconstructing the Nineteenth Century Lunatic Asylum, Housing, Theory and Society, 19 (3), 170–184.
51. Moses, Sarah (2015) Stigmatized space: Negative Heritage in Historic Preservation, thesis submitted for Graduate Program in Historic Preservation, University of Pennsylvania.

52. Sneikers, Maloe and Reijnders, Stijn (2011) An ethnography of guilty houses in Belgium, Intellect Limited: Northern Lights, 9: 27–44.
53. Gibbeson, Carolyn (2018) After the Asylum: Place, value and heritage in the redevelopment of historic former asylums, PhD thesis Newcastle University.
54. Stromberg, Per (2012) 'Funky Bunkers: The Post-Military Landscape as a Readymade Space and a Cultural Playground', in Linehan, Denis and Boyd, Gary A (2013) Ordnance: War + Architecture and Space, London, Routledge.
55. Scull, Andrew (1979) Museums of Madness: The social organisation of insanity in 19th century England, London, Penguin Books.
56. Scull, Andrew (2006) The Insanity of Place/ The Place of Insanity: Essays on the history of psychiatry, London, Routledge.
57. Taylor, Barbara (2015) The Last Asylum: A Memoir of Madness in our Times, London, Penguin.
58. Scull, Andrew (2006) The Insanity of Place/ The Place of Insanity: Essays on the history of psychiatry, London, Routledge.
59. Harrison, Rodney (2012) Heritage: Critical Approaches, London, Routledge; Harrison, Rodney (2013) Forgetting to remember, remembering to forget: Late modern heritage practices, sustainability and the 'crisis' of accumulation of the past, International Journal of Heritage Studies, 19 (6), 579–595.
60. Massey, Deborah (2005) For Space, London, Sage.
61. Harrison, Rodney (2013) Forgetting to remember, remembering to forget: Late modern heritage practices, sustainability and the 'crisis' of accumulation of the past, International Journal of Heritage Studies, 19 (6), 579–595.
62. Layton, Robert (2008) 'Conflict in the Archaeology of Living Tradition' in in Fairclough, Graham, Harrison, Rodney, Jameson Jnr, John H, Schofield, John (2008) (eds) The Heritage Reader, London, Routledge.
63. Uzzell, David and Ballantyne, Roy (2008) Contemporary issues in heritage and environmental interpretation, London, The Stationary Office.
64. Bartlett, Peter, Wright, David, (1999) Outside the Walls of the Asylum, the history of care in the community 1750–2000, London, The Athalone Press: Smith, Cathy (2006) Family, community and the Victorian asylum: A case study of the Northampton General Lunatic Asylum and its pauper lunatics, Family and Community History, 9 (2), 109–124.
65. Adargh-Walter, Nick, Naik, Prakash, Tombs, David, (1997) Staff attitudes to a psychiatric hospital closure, Psychiatric Bulletin, 21, 139–141; Rossun, Saira and McLeod, John (1994) Evaluation of Client and Staff Experiences of resettlement from Lancaster Moor Hospital, Keele University.

66. Kucik, Lisa M (2004) Restoring Life: the adaptive reuse of a Sanatorium, thesis submitted for Master of Architecture, University of Cincinnati; Moons, Graham, Kearns, Robert and Joseph, Alun (2015) The Afterlives of the Psychiatric Asylum. Recycling concepts, sites and memories, Farnham, Ashgate.
67. Portas, Mary (2011) The Portas Review of the High Street, London, Department for Business, Innovation and Skills.
68. Ludwig, Jens and Kling, Jefffrey R (2007) Is Crime Contagious? Journal of Law and Economics 50 (3). 491–518; Wilson, James Q and Kelling, George L (1982) The police and neighbourhood safety. Broken Windows, Atlantic, 249 (3).
69. Wassenberg, Frank (2004) Large housing estates: From stigma to demolition? Journal of Housing and the Built Environment, 19, pp. 223–232.
70. Lynch, Kevin (1990) Wasting Away, San Francisco, Sierra Club Books.
71. Cairns, Stephen, Jacobs, Jane M (2014) Building Must Die. A Perverse View of Architecture, Cambridge Massachusetts, The MIT Press.
72. Lynch, Kevin (1990) Wasting Away, San Francisco, Sierra Club Books.
73. Cairns, Stephen, Jacobs, Jane M (2014) Building Must Die. A Perverse View of Architecture, Cambridge Massachusetts, The MIT Press.
74. Lynch, Kevin (1972) What time is this place? Cambridge Massachusetts, The MIT Press.
75. Stromberg, Per (2012) 'Funky Bunkers: The Post-Military Landscape as a Readymade Space and a Cultural Playground', in Linehan, Denis and Boyd, Gary A (2013) Ordnance: War + Architecture and Space, London, Routledge.
76. Devine-Wright, Patrick (2009) Rethinking NIMBYism: The Role of Place Attachment and Place Identity in Explaining Place Protective Action, Journal of Community and Applied Social Psychology, 19, 426–441; Gibbeson, Carolyn (2018) Not always nice: The effect of a whole life perspective on heritage and redevelopment, Journal of Urban Regeneration and Renewal 12 (1), 32–42; Kalman, Harold D (2014) Heritage Planning, Principles and Process, London, Routledge; Larkham, Peter (1992) Conservation and the Changing Urban Landscape, Progress in Planning, 37, pp. 83–181.
77. Howard, Peter (2003) Heritage Management, Interpretation, Identity, London, Continuum.
78. Smith, L (2006) Uses of Heritage, London, Routledge.
79. Smith, L (2006) Uses of Heritage, London, Routledge.
80. Harrison, Rodney (2013) Forgetting to remember, remembering to forget: Late modern heritage practices, sustainability and the 'crisis' of accumulation of the past, International Journal of Heritage Studies, 19 (6), 579–595.

81. Harrison, Rodney (2013) Forgetting to remember, remembering to forget: Late modern heritage practices, sustainability and the 'crisis' of accumulation of the past, International Journal of Heritage Studies, 19 (6), 579–595.
82. Smith, L (2006) Uses of Heritage, London, Routledge.
83. Olsen, Bjørnar and Pétursdóttir, Þóra (2014) (eds) Ruin Memories. Materialities, Aesthetics and the Archaeology of the Recent Past, London, Routledge.
84. Edensor, Timothy (2005) Industrial Ruins: Space, Aesthetics and Materiality, Oxford, Berg; Mah, Alice (2012) Industrial Ruination, Toronto, University of Toronto Press.
85. Edensor, Timothy (2005) Industrial Ruins: Space, Aesthetics and Materiality, Oxford, Berg.
86. Edensor, Timothy (2005) Industrial Ruins: Space, Aesthetics and Materiality, Oxford, Berg.
87. Bangstad, Tongeir. R. (2014) 'Industrial heritage and the idea of presence' in Olsen, Bjornar and Petturdoir, Pora (2014) (eds) Ruin Memories. Materialities, Aesthetics and the Archaeology of the Recent Past, London, Routledge.
88. Bangstad, Tongeir R. (2014) 'Industrial heritage and the idea of presence' in Olsen, Bjornar and Petturdoir, Pora (2014) (eds) Ruin Memories. Materialities, Aesthetics and the Archaeology of the Recent Past, London, Routledge.
89. Gittins, Diane (1998) Madness in its place: Narratives of Severalls Hospital 1913–1997, London, Routledge.
90. Bartlett, Peter, Wright, David, (1999) Outside the Walls of the Asylum, the history of care in the community 1750–2000, London, The Athalone Press; Mooney, Graham, Reinarz, Jonathan (2009) Permeable Walls: Historical Perspectives on Hospital and Asylum Visiting, Amsterdam, Rodopi; Smith, Cathy (2006) Family, community and the Victorian asylum: a case study of the Northampton General Lunatic Asylum and its pauper lunatics, Family and Community History, 9 (2), 109–124.
91. Moons, Graham, Kearns, Robert and Joseph, Alun (2015) The Afterlives of the Psychiatric Asylum. Recycling concepts, sites and memories, Farnham, Ashgate.
92. Bynum, William F., Porter, Roy and Shepherd, Michael. (1989) (eds), The Anatomy of Madness: Essays in the History of Psychiatry London, Routledge.
93. Franklin, Bridget (2002) Hospital-Heritage-Home: Reconstructing the Nineteenth Century Lunatic Asylum, Housing, Theory and Society, 19 (3), 170–184.

94. Ellis, Robert (2013) 'A constant irritation to the townspeople?' Local, Regional and National Politics and London's County Asylums at Epsom, Social History of Medicine, 26 (4), 653–671; Mooney, Graham, Reinarz, Jonathan (2009) Permeable Walls: Historical Perspectives on Hospital and Asylum Visiting, Amsterdam, Rodopi; Bartlett, Peter, Wright, David, (1999) Outside the Walls of the Asylum, the history of care in the community 1750–2000, London, The Athalone Press; Walton, John K. (1989), 'Casting Out and Bringing Back in Victorian England: Pauper Lunatics, 1840–70', in Bynum, William F., Porter, Roy and Shepherd, Michael. (eds), The Anatomy of Madness: Essays in the History of Psychiatry London, Routledge.
95. Gittins, Diane (1998) Madness in its place: Narratives of Severalls Hospital 1913–1997, London, Routledge.
96. Ellis, Robert (2013) 'A constant irritation to the townspeople?' Local, Regional and National Politics and London's County Asylums at Epsom, Social History of Medicine, 26 (4), 653–671.
97. Bartlett, Peter, Wright, David, (1999) Outside the Walls of the Asylum, the history of care in the community 1750–2000, London, The Athalone Press.
98. Mooney, Graham, Reinarz, Jonathan (2009) Permeable Walls: Historical Perspectives on Hospital and Asylum Visiting, Amsterdam, Rodopi.

PART IV

Mad Studies and Activism

CHAPTER 14

Brutal Sanity and Mad Compassion: Tracing the Voice of Dorothea Buck

Elena Demke

for this is the dooming: from now on she [the patient] is estranged from herself, all you have experienced is sick and an error!

—Dorothea Buck, 1974 (Letter to Hans Krieger by Dorothea Buck, 12.1.1974; this one as well as the following quotations are my translations from German originals)

On Voice and the Obstacles to Voicing Madness

Voice is neither static nor linear; in fact, any voice can be seen as multi-voiced at any given time—indebted to the intertextual nature of meaning-making and depending on historical constraints of discourse. Experiencing and presenting such a multi-voiced construct as an individual voice is a matter of narrative and performance. This is not a solitary act but happens in interaction. An unheard voice remains non-existent. Establishing an individual voice thus requires the narrative to be deemed plausible and the

E. Demke (✉)
Medizinische Hochschule Brandenburg, Neuruppin, Germany

R. Ellis et al. (eds.), *Voices in the History of Madness*, Mental Health in Historical Perspective,
https://doi.org/10.1007/978-3-030-69559-0_14

performance to be considered adequate—not by everyone or all the time, of course, but at least in the light of some socially shareable context.[1] 'Voices of madness', as understood here, are not a synonym of the 'language of the other'.[2] They are not what psychiatry says about those diagnosed as mentally ill, nor are they bound to be a murmur intractable to the historian.[3] They are not necessarily to be found in 'patient accounts' since madness does not see itself as an illness. 'Voices of madness' are unlikely to come into being since identifying the mad, and denying them voice is one and the same act.[4] It is the very narratives and performances of the mad that are classified as symptoms of illness. The mad have tales to tell about being multi-voiced and yet not having voice.

As long as historians are prepared to use 'madness' and 'psychiatry' as interchangeable terms, these tales will scarcely be retrieved. While the former is not uncommon in the historiography of psychiatry, it seems unthinkable in the context of Mad History.[5] This chapter subscribes to the latter, focusing on the struggles of those deemed mentally ill to redress the silencing implied in this label.

Dorothea Buck succeeded in establishing her 'voice of madness' in the 1990s. Her memoirs of psychiatric treatment during the 1930s, 1940s and 1950s and personal recovery were published in 1990 (first under the pseudonym Sophie Zerchin, an anagram of the German term for 'schizophrenia') and soon reprinted. During the same time, as a co-founder of the German association of psychiatric survivors[6] (BPE e.V.), her long-established activism gained nationwide scope, and she became a much sought-after speaker at conferences.

This chapter will trace the genealogy of Dorothea's voice during the preceding decades. Dorothea, who died on 9 October 2019, just after this chapter had been drafted, had granted me access to her—then premature—legacy, containing more than 40 folders of letters and manuscripts. Together with published sources, they allow for a reconstruction of barriers and conflicts she experienced, as well as the strategies she developed in dealing with them and the effects these had on the emergence of her voice. This entails looking at performative aspects such as collaborations, conflicts and gestures of inscribing herself into certain discourses as well as analysing narrative structures.

Historiography and Framing the Study of the Voice of the Mad

Numerous magazines and newspapers, including the *New York Times* on the occasion of her death, have covered Dorothea as a Nazi and psychiatric survivor 'fighting for a more humane psychiatry'. She appears in a number of documentaries, among them a one-hour portrait of her life and work.[7] However, unlike its counterparts in English-speaking countries,[8] the German movement of psychiatric survivors, including Dorothea and her work, have barely been addressed by historiography so far.

Brückner offers a rough chronology of psychiatric reform, self-help and the evolving survivor movement in Germany, 1970–1990.[9] The 'socialist patient collective', founded in Heidelberg in 1970, attracted special attention due to its extremist legacy, but despite its name, this was in fact an initiative run by a renegade doctor.[10] A long-term analysis by Brink puts psychiatry into a broader societal context and examines contestations of psychiatric practice, including protests by patients in the late nineteenth century; however, the modern survivor movement does not come into closer focus.[11] This is also due to matters of timing, since the late 1970s appear as a period of declining interest in psychiatry in terms of public discourse[12] but were arguably a formative phase of the survivor movement.

One obstacle to scholarship on the survivor movement in Germany is its conflation with 'antipsychiatry', which tends to be treated as a terminological bin rather than being analysed in terms of overlapping and contradictory movements questioning mainstream psychiatry—including the particular uses of the term by activists as a self-identifier.[13] Geyer may serve as an illustration of the resulting historiographical silencing of psychiatric survivors: 'Doubtlessly, aversions against psychotropics contributed to the fact that the antipsychiatric movement survived the millennium, with "lunatics' offensives", committees of psychiatric survivors, runaway-houses.'[14] The plural here is a figure of derogative speech since there is only one 'lunatics' offensive' ('Irrenoffensive', founded in Berlin in 1980)[15] and one Runaway House ('Weglaufhaus', a survivor-run crisis centre, opened in Berlin in 1996)[16]—a rhetorical device suggesting the irrelevance of the subject by demonstrating that it is not worth any precision. Furthermore, calling the criticism of neuroleptics an expression of 'aversion' amounts to writing out of history the political objectives of the movement in terms of fighting for autonomy and choice. Framed this way, there is no need to study a figure like Dorothea Buck.

A recent exception is Schmitt, who compares Dorothea's memoirs with first-person accounts from English-speaking countries and positions them in the context of changing ways of inventing and presenting the self in the second half of the twentieth century. Schmitt identifies a suggestion by Dorothea's editor to focus on personal experience rather than theory, alongside the impact of psychoanalytic literature as being decisive for Dorothea's subjectivation, and the transforming of her experience into a narrative.[17] This interpretation, supported by the introduction and by frequent references to psychoanalytic literature in the last part of Dorothea's memoirs, overlooks significant contradictions. While she presents the editor, in the introduction, as the one encouraging her to write down her personal story, she relates in the text that she had begun writing what she ironically called her 'medical history' ('Krankengeschichte', brackets in the original) more than a decade before getting in touch with him and nearly three decades before the book eventually came out. Such a contradiction is notable and asks for an explanation. In this chapter, it will be interpreted as a result of the complexities involved in the ongoing work of reframing experience under the challenge of not having voice (in the above sense). In order to understand these complexities, power relations have to be taken into account. Being a woman, not being formally trained in a relevant field and being diagnosed as a 'severe case of schizophrenia', Dorothea stood little chance of being heard.

How did she go about this challenge, what resources came into play, what collaborations and conflicts had to be negotiated, how did madness figure in this strife, and what voice emerged from this?

Biographical Aspects

Considered biographically, Dorothea's voice was not a likely one. Born in 1917, her history of patienthood included stays in German psychiatric wards in 1936, 1938, 1943, 1946 and 1959.[18] Thus, she experienced psychiatry under Nazism, which saw the murdering of 300,000 patients and disabled people,[19] and in the post-war period, during which psychiatric patients were more likely to die from starvation than the average population;[20] as well as being a patient of West German psychiatry after the introduction of neuroleptics.[21] In 1936, she was taken to one of the psychiatric wards at Bethel—a foundation of the Protestant Church comprised of several institutions for people with disabilities, the main part of which were (and are still today) situated in the town of Bielefeld. There, at 19 years old, she was sterilized without her knowledge. In 1943, she heard rumours about 'tragic' referrals of fellow patients from a Frankfurt psychiatric ward. Much later she learnt that those referrals meant selection for the so-called 'wild euthanasia'—killings through medically supervised starving and lethal injections as it was applied when the gassings of patients had been officially stopped in 1941.[22] Sterilization led to massive stigmatization and being legally barred from higher education and marriage outside the circle of sterilized persons. To Dorothea, her goals in life seemed destroyed: becoming a kindergarten teacher, a wife and a mother. It was a common experience of those sterilized that the effects of gender roles and prejudice extended the effects of legal restrictions.[23] In her memoirs, Dorothea describes how the resulting urge to kill herself had been massive and long-lasting.

Her upbringing in a Protestant family entailed elements of patriarchal discouragement as well as resources for viewing herself as a person with a say. Even when she was well into her 40s, her uncle, a theologian she turned to for intellectual exchange and discussion of plans to emigrate, replied to her letter in a tone of telling off a silly child.[24] On the other hand, as a daughter of a man whose career had included positions abroad, thus in Cardiff and Alexandria, and in the German towns of Naumburg and Oldenburg before retreating as a parish minister to an island in the North Sea in 1935, she had been familiar with the air of entitlement and the art of speaking publicly.[25] Her parents valued Dorothea's gifts in music and fine art, supporting her accordingly in finding a new prospect for life after sterilization.

And while psychiatry had nearly muted her, madness had sparked her will to speak out. One of the intuitions which she experienced as an overpowering shock as a young woman was the conviction that one day she was going to 'have something to say and the words would just come to me'.[26] Another foreboding—an impending massive war—proved to be utterly true. Her later references, to the very perceptions and thoughts which psychiatry classified as symptoms of early psychosis, made clear that she granted them a kind of validity from which she derived determination and hope, contributing to her eventually gaining a powerful voice.

In the telling of her biography, Dorothea made a point of suggesting that transforming experiences that are usually pathologized into instruments of self-empowerment had been a recurring strategy. Thus, she also turned her suicidal urge into goals for every other year and thereby transformed it into an aid to live by.

After training in pottery and wood carving, qualifying as an organist, and studying art in the 1940s and early 1950s, Dorothea made a living as a sculptor throughout the 1950s and early 1960s. From 1961 onwards, she became increasingly preoccupied with Germany's dealing with perpetrators of the Nazi era. She also began to write up accounts of her experiences and to pursue extensive reading in the fields of psychiatric history as well as psychiatric and psychodynamic theorizing on psychoses. During the same decade, she gave up her career as a sculptor and was employed as an art teacher for a school.

During the 1970s and 1980s, she became involved in the emerging self-help movements of former psychiatric patients and of victims of eugenic sterilization. While victims of forced sterilization were far from being legally recognized as victims of Nazi persecution in Germany, their fight for recognition and compensation won new momentum in the 1980s, when public awareness of various groups of 'forgotten victims' grew. Social psychiatrist Klaus Dörner, with whom Dorothea stayed in close contact, supported their cause in particular.[27] Dorothea promptly tried to extend the newly emerging moral authority and right to be heard, based on her Nazi survivorship, to her agenda as psychiatric survivor. Thus, in the context of lobbying for victims of sterilization, she had been involved in a hearing at government level in 1987 and met the Minister of youth, family, women and health. A year later, and referring to this first meeting, Dorothea sent to the minister a resolution suggesting the creation of a joint committee of psychiatric survivors, their relatives and psychiatric professionals, with the aim of overcoming the somatic interpretation of psychoses and reforming psychiatry in this light.[28] In 1990, after nearly three decades of working on it, she published her memoirs under the title 'Tracing the morning star. Psychosis as self-discovery'. In the same year she began to collaborate with the Hamburg psychologist Thomas Bock, setting up 'psychosis seminars' and campaigning for what they named as a 'trialogue', bringing together (ex-)patients, relatives and professionals. However, unlike the envisioned committee at governmental level, 'trialogue' was not a powerful political body but rather about interpersonal encounter and personal growth.[29]

From 1990 onwards, Dorothea was an invited speaker at various conferences and was highly decorated, including the Federal medal of merit. In 1991, she co-convened a conference which led to the drafting of the statute of the German association of psychiatric survivors, formally founded in 1992. Since then, she stayed in close contact with a growing number of survivors of psychiatry, giving encouragement for recovery through finding personal meaning in psychotic experiences,[30] as well as discussing strategies of the movement; but also with those psychiatrists and social workers whom she considered allies. She carried on criticizing the use of force and the focus on somatic explanations in psychiatry, first as a member of the board of the BPE and later as its honorary chairwoman. The politics which she pursued in this context, well into her 90s, would require a chapter in its own right, due to the multifold nature of her activities and because the ways in which Dorothea used her voice once she had established it, and the ways in which it was used by others, would need to be differentiated and analysed. Instead, this chapter is dedicated to the preceding decades, during which Dorothea was striving to gain voice.

Towards a Genealogy of Dorothea's Voice

For the purpose of reconstructing the genealogy of her voice, those arguments which were central to her publications and public speeches from the 1990s onwards[31] are identified as the 'propositional core of her voice': a) contents of psychoses are meaningful expressions of inner conflicts; b) somatic interventions, including neuroleptics, block the curing potential of psychosis; c) somatic explanations of psychoses imply a 'speechless psychiatry'—where doctors do not even try to have meaningful conversations with their patients about their experiences; d) the mass killings of patients in 1939–1945 had become possible because of this speechlessness; e) people who have experienced psychosis are the foremost experts of it; f) therefore, not only personal meaning-making but also academic insight should be gained by building upon survivors' knowledge.

How do these assumptions emerge and evolve in her writing and activities before the publishing of her memoirs?

Past and Present Intertwined: Researching Literature and Searching for Allies

The 1960s and 1970s saw Dorothea's transformation from a freelance sculptor with a successful record of competing for public commissions to an activist who earned her bread and butter as a teacher at school and dedicated her life to writing and activism. This change was sparked off by two closely intertwined developments: her intellectual departure from psychiatric views on mental distress and her rising interest in how Germany was dealing with Nazi crimes.

In her memoirs, she describes how during her last hospitalization, in 1959, inspired by experiencing her fellow-patients and contrary to what doctors kept telling her, she came to embrace psychoses as meaningful expressions of inner conflict. This she considered her moment of 'healing'.[32] Soon after, she began writing up her experiences. A first manuscript appears to have been completed in 1960.[33] However, these were not yet extensive memoirs. Thus, she mentioned in retrospect that she had to stop writing in 1962 because of the sheer anger this work released.[34] This highlights the fact that gaining voice against the background of oppression is not just about making—acceptable—sense but also about tackling the pain of talking about traumatic memory.[35]

The synchronicity of her first writings, on her experiences as a patient, with a new media focus on the 'euthanasia' crimes, framed Dorothea's path to gaining voice in a double way. On the one hand, public interest in the field opened up a dialogical dimension to her experience transcending the immediate group of former fellow-patients. On the other hand, reading details about crimes committed, and the cynicism and stigma often documented in the reporting, intensified Dorothea's anger. Prosecution of the 'euthanasia' crimes had seemed to gain momentum in West Germany during the first half of the 1960s: one of the main perpetrators, Dr Heyde, was exposed in 1959, and Fritz Bauer, state attorney for the state of Hessen and a central agent in prosecuting Nazi criminals, worked with his colleagues towards what could have become a trial of outstanding significance, highlighting the roles of doctors and lawyers in the murdering of patients. In the end, however, the trial did not take place because of the suicide of the main culprit in 1964.[36] Nonetheless, its preparation had triggered a new quality of media coverage, as had the trials of, A. Eichmann (Jerusalem, 1961), and of Auschwitz personnel (Frankfurt, 1963–1965).[37] However, German society in general and the psychiatric profession in particular were far from facing up to their guilt and responsibilities. Arguments used by lawyers and psychiatrists to defend their deeds implied that ending the lives of those declared severely mentally ill could not be considered murder and thus gave witness to the continual massive stigmatizing and dehumanizing of this group of victims.[38] Dorothea followed up on these discussions, as documented by her collections of articles and newspaper clips. At the same time, she read a broad range of psychiatric literature, past and present, developing her own understanding of the historical origins of the 'euthanasia' murders.

During the second half of the 1960s, Dorothea wrote 'the tragedy of euthanasia' and, in connection with it, a 'satyr play' covering contemporary psychiatry.[39] Her choice of genre can be interpreted as a reaction to the cancelling of the trial against Dr Heyde and his collaborators. A trial would have provided a stage for crimes to be named and survivors to speak out, as famously happened at the Eichmann trial with respect to the Holocaust, and Dorothea stressed the impact the latter had had on her.[40] The fact that the characters of her play are patients, medical experts, theologians and lawyers, including the names of actual perpetrators, and the dramatic action resembling a sequence of hearings, supports this interpretation.

Past and present, the public and the personal, were closely intertwined in the emergence of Dorothea's voice addressing inhumane psychiatry. On the basis of having found her path to recovery in rejecting the teachings of mainstream psychiatry, and informed by her readings, she identified those teachings as central to both the past murders of patients and the detrimental effects of current treatments. Thus, the 'propositional core' of her voice had been formed during the 1960s, but if one assumes that an unheard voice remains inexistent, as suggested in the introduction, it was still a long way for Dorothea to actually gain a voice.

Seeking Allies

Throughout the three decades preceding the publication of her memoirs, Dorothea tried to find allies sharing her goal of disseminating alternative views on psychoses. Thus, she wrote to psychodynamically oriented authors. Only one of those letters has been accessible for the purpose of this chapter, but together with later references she made to it, it illuminates her strategies for making herself heard.

Written in 1960, this letter was addressed to neurologist Theodor Bovet. In it, Dorothea summarized her view on psychosis as a breaking open of the unconscious, similar to religious crises and talking in tongues, and she attached a manuscript of her personal story. In the opening sentence, she staged herself as a person entitled to judge: 'I read your book … and I'm very impressed by the fact how much your views divert from those of the psychiatrists I came across.'[41] Bovet replied in the tone of an academic competition for novelty, affirming Dorothea's views but stressing that they were not original since authors like Benedetti had developed similar theories about a decade earlier.[42] Thirty years later, in the introduction to her memoirs, Dorothea mentions this exchange as encouraging and helpful. However, one of her letters throws a very different light on the impact this contact and similar ones had on her. Thus, she wrote to the man who eventually became her editor:

> The psychotropic suffocation of all this developmental potential [in psychoses] is one of my most harrowing experiences as an inpatient. But survivors have to remain silent. Over the last 13 years, I have sent my essays and later on the manuscript of my book to seven well-known psychiatrists, in order to point out that it is necessary for patients to develop their own understanding of their psychoses … my pleading for supporting a publication was unsuccessful. You can think how discouraging it is for us [sic!] to have no chances to be published.[43]

Here, contacts such as the one with Bovet appear as instances of discouragement. Staging herself publicly as the willing pupil of established medical authors while disclosing frustration from interaction with these authors when addressing a potential supporter can be interpreted as two sides of the same coin. The very practice of sending letters to doctors and journalists appears to have been not just about seeking confirmation but also about searching for allies. Seen this way, personal discouragement and public talk of encouragement belonged together in her strife for gaining voice. Dorothea needed allies in order to be published, and she framed her views as supported by authorities in order to gain credibility.

Hans Krieger, a journalist frequently covering psychiatry and psychoanalysis for the weekly magazine *DIE ZEIT* and to whose analysis of pharmaceutical advertisements Dorothea had replied in her letter quoted above, became a key ally. Concerning the expertise of the survivor, in the same letter, she insisted on the 'necessity of an understanding of psychosis, developed by the survivor herself and in her sense'. She also suggested the production of a textbook about the meaningfulness of psychoses, by survivors and for survivors, in collaboration with psychiatrists.[44]

When asking for the significance of this contact in terms of Dorothea's subjectivation, the answer may lie in being able to perform the kind of eye-level contact which she had sought for so long, rather than in being acquainted with relevant literature. In fact, it was Dorothea who attached articles and manuscripts on the history of the 'euthanasia' crimes as well as on psychodynamic treatments of psychosis to her letter to him. A long-lasting collaboration ensued. Throughout the 1970s and 1980s, they worked towards the publication of Dorothea's memories. Krieger made editorial suggestions and contact with publishers, they discussed possible authors of a foreword, and Dorothea confided in him about the emotional labor this process implied for her.

Voice and Emotional Labour: Dealing with the Challenge of Power Structures

As mentioned earlier, the anger triggered when writing about her experiences constituted a challenge to Dorothea's striving to gain voice; facing up to feelings of powerlessness was another one. In 1979, after the famous psychoanalyst H.E. Richter had agreed to write a foreword, Dorothea felt confident about the acceptance of her book. She admitted to dreaming of investing fees from its sale into a survey of psychiatric hospitals informing potential patients on 'whether they had to expect psychotropic repression of symptoms or such talks' [i.e. about contents of psychoses]. When the publisher declined, to Dorothea this 'made, once again, all our powerlessness fall into my soul'.[45]

Dorothea seemed to take it for granted that her voice stood for a collective—her switching from 'I' to 'us' comes frequently and without explication throughout her letters, and later her publications and speeches. Gaining voice was not a purpose in itself—not only did she hold high hopes for a psychiatry reformed through survivors' voices but her insistence was built upon conceptual reasoning. To Dorothea, having voice was different from being quoted, since only the former implied the redressing of stigma.

This is what Dorothea tried to negotiate with Ernst Klee, who had become a well-known author on marginalized groups such as psychiatric patients, the homeless and disabled in the 1970s.[46] In 1978, Dorothea drew his attention to the forthcoming thirtieth anniversary of the beginning of the murdering of patients under Nazism. However, Klee—today remembered in particular for his work on the 'euthanasia' crimes—became interested in collaborating with her only in the 1980s. When Klee refused Dorothea's suggestion to include parts of her above-mentioned tragedy in his book, she tried to convince him of the significance of the voice of former patients in addressing these crimes, since 'They believe us to be incapable of it' and 'If once more we are objects for whom and about whom you write, we will not achieve the redressing of our devaluation… They will say, he, Ernst Klee has dug up the 'euthanasia' [topic] and patients instrumentalize this'.[47] This was both a plea for support and a criticism of the paternalism implied in taking up Dorothea's suggestion to work on this topic and the information she provided, while not being ready to use his influence to help her gain voice and visibility. Klee was outraged and spoke of her 'evil letter'.[48] They re-established some working contact, after Dorothea seemed to have accepted that the power issues involved could not be discussed and decided to term this conflict a 'misunderstanding'.

Dorothea was familiar with similar kinds of power dynamics. Thus, she had been active in 'Club 70', a self-help group initiated by a psychiatric survivor in Hamburg in 1970. She noted that in the course of the 1970s, meetings and activities lost their vividness after professional helpers got involved, and eventually, survivors lost their voice in representing the Club publicly.[49]

In the context of survivor research, this type of conflict—psychiatric survivors developing concepts or initiatives which then are taken over and changed in terms of aims and character by more powerful agents—has been analysed as co-optation.[50] Dorothea took a pragmatic stance on it, striking a conciliatory tone and emphasizing hope that unequal access to power will not preclude genuine solidarity. Thus, she commented on the publication of a study on self-help groups by a political scientist and a sociologist:[51] 'A real partnership and collaboration, giving our cause more publicity and thereby more weight, will only make us stronger.'[52]

Concluding from the analysis of her letters, the influence of her reading and contacts with authors on the formation of her voice was a complex one. She sought to bolster the credibility of her arguments, and sometimes strategically attributed her own insights to male academic authorities. She searched for allies who appreciated her view on the importance of speaking for herself, but accepted editorial advice as how to present her experiential expertise. She traced the history of psychiatric practices that had harmed her and interpreted their interrelatedness in a way that made her outrage about the sterilizations and murders of patients and her criticism of somatic views on psychoses a combined argument, thus extending her moral authority as a Nazi survivor to her claim to expertise from having lived through psychoses. She advertised the usefulness of her ideas and negotiated access to means of being heard publicly. This process seems to have been at least as much about making her voice palatable as about her story becoming narratable. The last paragraphs of this chapter will turn to the emergent narrative, as finally published in 1990.

Framing in Terms of Contradictions and Paradoxes: Her Memoirs

Literary scholar Woods characterized first-person narratives of people labelled 'schizophrenic' as written from the 'edge of meaning',[53] given the medical view of madness as characterized by incoherent thinking. In the introductory lines to this chapter, the latter was conceptualized as the simultaneous identification of the mad and denial of voice, implying an understanding of this 'edge' as one created by and charged with power relations. The analysis so far has shown Dorothea negotiating these power relations on various levels. However, while the resulting strategies had effects on the framing of her narrative, such as presenting it as supported and partly facilitated by other experts, they do not concern the way she made sense of her experience. The latter is put into a nutshell in the subtitle to Dorothea's memoirs: 'psychosis as self-discovery'.

This seems to fit well with what Davies identified as one out of three key narrative of patients accounts: 'tales of survival and self-discovery',[54] alongside 'stories of loss' and those of 'the self as a patient'. However, Davies' typology of narratives of (former) psychiatric patients, based on an oral history project focusing on Oxfordshire in the UK in the second half of the twentieth century, separates narrative structure from semantics, subsuming 'surviving the illness, the mental health system or treatments' under one type of key narrative frame. However, structural analysis at the cost of semantics precludes meaningful encounter.[55] Given the understanding of voice pursued in this chapter, neglecting semantics may amount to its silencing. As applied to Dorothea: 'Surviving the illness' contradicts her core propositions and subsuming her voice under such a 'key narrative' would mean to miss the point she makes.

Instead, the following analysis points towards a 'key structure' of her narrative and asks for its heuristic and semantic implications. This analysis starts from logical inference. Any structuring of experience depends on comparisons, on relating events to one another and instances to rules. Dorothea had lived through five psychoses and hospital stays. She was in a position to compare the effects of varying circumstances and interventions and to observe her own experiences in relation to that of fellow-patients. If one looks at comparisons in Dorothea's narrative, the central role of contradictions and paradoxes is conspicuous.

She describes the circumstances of her first stay in hospital as having lent themselves right from the beginning to perceiving things in terms of contradictions and paradoxes. The name of the church-run hospital of Bethel had long been familiar to her. When she was a child, her family had even economized on food in order to donate to Bethel. Now she witnessed the abuse of patients at this very place and wondered: 'Had it all been totally different from what we had learned?'[56] One situation made an especially strong impression on her. While Dorothea observed a deaconess who had pushed a patient to the ground and pulled her over the floor, grabbing her by her hair, Dorothea simultaneously read words from the gospel on the wall in front of which this scene was happening: 'Come to me all you who are weary and burdened, and I will give you rest',[57] and she concluded: 'We learned to fear this kind of sanity.' Outrage framed in terms of contradiction and paradoxes had heuristic consequences, and opened a path to think in terms of well-reasoned madness: 'I swore to myself rather to stay mentally ill than to appropriate the "mental sanity" which was exemplified to us here.'[58]

Dorothea also brings in history in ways that counteracts black-and-white narratives, but confirms the principle of contradiction and paradoxes. Thus, while describing the Bethel hospital of 1936 as the harshest place she experienced in terms of day-to-day treatment and sterilization, she includes the information that Bethel's manager had tried to resist 'euthanasia' killings which commenced three years later and that in contrast principals of friendlier hospitals she experienced had been willing collaborators.[59]

Thus, interest in differentiation and adhering to the key structure of contradictions and paradoxes went together, and it can be argued that the latter was central to her making sense of her experience.

Voicing Mad Wisdom

Dorothea goes into detail describing behaviour that appears senseless to the outside observer but elaborates on its meaningfulness. Even repelling digressions such as keeping excrements in her hospital bed were meaningful—in this instance, she hoped they could facilitate protection: the smell keeping away intruders.[60] Thus, she shows how supposedly crazy behaviour made sense, under the restrictions of the ward and the rule of symbolism over her inner world. Apart from the discussion of one particularly intense perception[61]—seeing a burning dot on her bed linen and being able to feel it—Dorothea does not use psychoanalytic or psychiatric explanations in those passages. She rather follows a kind of ethnographic approach: observing the tension between incompatible systems of meaning-making and inferring from it. Since the approach of doctors and nurses seemed utterly strange to her—especially the refusal to communicate with patients—and supranatural explanations came natural to her mad reasoning, she concluded that doctors and nurses were under a spell without knowing.[62] Dorothea makes these thoughts, and her resulting unusual questions and gestures appear plausible to the reader and thereby brings to life the absurdity—and cruelty—of the ensuing interactions. To the doctors, her actions and utterances were signs of the severity of her supposed illness, justifying her sterilization.

Understanding her experience along the lines of paradoxes and contradictions, and structuring her narrative accordingly, enables Dorothea to juxtapose brutal sanity and mad compassion. Against this background, she establishes a proud voice that has command over something I'd like to term 'mad wisdom'. It draws on her ability—mentioned in the context of her biography—to turn what is usually pathologized into means of self-empowerment. Thus, she relates that on some occasion, she felt compelled to stress words differently. She moves on to explain that this gave her insight into a different view on psychosis: reality is still accessible, but spelled out differently. She also describes having conceived of an alternative word for psychosis: 'Zentralerleben',[63] which might be translated as, 'centralized way of perceiving and experiencing'. When everything appears as connected, Dorothea argues, the so-called delusions are a logical consequence. To her, this experience of connectedness held a great potential of healing—not from an illness, but from psychological pain.

In Conclusion: Emergence of a New Expertise

Contradictions and paradoxes seem to have been essential in the emergence of Dorothea's voice. They come up as ways of structuring her experience, as rhetorical means, and on a more abstract level, they appear central to the mere thinkability of her core propositions, questioning psychiatric doctrines and practices. However, Dorothea also tended to be diplomatic, choosing the cloak of medical language and sometimes disguising her agency by staging male professionals as the authorities motivating her thought and action. For contradicting psychiatry was not an end in itself. It was a corollary of her views on the meaningfulness of psychoses. She argued that every survivor had to find this meaning in her own terms, and appears to have believed in the possibility of a psychiatry supporting people to do so. Her hope was for her views to be spread for the benefit of a larger community.

While the role of shared activism from the 1970s onwards cannot be covered within the limits of this chapter, the significance of interactions with fellow patients as related in her memoirs shall at least be mentioned briefly. Thus, Dorothea relates how during her last stay in hospital, in 1959, patients helped themselves. 'In a group of eight patients …we talked about what had been especially impressive from our psychotic experiences. Thus we were able to encourage each other in the notion that our experience was meaningful and overcome the devaluating psychiatric judgement which undermines our confidence … It is the fellow patients who can make the time as an inpatient valuable since they know first hand what a psychosis is and thus they know more than those experts by profession who have neither experience [sic!] nor are they ready to get more knowledgeable from talking to their patients.'[64] This passage can be read as a description of a momentary 'safe space',[65] and the effects it has in terms of validating knowledge and allowing for the emergence of experiential expertise.

Gaining voice thus was about making known and strengthening the validity of an expertise which Dorothea did not consider just her individual one. This expertise had the potential to redress what in her initial quote is termed as psychiatric 'dooming'—a 'self-estrangement' brought about by an act of labelling which deprives the person thus labelled of the chance to voice her experience. In consequence, gaining voice and becoming a self that embraces her mad expertise were two closely intertwined aspects of one and the same process.

Notes

1. The literature on performative and narrative aspects of the construction of identity, and hence of voice, is multifold, influenced, among others, by Goffman, Erving. *The Presentation of Self in Everyday Life*. New York: Anchor Books, 1959 and Ricoeur, Paul. *Onself as another*. Chicago: University of Chicago Press, 1992 (1990).

2. *Die Sprache des Anderen*—language of the other—is the title of a book on language and schizophrenia by leading German social psychiatrists of the 1970s: Hofer, Gunter and Karl Peter Kisker, eds. *Die Sprache des Anderen.* Gedenkschrift für Theodor Spoerri. Basel: S. Karger, 1976.
3. Foucault, Michel, *Wahnsinn und Gesellschaft. Eine Geschichte des Wahnsinns im Zeitalter der Vernunft.* Frankfurt: Suhrkamp 1973, Introduction.
4. Alison Faulkner's chapter in this book, in particular her paragraph on 'finding our voices', elaborates this argument; the quote by Grant-Smith cited there strongly resonates with Dorothea's experience.
5. Geoffrey Reaume, author of the following chapter, has been a pioneer and prolific scholar of Mad History in Canada. On the historical and personal background, see Reaume, Geoffrey. Creating Mad People's History as a University Credit Course since 2000: *New Horizons in Adult Education & Human Resource Development* 31, no.1 (2019): 22–39. For the Scottish and English projects of writing history from within the survivor movement see the chapter by Mark Gallagher.
6. Throughout the chapter, 'survivor' is used for the German term 'Betroffene'. Literally, 'Betroffene' is someone affected by something. The word does not have the same connotation as 'survivor'. However, in terms of linguistic usage, in particular as a self-identifier, 'psychiatric survivor' and 'survivor movement' come closest to 'Psychiatriebetroffene' and 'Betroffenenbewegung' in German.
7. Pohlmeier, Alexandra. *Himmel und mehr* Berlin: Alexandra Pohlmeier-Filmproduktion, 2015.
8. On Canada and Great Britain, see the chapters by Reaume and Faulkner, respectively, and the references given there.
9. Brückner, Burkhart. 'Nichts über uns ohne uns!' Psychiatrie-Erfahrene im Prozess der deutschen Psychiatriereform, 1970–1990. In *40 Jahre Psychiatrie Enquete – Blick zurück nach vorn*, edited by Jürgen Armbruster et al., 138–47, Köln: Psychiatrie Verlag, 2015.
10. Pross, Christian. '*Wir wollten ins Verderben rennen*': *die Geschichte des Sozialistischen Patientenkollektivs Heidelberg 1970–1971.* Köln: Psychiatrie Verlag, 2016.
11. Brink, Cornelia. *Grenzen der Anstalt: Psychiatrie und Gesellschaft in Deutschland, 1860–1980* Göttingen: Wallstein, 2010.
12. Ibid., 452.
13. As an example, see Peter Lehmann, prolific author and influential activist who named the publishing house run by him 'Antipsychiatrieverlag'; see www.antipsychiatrieverlag.de [accessed 20.8.2020].
14. Geyer, Dietrich. *Trübsinn und Raserei: die Anfänge der Psychiatrie in Deutschland.* München: C.H. Beck, 2014.

15. Stöckle, Tina. *Die Irren-Offensive. Erfahrungen einer Selbsthilfe-Organisation von Psychiatrieopfern.* Frankfurt a.M. Extrabuch Verlag, 1983.
16. Kempker, Kerstin, (ed.). *Flucht in die Wirklichkeit. Das Berliner Weglaufhaus.* Berlin: Antipsychiatrieverlag 1998.
17. Schmitt, Sandra. *Das Ringen um das Selbst: Schizophrenie in Wissenschaft, Gesellschaft und Kultur nach 1945*, Berlin: De Gruyter Oldenbourg, 2018, 397.
18. Unless stated otherwise, biographical information is based on Zerchin, Sophie [Buck, Dorothea]. *Auf der Spur des Morgensterns: Psychose als Selbstfindung; ein Erlebnisbericht.* München: List, 1990, and Pohlmeier, *Himmel.*
19. This estimate applies when victims from occupied territories are included, see e.g. Brink, *Grenzen*, 259 and for a very short overview in English: https://www.stiftung-denkmal.de/memorials/place-of-remembrance-and-information-for-the-victims-of-the-national-socialist-euthanasia-murders/ [accessed 20.08.2020].
20. Faulstich, Heinz. *Hungersterben in der Psychiatrie 1914–1949. Mit einer Topographie der NS-Psychiatrie* Freiburg: Beck 1998.
21. Balz, Viola. Zwischen, Wirkung und Erfahrung. Eine Geschichte der Psychopharmaka. Neuroleptika in der Bundesrepublik Deutschland, 1950–1980, Bielefeld: transkript, 2010.
22. On her perception of rumours about the referrals: Zerchin, *Auf der Spur*, 145; out of the numerous regional studies on the 'wild euthanasia', Sandner, Peter. *Der Eichberg* im Nationalsozialismus. In *Wissen und Irren*, edited by Landeswohlfahrtsverband Hessen, 164–220. Kassel: Eigenverl. des LWV Hessen, 1999, deals with the hospital mentioned by Dorothea.
23. Westermann, Stefanie. *Verschwiegenes Leid: der Umgang mit den NS-Zwangssterilisationen in der Bundesrepublik Deutschland.* Köln: Böhlau, 2010.
24. Letter to Dorothea Buck by her uncle Günther, 29.03.1960.
25. Newspaper clip from Dorothea's legacy: Kirchenrat Buck zum Pfarrer in Wangerode ernannt. In *Nachrichten für Stadt und Land: Oldenburger Zeitung für Volk und Heimat*, 9.10.1934.
26. Zerchin, *Auf der Spur.*
27. Inspired by Dörner, the German head of state, Richard von Weizsäcker, addressed the suffering of the victims of forced sterilizations in his famous speech on occasion of the 40th anniversary of the end of World War II: https://www.bundespraesident.de/SharedDocs/Downloads/DE/Reden/2015/02/150202-RvW-Rede-8-Mai-1985-englisch.pdf?__blob=publicationFile [accessed 20.8.2020].

28. Buck, Dorothea S. *Ermutigungen. Ausgewählte Schriften.* Neumünster/ Norderstedt: Paranus/Anne Fischer Verlag, 2012, 48–79.
29. Bock, Thomas, Joachim Meyer, and Tuula Rouhiainen. *Die Entwicklung des Subjekts: Trialog und Empowerment.* In *40 Jahre Psychiatrie Enquete – Blick zurück nach vorn*, edited by Jürgen Armbruster et al., 489–499, Köln: Psychiatrie Verlag, 2015.
30. Buck, Dorothea S., Hartwig Hansen, and Fritz Bremer, eds. *Mit meinen herzlichen Grüßen! Der Gartenhaus-Briefwechsel.* Neumünster: Paranus-Verlag, 2016.
31. Five books, and more than 20 chapters or articles have been published; for an overview, see http://www.bpe-online.de/buck/ [accessed 7.10.2019]; a speech by Dorothea with English dubbing can be watched under: http://ki-art-multimedia.de/dresden/doro-english.htm [accessed 7.10.2019].
32. Zerchin, Auf der Spur, 226ff.
33. Mentioned in her letter to Theodor Bovet, 31.5.1960.
34. Zerchin, *Auf der Spur*, 122.
35. Emcke, Carolin. *Weil es sagbar ist. Über Zeugenschaft und Gerechtigkeit.* Frankfurt a.M.: Fischer 2013.
36. Godau-Schüttke, Klaus-Detlev, *Die Heyde/Sawade-Affäre.* Baden-Baden: Nomos, 2001.
37. Krause, Peter, *Der Eichmann-Prozess in der deutschen Presse*, Frankfurt am Main: Campus 2002.
38. DER SPIEGEL (author not named). Euthanasie. Die Kreuzelschreiber. *Der Spiegel* 19/1961, 1961/05/03, 35–44, https://www.spiegel.de/spiegel/print/d-43160977.html [accessed 2012.2019.
39. Die Tragödie der Euthanasie. Ein Spiel der Geisteskranken zur 30. Wiederkehr des Euthanasiebeginns im Herbst 1969 und ihrer seither ausgebliebenen Wandlung zur Hilfe und Menschlichkeit, unpublished manuscript, an abbrieved version published in: Buck, *Ermutigungen*, 12–44.
40. Zerchin, *Auf der Spur*, 14.
41. Letter to Theodor Bovet by Dorothea Buck, 31.5.1960.
42. Letter to Dorothea Buck by Theodor Bovet, 10.7.1960.
43. Letter to Hans Krieger by Dorothea Buck, 12.1.1974.
44. Letter to Hans Krieger by Dorothea Buck, 12.1.1974.
45. Letter to Hans Krieger by Dorothea Buck 9.10.1979.
46. E.g. Klee, Ernst. *Die im Dunkeln ... Sozialreportagen* Düsseldorf: Patmos, 1971; Klee, Ernst. *Behinderten-Report.* Frankfurt a. M.: Fischer, 1976.
47. Quotation from a letter to Ernst Klee, in a letter to Hans Krieger by Dorothea Buck, 17.01.1982.
48. Ibid.
49. Letter to Monika Dobler by Dorothea Buck, 18.1.1984.

50. For example, Penney Darby, and Prescott, Laura. The co-optation of survivor knowledge: The danger of substituted values and voice. In *Searching for a rose garden: Challenging psychiatry, fostering mad studies*, edited by Jasna Russo and Angela Sweeney, 35–45. Ross-on-Wye: PCCS Books, 2016, see also the discussion of the effects of co-optation in the chapter by Faulkner.
51. Kickbusch Ilona, und Alf Trojan. *Gemeinsam sind wir stärker: Selbsthilfegruppen und Gesundheit: Selbstdarstellungen, Analysen, Forschungsergebnisse*. Frankfurt am Main: Fischer Taschenbuch Verlag, 1981.
52. Letter to Monika Dobler by Dorothea Buck, 18.1.1984.
53. Wood, Mary Elene. *Life writing and schizophrenia: encounters at the edge of meaning*. Amsterdam; New York: Rodopi, 2013.
54. Davies, Kerry. 'Silent and Censured Travellers'?: Patients' Narratives and Patients' Voices: Perspectives on the History of Mental Illness since 1948'. *Social History of Medicine* 14, no. (2001): 267–92, 281.
55. This line of criticism was famously expressed by Ricoeur in relation to Lévi-Strauss' method of structural analysis, for example documented in the proceedings of a 1963 radio discussion, In Lévi-Strauss, Claude. Das wilde Denken. Eine Diskussion mit Paul Ricoeur, et al., In Lévi-Strauss. Mythos und Bedeutung, 71–112, Frankfurt. Suhrkamp 1980.
56. Zerchin, *Auf der Spur*, 75.
57. Ibid., 66.
58. Ibid., 86.
59. Ibid., 129–134 and 173–175.
60. Ibid., 63.
61. Ibid., 80. The psychiatrist Ernst Kretschmer, whose theories she quotes as helpful at this point, was also an agent of forced sterilizations and involved in the supervision of 'euthanasia' mass murders.
62. Ibid., 77.
63. Ibid., 207.
64. Ibid., 220.
65. See the chapter by Faulkner, especially the paragraphs on 'Letting stories breathe. The power of personal narratives' and 'Finding safe spaces'.

CHAPTER 15

Mad Activists and the Left in Ontario, 1970s to 2000

Geoffrey Reaume

Introduction: Mad Activists, Identity Politics and the Left

In 1996, David Oaks, editor of the American magazine *Dendron*, wrote: "Since the very origins of psychiatry, psychiatric survivors have individually resisted human rights violations and sought humane alternatives. In the past 25 years [since 1971], however, a small wave of diverse organized groups, networks, publications, have sprung up and connected internationally… In the family of social change movements this past 25 years, the psychiatric survivors liberation movement has been the 'aunt in the attic' who is usually ignored."[1] Oaks' comments are particularly relevant when considering whose voice is listened to among those who seek to represent marginalized communities in social activism. Voice in this context refers to

This chapter is dedicated to the memory of Kevin Jackson (1969–2019), activist and scholar in Toronto's mad and disability community.

G. Reaume (✉)
Critical Disability Studies, York University, Toronto, ON, Canada
e-mail: greaume@yorku.ca

R. Ellis et al. (eds.), *Voices in the History of Madness*, Mental Health in Historical Perspective,
https://doi.org/10.1007/978-3-030-69559-0_15

first-person perspectives of people who had been confined in mental institutions and who were publicly active as current or former psychiatric patients, whose views were generally marginalized among contemporary social justice activists among the broader left. Thus, the concept of voice refers to spoken words, written accounts and direct involvement in social activism by people deemed mad by their contemporaries. It also relates to whose voices were and were not privileged within left-wing community activist efforts at a time when newly organized groups sought wider recognition and support from potential allies.

When referring to mad activists and the mad movement, it is important to emphasize that the politicization of this term from the perspectives of people deemed mad happened during the last decades of the twentieth century and into the twenty-first century.[2] It should also be mentioned that the term 'mad activists' is itself a term many of the people being discussed in this chapter would not recognize as a self-descriptor. While the history of changing terminology is important in that it reflects the political orientation of activists, ranging from ex-patient, ex-inmate, psychiatrized, survivor and consumer, among other terms, it suffices to say that, in relation to the wider world, all such activists were considered 'mad', a term which more recently has been reappropriated by some people as a positive self-identity. This in turn influenced responses to activists, and thus the term 'mad' will be used generally, whilst some of the other identities will also be included.[3] 'Non-psychiatrized' leftists refers to political activists on the left who do not identify as being mad or having had psychiatric treatment.

The development of the mad movement in North America during the 1970s reflected wider developments in what has come to be called 'new social movements'.[4] While mad people had been active in North America demanding rights and better treatment since the nineteenth century, the most widely organized protest movement of ex-psychiatric patients in Canada and the United States developed out of the social protests of the 1960s with demands for greater rights of Blacks, Indigenous people, women, gays, lesbians and the student movement, as well as the anti-Vietnam War movement.[5] This period also saw the rise of the disability rights movement in North America, which had some of the closest ties with the mad movement of all the groups considered here.[6] While mad activists during this period were definitely not the first ex-inmates of asylums to call public attention to issues affecting people variously described as mad, mentally ill, insane, psychiatric patients, and a host of other terms, they did establish organizations and international contacts to a greater extent than before.[7] It is these identities, chosen and imposed, that impact on so much of this history. At the most basic level, people identified as mad have long been regarded by those who are not so labelled, as devoid of reason, having nothing to say that is worth taking seriously, or for those who adhere to the medical model of mental illness, lacking insight into their mental world, if an individual rejects a diagnosis of illness.[8] Thus, when discussing self-identity, it is essential to stress this basic point to place in context wider social stereotyping of mad people as lacking mental competence. Their identities were contested from the start.

As Lennard Davis notes, the advent of the disability rights movement, of which mad activists were a part as time went on, included a "grand reexamination" around race, gender and sexual orientation with disability being "the most recent identity group on the block".[9] Mad activists, being part of this "most recent identity group", tried to establish themselves both by organizing conferences to discuss their concerns and political direction, and also by trying to forge solidarity links with fellow leftists. Finding a common political orientation had to go beyond a general philosophical orientation as a 'leftist', with all the variations in goals, strategies and beliefs that this involved. It also involved, for mad activists, an understanding of working with each other in a way the put aside the therapeutic condescension that mental health professionals believed they knew best.

This idea of who knows best between mental health professionals and early mad activists was expressed more broadly in interpretations of the medical model of mental illness. An example of this can be found in the US Marxist newspaper *The Guardian*, in which there appeared a series of articles between December 1982 and May 1983 dealing with anti-psychiatry and the concept of mental illness. The first article was a strong attack on the medical model by Lenny Lapon, a widely known and respected activist based in Massachusetts and one of the first historians of the mad movement.[10] Richard Morrock, a non-psychiatrized Marxist, wrote an attack on Lapon's piece in which he criticized Lapon's views as a rehash of the "conservative" anti-psychiatry views of Thomas Szasz, a form of right-wing libertarianism. Steve Holochuck, described as a "former 'mental patient' and a Massachusetts-based activist in the psychiatric inmates' liberation movement", wrote in response to the attack on Lapon that most of the people who make up the psychiatrized are disenfranchised poor people who do not suffer from mental illness but from alienation rooted in their material and social circumstances. Holochuck continued:

> The psychiatric inmates' liberation movement is one front where people are struggling to overcome their alienation and change social structures. And though indebted to the pioneering work of Szasz, Laing, Cooper, and others, it has used the experiences of real, live psychiatric inmates to go beyond the ideas of these original thinkers to arrive at a higher theoretical synthesis. Our movement is not the only front on which to struggle to ease the emotional pain of intense alienation.... Other dimensions must be confronted through unions, political parties, women's groups, third-world organisations, etc.... Like other oppressed groups we feel that we are the ones best able to theorise about our particular oppression and to formulate the specific strategies for our liberation struggle. Many of us see ourselves as part of a wider movement for the total liberation of workers and all oppressed people, the struggle for world socialism. We earnestly desire to join in common struggle with those in the wider movement. We extend our hand, seeking solidarity, not diagnoses.[11]

This debate reflects how the efforts to forge some kind of inclusion into the older, more established left by new identity formations led to differences about the relevance, or lack thereof, of a new identity—new, that is, in the sense of wanting to be taken seriously as political activists in their own right. This contention arises partly due to the "existing welter of identities", as Davis has noted with respect to disability more broadly, a process by which older, established left-wing identity formations worry that newer groups advocating for inclusion "dilutes the general category of identity".[12] Expanding the category of oppressed identities to mad people, as was being proposed and critiqued in the pages of *The Guardian*, challenged a way of thinking amongst activists who were part of this practice of exclusion. To acknowledge the justice of including mad people as an equity-seeking group would mean that some left-wing activists would have to acknowledge the oppressiveness of their own practices and attitudes, a theoretical and practical readjustment too far for some to take. As will be discussed in the pages that follow, between the 1970s and the close of the twentieth century prejudices towards and among mad activists were part of the reason for the difficult relations between mad activists and the left in Ontario, as well as within the mad community itself.

Of course, new social movements during this period were not monolithic in regard to how they responded to mad activists. Emerging political formations—the disability rights movement, gays and lesbians, for example—were more likely to find common cause with mad activists given their status as being relatively new to organized political action and in need of allies themselves. Other, well-established political formations—such as unions—were less inclined to support the civil rights agenda of mad activists, particularly when it threatened their own jobs and positions of power over mad people in the mental health system. More established political formations on the left, who already had their territory marked out in relation to their job, were less willing to take seriously activists whose mental competence had for so long been derided in broader society.[13]

From the 1970s, when the mad movement in North America in more recent times began to take shape, efforts were made to form working political alliances between mad activists and non-psychiatrized leftists, usually at the instigation of the former.[14] This chapter will examine the relationship between activists who self-identify as having experienced psychiatric treatment in some way and leftists who do not identify as such. The goal here is to interpret how activists who identified in some way as 'mad', or as current or former psychiatric patients, sought to establish political legitimacy within the activist left while also seeking to expand representation in relation to existing and emerging political groups, such as trade unions, political parties, anti-poverty organizations and equity-seeking groups focused on rights for women, racialized people, sexual minorities and disabled people, among others.

Although the first part of this chapter will include examples from both Canada and the United States—which, given both country's geographical proximity, led to regular cross-border connections—most of the history for this period focuses on Ontario, and in particular the province's biggest city, Toronto. What little research has been published on the history of mad activism by current and former patients in North America has included virtually no detailed discussion of how the objectives and views of mad people were received by other left-wing community organizers. This chapter also avoids the simplistic division between anti-psychiatry versus psychiatry which is only one part of a much broader and more complex story of how current and former patients engaged in community politics during the deinstitutionalization era. As Elena Demke eloquently points out in her chapter in this volume about Dorothea Buck, among academics "anti-psychiatry" has become a "terminological bin rather than being analyzed in terms of overlapping and contradictory movements questioning mainstream psychiatry".[15] This chapter contributes to documenting how 'anti-psychiatry' is only one of numerous identities which left-wing mad activists were grappling with that cannot be subsumed under one tidy category.

Left-wing here refers to political beliefs based on promoting the redistribution of resources and implementing public policies in a way that promotes equity and social inclusion of historically marginalized groups in capitalist economies. Such views were espoused by people who adopted a variety of perspectives ranging from social democrats, Marxists, socialists, anarchists, religious and politically unaffiliated activists. Left-wing mad activists included those who espoused some of the political orientations noted above, as well as critical perspectives about psychiatry ranging from anti-psychiatry to wanting to work within the mental health system; they sought alliances with other activists on issues related to equity and rights advocacy for marginalized groups.[16] Ultimately, this chapter argues that being accepted as having a legitimate claim to left-wing civic engagement was very much a matter of whose voice was considered worth listening to and why among equity-seeking groups.

Deinstitutionalization in Canada

To begin to understand this history, it is first necessary to outline the deinstitutionalization era in which it took place. When deinstitutionalization began in Canada during the mid-1960s, the impact on the number of people in mental health facilities was significant: in the country overall, the 'bed capacity of operating institutions' fell by 70.6 per cent between 1965 and 1981; in Ontario, the total decrease in the number of in-patients fell during this period by just under 67 per cent.[17] In stark numbers, this was a decrease of 16,033 people in the province's psychiatric institutions during this sixteen-year period. When this change is calculated on the basis of the 'rate per population' for each year, the decline registers at 71.4 per cent for Canada overall and 75 per cent for the province of Ontario from 1965 to 1981.[18] Harvey Simmons has shown that this development in Ontario was due to the haphazard confluence of circumstances, including government cost-cutting and the advent of neuroleptic drugs, rather than any coordinated systematic policy.[19] This process continued throughout the period under consideration. Days of care in both general hospital psychiatric units and provincial psychiatric hospitals declined between 1985 to 1999 per 1000 population by over 38 per cent in Canada overall and in Ontario specifically by over 45 per cent; this percentage, however, declined less dramatically in regard to psychiatric hospitals on their own during this same period which witnessed a reduction of in-patients by 5.3 per cent in Canada and 15.3 per cent in Ontario.[20] These latter figures indicate that deinstitutionalization represented much more than the reduction of beds in large-scale psychiatric hospitals—it was also a process of shifting people out of large-scale institutions into smaller facilities, such as general hospital psychiatric units, and nursing homes.[21]

These developments gave more individuals than ever before who had been released from psychiatric institutions the chance to engage in activist efforts affecting themselves and their peers. As a result, the first activist group founded by ex-psychiatric patients in Canada began in Vancouver in 1970, the Mental Patients Association. In Ontario, the first groups by ex-patients were founded in the mid-to-late 1970s.[22] The far-reaching demographic changes which led to the establishment of such groups, along with the social and political climate of the times, led to a greater sense of community amongst like-minded activists. With this emerged a greater expectation that a wider level of support would develop among those on the left for mad activism. This usually did not materialize, however, primarily due to discriminatory views towards people with a psychiatric history by activists who had no such experience as well as due to the tensions between activists promoting civil rights for people with a psychiatric diagnoses and hospital staff threatened by job losses and being held accountable by rights advocates as will be discussed below.

Disability and Mad Movement Activists in Ontario

Among the earliest and most consistent allies of mad activists have been activists in the broader disability rights community. Much of this support was due to the fact that people from both communities had multiple experiences of being categorized as disabled and confined. Thus, there was a common history of discrimination and exclusion. For example, Mike and Cathy Yale, two of the original four-person editorial collective on the anti-psychiatry magazine *Phoenix Rising* (1980–1990), were ex-inmates of mental institutions and were also blind. In the second issue of this magazine in 1980, Mike Yale wrote an article about people who were blind. It was also mentioned in this same issue that copies of the magazine were tape-recorded "for the use of blind readers" with a contact number to call, the point being to broaden the readership beyond sighted people and thus to try to build links with the blind community.[23] To address some of these common issues, a broad-based group of disability rights activists founded the Ontario-based Coalition on Human Rights for the Handicapped in 1980. Their purpose was to fight against the exclusion of people labelled handicapped from the new Ontario Human Rights Code who were not covered in the anti-discriminatory provisions of this law. Mad activists from an ex-patient-run community centre in Toronto, called On Our Own, joined forces with various other groups representing people with sensory, intellectual and physical disabilities. Their definition of handicap included people undergoing psychiatric treatment, a position which the Ontario government initially opposed only to relent and agree that "mental handicap" should be included as a protected group.[24]

A similar group was founded in 1977 called the Coalition of Provincial Organizations of the Handicapped (COPOH), which spread across Canada over the next decade.[25] Their original focus was on prejudices towards people with physical disabilities but this expanded to include:

> prejudice against the psychiatrized. In the struggle to make discrimination against all disabled people illegal under federal jurisdiction, COPOH-member provincial councils were shocked to hear that a major stumbling block was an objection from the Federal Department of Finance, which was concerned that hiring a psychiatrized employee might jeopardize its security.[26]

The creation of legal aid centres in Ontario during the 1970s and 1980s was also essential to promoting mad people's rights, public funding for which in 1985 was extended to involuntary patients.[27] Legal aid clinics facilitated more widespread involvement of left-wing lawyers and legal aid workers who fought for civil rights of patients together with ex-inmate activists. This included public forums such as a 'Patients' Rights Symposium' held in Toronto in February 1982 which discussed a broad range of issues, including psychiatric patients' rights and was attended by lawyers, health care professionals and current and former patients.[28] Some of these legal workers were themselves formerly psychiatrized people such as Carla McKague, who became a prominent disability rights lawyer in Toronto.[29] In the mid-1980s, lawyers with the Advocacy Resource Centre for the Handicapped (ARCH), including McKague, along with activists from an ex-patient-run community centre, On Our Own, made representations at public hearings to advocate for people in mental institutions to have the right to vote in elections. This right was legalized for psychiatric patients in Ontario for the first time in the 1985 provincial and municipal elections.[30] The 1985 provincial election also saw David Reville become the first public ex-psychiatric patient elected as a Member of Ontario's

Provincial Parliament for the New Democratic Party, having been previously elected to Toronto City Council during which time he went public with his own history of madness.[31]

Fighting for institutionalized people's enfranchisement took longer at the federal level, due not least to the resistance of the Conservative Canadian federal government of Brian Mulroney (1984–1993). On 17 October 1988, an Ottawa court struck down a law that excluded people in mental institutions from being able to vote in federal elections, thus assuring that all psychiatric patients and people with intellectual disabilities forthwith had the right to vote in national elections beginning with the federal election the following month. This legal change at that time covered 50,000 people who were labelled incompetent and who had been previously disenfranchised across Canada.[32] These efforts continued on other legal fronts such as on Human Rights Day, 10 December 1987, when the Ontario Coalition to Stop Electroshock held a joint news conference at the provincial legislature with the Blind Organization of Ontario with Self-Help Tactics (BOOST), where they criticized the Ontario government for stalling on passing an amendment to the provincial human rights code that would protect people defined as disabled from discrimination in the housing market and to protect the rights of people in psychiatric facilities.[33]

It must also be noted that some activists with physical and sensory disabilities have at times not wanted to be associated with people who have had experiences as psychiatric patients, and some mad activists do not see themselves as disabled and reject the idea that they have a psychiatric disability.[34] Yet people involved in these efforts needed allies to accomplish their objectives, and people who fell under the common category of disability—physical, sensory and mental—made working together more likely than any other identity group. There was an appreciation that people also had multiple disabilities; thus, neat distinctions in categories existed more on paper than in reality. Whatever differences existed did not obscure the common need to push for inclusion as citizens in human rights legislation and voting rights, a major legal and psychological victory for all people defined as disabled. As the following section will indicate, this push for greater civil rights did not automatically translate into a broader cross-representation of mad activists.

Race, Gender, Sexual Orientation and Ontario's Mad Movement

During the last three decades of the twentieth century, the domination of the North American mad movement by white people has been the most significant example of the lack of representation of the wider community. While people from racially and ethnically diverse backgrounds were involved at the local levels during this period, including in the organizing of Psychiatric Survivor Pride Day events beginning in 1993 in Toronto, the majority of mad activists during the thirty-year period examined here were white in Ontario, as elsewhere (including the author of this chapter).[35] Criticism from within the movement about this under-representation goes back to the early years of organizing. In May 1983, eight Canadians, including five activists from Ontario and three from Quebec, attended the annual ex-inmate human rights and psychiatric oppression conference, which was held in Syracuse, New York. In a report published afterwards, Toronto-based activist Don Weitz noted that two well-attended workshops on racism at the conference discussed why "our Movement has failed to attract black people and other people of colour". It was noted that the "presence and key contributions of three black people made this workshop more credible and relevant than ones held at previous conferences". Issues discussed included racism within the movement, lack of solidarity work in areas of common concern such as housing and welfare, integrating "an anti-racist analysis into our antipsychiatry ideology and reaching out" to racialized people, and supporting a National Anti-Klan Coalition in the United States.[36] These issues, while discussed at a conference across the border, of course had relevance in Canada where racism has always been endemic and Indigenous people have been subjected to centuries of colonization.[37] In publications during this period, some writing by racialized people were included, such as by Lionel Vermette and Vern Harper on racism experienced by Indigenous Canadians in the mental health system.[38] Similarly, Bobbi Nahwegahbow was involved in Toronto mad pride organizing from 1993 until her death in 2007. Generally, however, the mad movement during this time remained primarily, though not exclusively, white.

The under-representation of racially diverse communities within the mad movement during this period reflected on the political emphases of activists. Denunciations of psychiatry included racism on the list of what was wrong with the profession, but it was one of a list of oppressions being denounced. Anti-racist solidarity work was not an actual priority of the mad movement itself even though statements were made supporting such efforts and some individuals were more seriously involved than others in this work. This reality was combined with generally white activists where racists at times made their presence known. In the 1990s, the author of this chapter heard an activist excuse racism among white patients towards psychiatric hospital staff members who were of Southeast Asian background, while another activist expressed sympathy for neo-nazis who were then organizing in Toronto. This bigotry was denounced by other white and racialized activists; however, prejudice like this led to an environment that was not conducive to making the mad movement a welcoming or relevant place for current and former patients who were not white, nor for activists of any colour who sought to build solidarity with people of all backgrounds. Given the history of police shootings of racialized people with a psychiatric history, people from diverse Black, Indigenous and Asian communities were and are less likely to be 'out' as mad as they face a greater likelihood of being killed than more privileged white activists.[39] As well, the long history of white people associating Black people with madness and social deviance further reduces the appeal of white-dominated mad activism.[40] There were, however, racialized people involved in mad activism in Toronto during this period. Likely the most significant activist effort in Ontario during this period involving anti-racist and mad activists was protesting and being involved in hearings about police shootings of psychiatrized people from racially diverse backgrounds in the Toronto area. This culminated in a conference on this topic in 2000. Organized by the Queen Street Patients Council and the Urban Alliance on Race Relations, this two-day conference, which also involved law enforcement officials, addressed the need to use alternatives to deadly force when relating to people from racially marginalized and psychiatrized backgrounds.[41]

While racially diverse communities were generally under-represented in Ontario's mad movement during this time period, issues around gender inequality were more consistently addressed, largely due to the involvement of women who protested sexism within and without the activist community. At the tenth Annual International Conference on Human Rights and Psychiatric Oppression, in May 1982, which was held in Toronto, a group of seven activists, including two women from Ontario, published a position paper on 'Mental health and violence against women'. They asked non-psychiatrized feminists to "recognize our experience and analysis as ex-inmate women rather than ignoring us, rejecting us as sick or crazy, or being embarrassed by us". In their analysis, they pointed out the differences regarding class, race and sexual orientation for women who needed support services and what was, and was not, available to them due to socio-economic inequalities. They also wrote: "We join the ex-inmate movement, and expect to find sexism, but will not accept the failure of members to recognize it and be accountable for it."[42] A year later at the next annual conference, perhaps in response to this position paper, twenty men, including representation from Toronto, held a workshop and issued a statement denouncing sexism.[43] As this evidence suggests, feminists were more extensively involved in the mad movement than anti-racist activists during this period. As a result, gender issues were addressed directly on a more frequent basis than was race, as can be seen from the thirty-two issues of the radical anti-psychiatry magazine *Phoenix Rising*, published in Toronto between 1980 and 1990.[44]

Relations between the gay and lesbian community and mad groups, similar to feminist activists, were greatly influenced by the cross-over of people in each group. The pathologization of homosexuality by psychiatrists until 1973–1974, when it was dropped as a 'mental illness' after years of protests by gays and lesbians, had an important impact on the growth of the mad movement.[45] As was pointed out in *Phoenix Rising*, however, "psychiatric homophobia" continued to persist through various renamed diagnostic labels such that an acquiescent gay and lesbian community was criticized by activists for being co-opted by psychiatry.[46] As with some disability rights activists, there were also some activists from both communities who would rather not be associated with either group. Lilith Finkler, one of the early organizers of what was originally called Psychiatric Survivor Pride Day starting in 1993, wrote that there was homophobia from some heterosexual mad activists. At the same time, she also wrote that "Some gays and lesbians did not want to be associated with 'crazies' and felt that we were 'stealing' their day [Gay and Lesbian Pride Day]. 'Name your day something else. Don't name it after us!'"[47] Nevertheless, gays and lesbians as well as transgender activists were among the strongest supporters in the mad activist community during this period.

While class issues were addressed more consistently than race among Ontario's mad activists, class fissures also opened when issues of power and jobs were at stake.

Class, Unions and Mad People's Civil Rights

As deinstitutionalization intensified from the late 1970s onwards, increasing numbers of people were discharged into boarding homes or nursing homes, or became homeless. It was therefore not surprising that the earliest organizing by mad activists in Toronto were in economically marginalized areas of the city where ex-patients were most likely to live. In one case, this was initially supported by a left-wing Christian leader. Reverend Norman Ellis, head of All Saints Anglican Church in Toronto in the downtown east end, supported the first meeting of the Ontario Mental Patients Association (OMPA) on 9 August 1977 which was attended by 150 people at this church.[48] Reverend Ellis also agreed to let OMPA use a room there as their first meeting place and community centre for a year, in 1977–1978, before it became On Our Own in 1980 and moved elsewhere until its demise in 1996. Activists engaged working-class ex-patients where they lived to organize some of the earliest mad groups and publications in the province. Pat Capponi and others who lived in boarding houses in Toronto's west end Parkdale neighbourhood, not far from the city's largest psychiatric hospital, produced a newsletter called *Cuckoo's Nest*. It was published from 1979 until 1986 to bring attention among the wider public and local politicians to living conditions endured by the poorest discharged psychiatric patients who lived down the street or across town.[49] Mad activists were also involved with 'angry roomers' who protested at the provincial housing ministry offices for protection from abusive and exploitative landlords and advocated for 'decent, affordable housing'.[50] From the earliest years of political activism by ex-patients, housing conditions were therefore a major concern. The reality of social isolation and poverty of current and former patients was an important impetus for mad activists, many of whom knew this experience only too well. Solidarity with the poorest of deinstitutionalized people was therefore essential for mad activists. This did not, however, mean that solidarity was possible or desired by mad activists with the most well established of all working-class organizations in Ontario—trade unions.

Probably nowhere else during this period was there as contentious a relationship as that which existed between mad activists and hospital unions. Much of this was due to the front-line nature of work for people on both sides in an era of deinstitutionalization, loss of hospital jobs, the extension of civil rights to people in mental institutions and conflicts between patients' rights advocates and unionized employees. Perhaps the most visible dispute between both groups in recent Ontario history was during the March 1996 Ontario Public Sector Employees Union (OPSEU) strike, which affected provincial mental hospitals. As Lilith Finkler, a Community Legal Worker in Toronto at that time has written, "The interests of workers conflicted directly with the needs of patients."[51]

Tension between hospital staff and patients have existed in Ontario's mental institutions since the nineteenth century over issues of power and abuse.[52] These tensions have taken on a more public form with the advent of widespread organized activism by ex-patients which has led to conflicts between unions representing staff and groups representing psychiatric patients. One of the earliest examples of political differences between organized patient activists and unions was expressed in an article in a 1981 issue of *Phoenix Rising* which discussed an OPSEU critique of the province's psychiatric system. First published as a pamphlet in 1980 and then, two years later as a book, this study was written in the wake of the closure of Toronto's Lakeshore Psychiatric Hospital in 1979 and focused on government layoffs and staff cutbacks.[53] Noting that the tone of the original 1980 booklet was one of "righteous anger", *Phoenix Rising* pointed out that union members "could lose their jobs for speaking out" about abuses. The article concluded: "The battle against institutional psychiatry must be waged chiefly by inmates and former inmates. OPSEU's 'mental health' workers are welcome to help in this struggle, providing they join us as *equals*."[54]

The difficult position which staff members faced when speaking out about abuse was evident in early 1981. Mavis MacKenzie, a nurse with twenty years of experience, was fired from Scarborough Centenary Hospital, located in a Toronto suburb, where she worked on the psychiatric ward after complaining about staff neglect of an elderly patient that led to the death of Jamila Tissawak, an elderly woman who spoke only Arabic. Though translators were available staff dismissed this woman's complaints that referred to her eventually fatal liver or kidney failure as having been "all in her head". Other staff did not support their fired colleague.[55]

There were episodes when unions did fight abuse and neglect of patients, such as at a nursing home in Toronto.[56] It was evident, however, that when mad people tried to initiate charges and were supported by individual staff members, solidarity between most other staff with patients was non-existent. A patient in the Ontario provincial hospital in St Thomas, named Leigh, wrote in 1987: "When we try to improve conditions, Robert Cunningham, our administrator, accuses us of being manipulative and trying to control the ward—that is wresting control from the 'pros'. A very small minority of the staff has been good. Some of these staff members have been hounded out of their jobs, falsely accused by other staff. Their crime: being supportive to patients like us: the 'personality disorders', 'schizos', and 'psychopaths'."[57] Thus, staff could oppress other staff who took the side of patients when it came to patient-initiated advocacy efforts. When organized staff members protested abuse of patients, this was far more likely to get widespread support than when patients and mad activists protested abuses even with the support of individual staff. Only when an isolated staff member went outside of the hospital that they worked at and reported abuse to outsiders were more rights violations able to get wider attention. Perhaps the most publicized example of such an occurrence during this period was in 1980 when nineteen-year-old Aldo Alviani died after being given a massive and ultimately lethal overdose of powerful drugs at Toronto's oldest psychiatric institution. The manner of his death thirty-six hours after admission was only made public three months later when an anonymous hospital staff member leaked part of Alviani's medical file to Mike Breaugh, health critic for the opposition New Democratic Party in the Ontario provincial legislature, who in turn made this information public. Hospital administrators afterwards responded by defending the use of forced medication on "aggressive" patients.[58] After his death was exposed, the first rally and march in Ontario led by ex-psychiatric inmates took place at the provincial legislature on 3 October 1980, attended by about thirty people. The rally ended with a march to the psychiatric facility where Alviani died with a five-minute vigil in memory of patients whose death was caused by over-drugging. An inquest was held in November 1980 which eventually led to the founding of a provincially funded advocate's office; however, this did not resolve the need for advocacy issues in the long run.[59]

Staff complaints of abuse by patients are an area where unions and psychiatric patients' advocates have had some of their sharpest differences. In a July 1991 newsletter for OPSEU Local 531, which represented workers at Queen Street Mental Health Centre, the lead article was entitled 'Campaign for the Prevention of Cruelty to Staff', in which it was noted that just under one staff person a day was injured by patients, though no figures were given on patients injured by staff. The article went on to state that the reasons for the injuries include the "undermedication" of patients; restraints were not used enough; "shrinks are intimidated by lawyers, patients advocates, etc."; "policies (e.g. on restraint) address patient welfare and rights, not staff safety as a priority". In addition to these comments in this July 1991 union newsletter, there was also on the front page, right next to the story about abuse, a cartoon which had four large angry-looking dinosaurs surrounding a cave from which a voice came out stating, "OK people, our safety meeting is over! Everybody back outside!"[60]

This newsletter's message was that safeguards which were in place to protect patients' rights were causing problems for the staff, to the point that patients were portrayed as dinosaurs right next to the story about staff being abused by patients (Fig. 15.1).[61] There was no indication in this newsletter that patients could also be victims of abuse from staff, and that the vast majority of patients did not abuse staff.

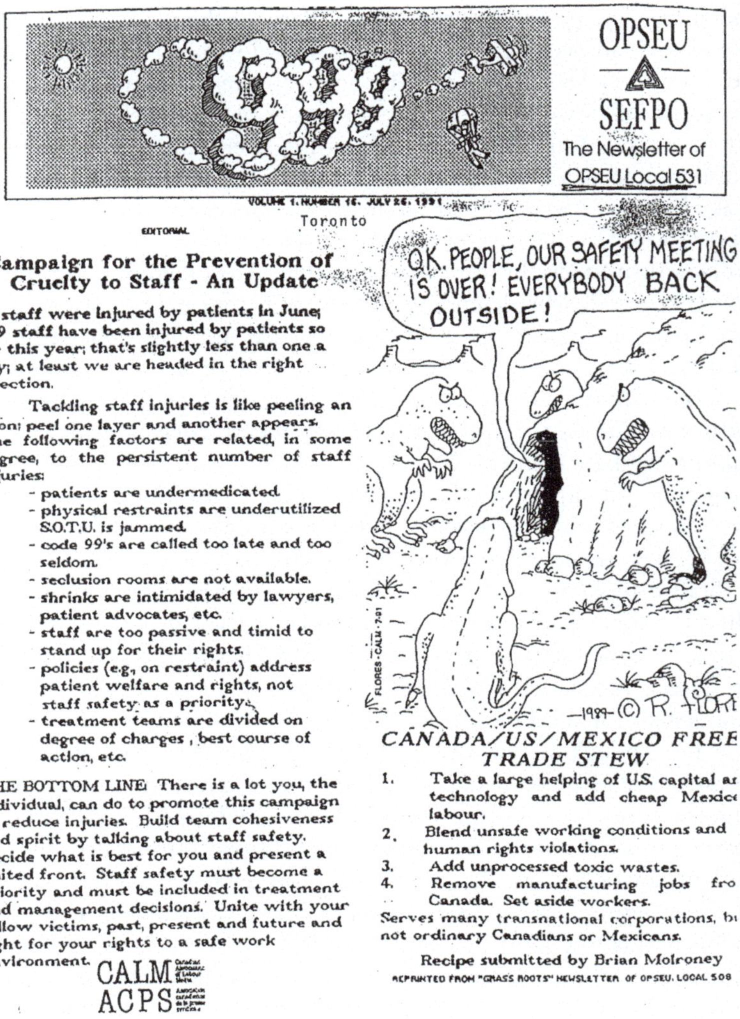

999
OPSEU
SEFPO
The Newsletter of
OPSEU Local 531
VOLUME 1, NUMBER 16, JULY 26, 1991
Toronto
O.K. PEOPLE, OUR SAFETY MEETING IS OVER! EVERYBODY BACK OUTSIDE!
FLORES · CALM · 7-91
—1989— © R. FLORE

EDITORIAL

Campaign for the Prevention of Cruelty to Staff - An Update

33 staff were injured by patients in June; 179 staff have been injured by patients so far this year; that's slightly less than one a day; at least we are headed in the right direction.

Tackling staff injuries is like peeling an onion: peel one layer and another appears. The following factors are related, in some degree, to the persistent number of staff injuries:

- patients are undermedicated.
- physical restraints are underutilized S.O.T.U. is jammed.
- code 99's are called too late and too seldom.
- seclusion rooms are not available.
- shrinks are intimidated by lawyers, patient advocates, etc.
- staff are too passive and timid to stand up for their rights.
- policies (e.g., on restraint) address patient welfare and rights, not staff safety as a priority.
- treatment teams are divided on degree of charges , best course of action, etc.

THE BOTTOM LINE: There is a lot you, the individual, can do to promote this campaign to reduce injuries. Build team cohesiveness and spirit by talking about staff safety. Decide what is best for you and present a united front. Staff safety must become a priority and must be included in treatment and management decisions. Unite with your fellow victims, past, present and future and fight for your rights to a safe work environment.

CALM
ACPS

CANADA/US/MEXICO FREE TRADE STEW

1. Take a large helping of U.S. capital ar technology and add cheap Mexic labour.
2. Blend unsafe working conditions and human rights violations.
3. Add unprocessed toxic wastes.
4. Remove manufacturing jobs fro Canada. Set aside workers.

Serves many transnational corporations, b not ordinary Canadians or Mexicans.

Recipe submitted by Brian Molroney

REPRINTED FROM "GRASS ROOTS" NEWSLETTER OF OPSEU, LOCAL 508

Fig. 15.1 Campaign Newsletter, 1991

When a former patient obtained of a copy of this newsletter and demanded an apology, the union local which produced it ignored this request. It was not until the story was reported two months later in a free weekly Toronto magazine that a union spokesperson claimed that the dinosaurs did not represent patients, though he said OPSEU would apologize. No such apology, however, was ever offered regarding this episode. Carla McKague, a former psychiatric inmate, and at that time a lawyer with the Advocacy Resource Centre for the Handicapped, noted that the staff were "very hostile about some of the civil liberties advances that have been made" by psychiatric patients.[62]

Along with ongoing disputes over patient advocacy, some of the most vocal differences between unions and civil rights advocates centred on deinstitutionalization and transferring large numbers of psychiatric patients to the community. The hospital workers' union, OPSEU, was vocal in protesting these policies. Advocates working with mad people have generally welcomed community-based approaches but also decried government funding cutbacks that have left many discharged patients with little or no supports once they leave the hospital, resulting in homelessness or living in wretched rooming houses.[63]

Hospital union activists criticized community-based funding as ineffective in which provincial governments wanted to save money by having municipalities and private agencies pay for them instead. Kingston OPSEU Local 431 president, Ron Lavigne, said in 1994, "The government likes to dress up these cuts as mental health reform, but it is just a money grab off the backs of the weak."[64] On the other hand, less than three months later another OPSEU leader, Warren Thomas, said the transferal of funding to the community was a good thing, so long as union jobs went with it.[65] However, due to the uncertainty of who would get these jobs, widespread resistance to community funding for mental health services from within hospital unions persisted. When the Ontario New Democratic Party Government Minister of Health Ruth Grier announced in 1993 that the mental health budget transferred to the community would rise from 20 per cent to 60 per cent over a ten-year period, she was met with 'audible anger' by union members at an OPSEU-organized symposium on mental health care who were angry because of potential job losses. At this same union event, June Beeby of the family-run Ontario Friends of Schizophrenics (OFOS) was given a standing ovation when she denounced a government that "was spending millions on a legalistic advocacy system for patients, and cutting the salaries of those who provide the care and treatment to these vulnerable people".[66]

The tension on the left between psychiatric patients and their advocates on one side and unions representing hospital employees on the other side could not have been starker than the divisions which this event illustrates. A representative of an organization, the Ontario Friends of Schizophrenics, that had been in the forefront of opposing patients civil rights advances is given a warm welcome by union members when she attacks the funding of a legal advocacy system for psychiatric patients and, by extension, for disabled people more generally through the then proposed Ontario Advocacy Commission. This was done by using key words such as referring to patients as "vulnerable people" even though the advocacy system which Beeby was attacking was essential to protecting these very same people from the vulnerability that so many institutionalized people have endured. By conflating the progressive advance of rights for psychiatric patients with staff cutbacks, the OFOS spokesperson linked both issues in an effort to curb these rights—why should patients get more rights through a wasteful legal system, she was saying, when staff were losing money? This anti-advocacy position, when advocacy was initiated by mad and disabled activists, was at the core of the dispute about whose voice was deemed most privileged in speaking on behalf of people with a psychiatric history: ex-patient advocates or hospital staff and family members. Linking up with the hospital union in trying to curtail mad people's advocacy was very much a strategy to isolate patients' rights advocates on the left. This linkage was not too difficult to create since historical differences already existed to foster this approach.

The organization whose representative was given a standing ovation at the hospital union workers' conference was, a few short years later, enthusiastically supporting the anti-union Ontario Conservative Government of Michael Harris, elected in 1995.[67] This government enacted some of the most draconian attacks on the civil rights of patients since the 1970s in the form of Community Treatment Orders (CTO). When mad activist efforts to oppose community treatment orders was in full swing in 2000, most of the well-established left in Ontario were silent with some exceptions, notably the grass-roots-based Ontario Coalition Against Poverty. The main opposition to CTOs among activists was due to their coercive nature, in which people who live in the community are forced by medical monitoring teams to take their drugs.[68] Mad activists and some allies protested the introduction of this new law as did some legislators from the provincial New Democratic Party on 1 December 2000 outside the provincial legislature in Toronto. As one of the speakers, Diana Capponi, observed that day, most left-wing social justice groups were notable by their absence.[69]

Conclusion

Efforts to establish working relationships between mad activists and other left-wing social justice groups met with some success during a period influenced by identity politics and, in the later years of the twentieth century, by government downloading of social services into local communities. Activists in the disability community forged links on issues affecting human rights protections and a mutual desire to advance civic involvement among all people labelled disabled. In a similar political alliance, feminists, gays and lesbians were all part of the mad movement from the earliest days of activism in Ontario. Their issues became the movement's issues in a joint effort to address identity politics and prejudices within and without activist groups. Yet, mad activism did not appeal as widely as activists had wanted. The significant lack of people from racialized communities in mad movement politics, though not uniform in every respect, was nevertheless generally acknowledged and reflected who could more safely identify as mad and who could not. Thus, the mad movement did not establish links with activist groups in racially diverse communities for most of the period studied here to build an effective coalition that represented wider constituencies, until such links began to be developed during the late 1990s following police killing of racially marginalized mad and disabled people.

In class terms, it is not surprising that the mad movement was widely represented by people from a broad socio-economic stratum, given the numbers of people discharged from public institutions during this period. This did not, however, translate into wider class identity solidarity beyond mad movement activists, as can be seen in regard to hospital unions. Relations between hospital workers' unions and psychiatric patient rights advocates were characterized by mutual mistrust. Unlike some other left-wing social justice activists where engagement with mad people was welcomed and sought, the significant power struggle between the rights of current and former psychiatric patients and the job security of hospital staff militated against common ground being found since both sides had such different objectives over whose rights deserved most protection and how and whose voice was most privileged in these debates. As well, power differentials were significant, both within the mental health system and among the established left where, in both instances, hospital workers and their union held greater influence than mad activists and their constituency. Unlike unions which are well established with a long history of fighting for workers' rights, organized psychiatric patients' activists, while dating back to the nineteenth century in the Western world, have generally not had the resources, long local history and clout of the more established non-psychiatrized left. Yet it is also clear that where support was obtained this was most achievable in those communities which had the most to gain from engaging mad activists on the left due to mutual interests and similar histories of being ostracized for who they were as people. This was particularly so where identity politics crossed over between different communities that intersected in so many personal and political ways. That these efforts were much less successful with people of colour, the most marginalized population in the mad community, raises questions about how identity politics worked to exclude as much as to include in Ontario's mad politics during the last three decades of the twentieth century.

Notes

1. David Oaks, "Editorial," *Dendron*, (1996) Vol. 37/38, 3.
2. Linda Morrison, *Talking Back to Psychiatry: The Psychiatric Consumer/Survivor/Ex-Patient Movement* (New York: Routledge, 2005); Duncan Scott Campbell, *Unsettled: Discourse, Practice, Context and Collective Identity among Mad People in the United States, 1970–1999* (PhD Dissertation, Faculty of Environmental Studies, York University, 2011).
3. Geoffrey Reaume, "Lunatic to Patient to Person: Nomenclature in Psychiatric History and the Influence of Patients' Activism in North America," *International Journal of Law and Psychiatry.* 25, no. 4 (July/August 2002): 405–426.
4. Barbara Everett, *A Fragile Revolution: Consumers and Psychiatric Survivors Confront the Power of the Mental Health System* (Waterloo, Ontario: Wilfrid Laurier University Press, 2000), 53–58.
5. Morrison, *Talking Back to Psychiatry*, 66–80.
6. Diane Driedger, *The Last Civil Rights Movement: Disabled People's International* (New York: St. Martin's Press, 1989); Doris Zames Fleischer and Frieda Zames, *The Disability Rights Movement: From Charity to Confrontation* (Philadelphia: Temple University Press, 2001); Sharon

Barnartt and Richard Scotch, *Disability Protests: Contentious Politics, 1970–1999* (Washington, D.C.: Gallaudet University Press, 2001); Sharon Barnartt, "Social Movement Diffusion? The Case of Disability Protests in the US and Canada," *Disability Studies Quarterly* 28, no. 1 (2008); Melissa Graham and Kevin Jackson, "Divided No More: The Toronto Disability Pride March and the Challenges of Inclusive Organizing," in *Mobilizing Metaphor: Art, Culture, and Disability Activism in Canada*, eds. Christine Kelly and Michael Orsini (Vancouver: University of British Columbia Press, 2016), 279–288; Diane Driedger, "Organizing for Change: The Origins and History of the Manitoba League of the Physically Handicapped, 1967–1982," in *Untold Stories: A Canadian Disability History Reader*, eds. Nancy Hansen, Roy Hanes and Diane Driedger (Toronto: Canadian Scholars' Press, 2018), 221–242; April D'Aubin, "The Council of Canadians with Disabilities: A Voice of Our Own, 1976–2012," in *Untold Stories: A Canadian Disability History Reader*, eds. Nancy Hansen, Roy Hanes and Diane Driedger (Toronto: Canadian Scholars' Press, 2018), 243–267.

7. Nicholas Hervey, "Advocacy or Folly: The Alleged Lunatics' Friends Society, 1845–63," *Medical History* 30:3 (July 1986): 245–275; Ann Goldberg, "A Reinvented Public: Lunatics' Rights and Bourgeois Populism in the Kaiserreich," *German History* 21:2 (May 2003): 159–182; Linda Carlisle, *Elizabeth Packard: A Noble Fight* (Urbana: University of Illinois Press, 2010); Neree St-Amand and Eugene LeBlanc, "Women in 19th-Century Asylums: Three Exemplary Women; A New Brunswick Hero," in *Mad Matters: A Critical Reader in Canadian Mad Studies*, eds. Brenda LeFrancois, Robert Menzies and Geoffrey Reaume (Toronto: Canadian Scholars' Press, 2013): 38–48.
8. Dale Peterson, ed., *A Mad People's History of Madness* (Pittsburgh: University of Pittsburgh Press, 1982); Roy Porter, *A Social History of Madness: Stories of the Insane* (London: Weidenfeld and Nicolson, 1987); Jeffrey Geller and Maxine Harris, eds., *Women of the Asylum: Voices from Behind the Walls, 1840–1945* (New York: Anchor Books, 1994); Allan Ingram, ed., *Voices of Madness: Four Pamphlets, 1683–1796.* (Gloucestershire: Sutton Publishing, 1997); Erick Fabris, *Tranquil Prisons: Chemical Incarceration Under Community Treatment Orders* (Toronto: University of Toronto Press, 2011), 80–84, 175–77
9. Lennard J. Davis, *Bending over Backwards: Disability, Dismodernism & Other Difficult Positions* (New York: New York University Press, 2002), 13.
10. Lenny Lapon, *Mass Murderers in White Coats: Psychiatric Genocide in Nazi Germany and the United States* (Springfield, MA: Psychiatric Genocide Research Institute, 1986).

11. Steve Holochuck, "Alienation, not mental illness," *Phoenix Rising*, 4:2 (1983), 44–45.
12. Davis, *Bending over Backwards*, 85, 101.
13. John Marshall, *Madness: An Indictment of the Mental Health Care System in Ontario* (Toronto: Ontario Public Service Employees Union, 1982).
14. Lapon, *Mass Murderers in White Coats*, 159–216; Judi Chamberlin, "The Ex-Patients' Movement: Where We've Been and Where We're Going," *Journal of Mind and Behavior* 11, no. 3 (Summer/Autumn 1990): 323–336; Irit Shimrat, *Call Me Crazy: Stories from the Mad Movement* (Vancouver: Press Gang, 1997); Everett, *A Fragile Revolution*; Morrison, *Talking Back to Psychiatry*; Nancy Tomes, "The Patient as A Policy Factor: A Historical Case Study of the Consumer/ Survivor Movement in Mental Health," *Health Affairs*, 25, no. 3 (May–June 2006): 720–729; Campbell, "Unsettled"; David Reville and Kathryn Church, "Mad Activism Enters Its Fifth Decade: Psychiatric Survivor Organizing in Toronto," in *Organize! Building from the Local for Global Justice*, eds. A. Choudry, J. Hanley, E. Shragge, (Oakland, CA: PM Press, 2012), 189–201; Erika Dyck and Alex Deighton, *Managing Madness: Weyburn Mental Hospital and the Transformation of Psychiatric Care in Canada* (Winnipeg: University of Manitoba Press, 2017), 200–228.
15. Elena Demke, "Brutal sanity and mad compassion. On the genealogy of the voice of Dorothea Buck: a survivor," in Rob Ellis, Sarah Kendal and Steven Taylor (eds) *Voices in the History of Madness: Personal and Professional Perspectives on Mental Health and Illness* (London: Palgrave Macmillan, 2021).
16. Lapon, *Mass Murderers in White Coats*; Shimrat, *Call Me Crazy*; Everett, *A Fragile Revolution*; Campbell, "Unsettled".
17. Patricia Sealy and Paul Whitehead, "Forty Years of Deinstitutionalization of Psychiatric Services in Canada: An Empirical Assessment," *Canadian Journal of Psychiatry* 49:4 (April 2004), 251, Table 1.
18. Sealy and Whitehead, Forty Years of Deinstitutionalization, 251, Table 1.
19. Harvey Simmons, *Unbalanced: Mental Health Policy in Ontario, 1930–1989* (Toronto: Wall & Thompson, 1990), 157–161; Megan Davies, Erika Dyck, Leslie Baker, Lanny Beckman, Geertje Boschma, Chris Dooley, Kathleen Kendall, Eugene LeBlanc, Robert Menzies, Marina Morrow, Diane Purvey, Neree St-Amand, Marie-Claude Thifault, Jane Melville Whyte, and Victor Willis, "After the Asylum in Canada: Surviving Deinstitutionalisation and Revising History," in *Deinstitutionalisation and After: Post-War Psychiatry in the Western World*, eds. D. Kritsotaki, V. Long, M. Smith, (Cham, Switzerland: Palgrave Macmillan, 2016), 75–95.
20. Sealy and Whitehead, Forty Years of Deinstitutionalization, 253, Table 4.
21. Sealy and Whitehead, Forty Years of Deinstitutionalization, 256; Everett, *A Fragile Revolution*, 38; Elizabeth Tobin LeBlanc Haley, "Transinstitutionalization: A Feminist Political Economy Analysis of

Ontario's Public Mental Health Care System" (PhD Dissertation, Department of Political Science, York University, 2017).

22. Lanny Beckman and Megan J. Davies, "Democracy is a Very Radical Idea," in *Mad Matters: A Critical Reader in Canadian Mad Studies*, eds. Brenda LeFrancois, Robert Menzies and Geoffrey Reaume (Toronto: Canadian Scholars' Press, 2013), 49–63. For developments in Toronto see: Don Weitz, "Notes of a Schizophrenic Shitdisturber," in *Shrink Resistant: The Struggle Against Psychiatry in Canada*, eds. Bonnie Burstow and Don Weitz (Vancouver: New Star Books, 1988), 291–292.
23. Mike Yale, "Blindness: More than meets the eye," *Phoenix Rising*, 1:2 (1980), 27.
24. "Rights for the Handicapped: Psychiatric inmates need not apply," *Phoenix Rising*, 1:1 (1980), 20; Nicholas Ignatieff, "Letter to the editor," *Phoenix Rising*, 1:2 (1980), 3–4; "New Ontario Human Rights legislation," *Phoenix Rising*, 2:2 (1981), 24–25.
25. Dustin Galer, *Working Towards Equity: Disability Rights Activism and Employment in Late-Twentieth Century Canada* (Toronto: University of Toronto Press, 2018), 82–86.
26. COPOH, *Phoenix Rising*, 8:1 (1988), 30.
27. "Where to go when you have a problem: General Legal Help – Free Advice and Assistance" [list of publicly funded legal clinics in Ontario], *Phoenix Rising*, 5:2&3 (1985), 38A; "Ontario extends legal aid for psychiatric victims," *Phoenix Rising*, 5:4 (1985), 41.
28. Don Weitz, "Symposium on patients' rights", *Phoenix Rising*, 2:4 (1982), 28.
29. Carla McKague, Obituary, *Toronto Star*, 26 September 2015.
30. "Revised Election Act lessens Voting Discrimination: Section 16(2)2 of Bill 17 excluded psychiatric inmates", *Phoenix Rising*, 5:2&3 (1985), 28A–30A; "Voting Rights Restored to Some Inmates", *Phoenix Rising*, 5:4 (1985), 43.
31. "Coming Forward: from Kingston Psychiatric to City Hall," *Phoenix Rising*, 2:1 (1981), front cover and inside story: David Reville, "Don't Spyhole Me," *Phoenix Rising*, 2:1 (1981), 22 page insert.
32. Don Weitz, "Inmates fought to exercise fundamental rights," *Phoenix Rising*, 8:2 (1989), 27–28.
33. "Human Rights Day Events," *Phoenix Rising*, 7:4 (1988), 28.
34. Peter Beresford, "What Have Madness and Psychiatric System Survivors Got to Do with Disability and Disability Studies?" *Disability & Society* 15, no. 1 (January, 2000), 167–172.
35. Morrison, *Talking Back to Psychiatry*, 78–79. See also: Geoffrey Reaume, "A History of Psychiatric Survivor Pride Day during the 1990s," *The Consumer/Survivor Information Resource Centre Bulletin* [Toronto], No. 374, July 14, 2008, 2–3: http://www.csinfo.ca/bulletin/Bulletin_374.pdf. Accessed on 10 August 2020.

36. Don Weitz, "11th Annual International Conference for Human Rights and Against Psychiatric Oppression," *Phoenix Rising*, 4:1 (1983), 14.
37. A few examples of the vast historiography of colonialism and racism in Canada include: Howard Adams, *Prison of Grass: Canada from a Native Point of View* (Rev. ed. Saskatoon: Fifth House, 1989); Constance Backhouse, *Colour-Coded: A Legal History of Racism in Canada, 1900–1950* (Toronto: University of Toronto Press, 1999); Afua Cooper, *The Hanging of Angélique: The Untold Story of Canadian Slavery and the Burning of Old Montréal* (Toronto: HarperCollins, 2006); John Lutz, *Makúk: A New History of Aboriginal-White Relations* (Vancouver: University of British Columbia Press, 2008); Karen Stote, *An Act of Genocide: Colonialism and the Sterilization of Aboriginal Women* (Halifax: Fernwood Publishing, 2015); Robyn Maynard, *Policing Black Lives: State Violence in Canada from Slavery to the Present* (Halifax: Fernwood Publishing, 2017).
38. Lionel Vermette, "The 33 Years of the Lost Indian Walk," in B. Burstow & D. Weitz, (eds), *Shrink Resistant: The Struggle Against Psychiatry in Canada* (Vancouver: New Star Books, 1988), 117–120; Vern Harper, "Them Crazy Indians," in B. Burstow & D. Weitz, (eds), *Shrink Resistant: The Struggle Against Psychiatry in Canada* (Vancouver: New Star Books, 1988), 121–125.
39. The targeting of Black people by Toronto police continues long past the period covered by this chapter: Wendy Gillis and Jim Rankin, "Black people far more likely to be arrested, charged, shot, and killed by Toronto Police, Ontario Human Rights Commission finds," *Toronto Star*, 10 August 2020. Available at: https://www.thestar.com/news/gta/2020/08/10/black-people-more-likely-to-be-arrested-charged-shot-and-killed-by-toronto-police-ontario-human-rights-commission-report-finds.html.
40. Mab Segrest, *Administrations of Lunacy: Racism and the Haunting of American Psychiatry at the Milledgeville Asylum* (New York: The New Press, 2020); Therí Alyce Pickens, *Black Madness: Mad Blackness* (Durham: Duke University Press, 2019); Wendy Gonaver, *The Peculiar Institution and the Making of Modern Psychiatry, 1840–1880* (Chapel Hill: University of North Carolina Press, 2019); Jonathan Metzl, *The Protest Psychosis: How Schizophrenia Became a Black Disease* (Boston: Beacon Press, 2010).
41. Ahmad Saidullah, et al., *Saving Lives: Alternatives to the Use of Lethal Force by Police – Report of a Conference Held in Toronto, June 23–24, 2000, Urban Alliance on Race Relations, Queen Street Patients Council* (Toronto: Urban Alliance on Race Relations, 2002).
42. Virginia Raymond, Dana Lear, Rene Bostick, Laurie Bradford, Judi Chamberlin, Susan Price, Jeanne Dumont, "Mental health and violence

against women: a feminist ex-inmate analysis," *Phoenix Rising*, 3:3 (1983), 43–47.
43. Don Weitz, "11th Annual International Conference for Human Rights and Against Psychiatric Oppression," *Phoenix Rising*, 4:1 (1983), 14–15.
44. Thirty-two issues of *Phoenix Rising* were published in Toronto during its ten-year existence from 1980 to 1990.
45. Barry Adam, *The Rise of a Gay and Lesbian Movement* (Boston: Twayne Publishers, 1987), 81–82.
46. Bonnie Burstow, "A History of Psychiatric Homophobia," *Phoenix Rising*, 8:3&4 (July, 1990), S38–S39.
47. Lilith Finkler, "Psychiatric Survivor Pride Day: Community Organizing with Psychiatric Survivors," *Osgoode Hall Law Journal* 35:3 & 4 (Fall and Winter 1997), 766.
48. Where we're coming from," *Phoenix Rising*, 1:1 (1980), 2–3.
49. *Cuckoo's Nest* was published in Toronto from 1979–1986. See also Capponi's book on this topic, Pat Capponi, *Upstairs in the Crazy House: The Life of a Psychiatric Survivor* (Toronto: Viking, 1992).
50. Irit Shimrat, "Angry Roomers Protest," *Phoenix Rising*, 6:4 (1987), 26.
51. Lilith Finkler, *Our Times*, 15 (1996), 13.
52. James Moran, "Keepers of the Insane: The Role of Attendants at the Toronto Provincial Asylum, 1875–1905," *Histoire Sociale/Social History* 28, no. 55 (May 1995): 51–75; Geoffrey Reaume, "Accounts of Abuse of Patients at the Toronto Hospital for the Insane, 1883–1937," *Canadian Bulletin of Medical History* 14, no.1 (1997): 65–106.
53. Marshall, *Madness.*
54. "Union attacks psychiatric system", *Phoenix Rising*, 1:4 (1981), 31.
55. "Nurse blows whistle on staff neglect," *Phoenix Rising*, 2:1 (1981), 17–18.
56. "Dumped & Drugged – a special report on the aged", *Phoenix Rising*, 2:4 (1982), 12.
57. Leigh [no last name], St. Thomas, Ontario, "Letter to the editor," *Phoenix Rising*, 7:1 (1987), 4.
58. "The Death of Aldo Alviani," *Phoenix Rising*, 1:3 (1980), inside front cover and inside back cover.
59. "On Our Own," *Phoenix Rising*, 1:3 (1980), 4–6; "Aldo: The Inquest and After," *Phoenix Rising*, 1:4 (1981), 5–7; Catherine Rodd, "A baffling death by misadventure," *Maclean's*, 8 December, 1980: https://archive.macleans.ca/article/1980/12/8/a-baffling-death-by-misadventure. Accessed, 10 August 2020; Ty Turner, "The Early Origin of the Psychiatric Patient Advocate Office," In *Mental Health and Patients' Rights in Ontario: Yesterday, Today and Tomorrow – 20th Anniversary Special Report, May 2003, Psychiatric Patient Advocate Office* (Toronto: Queen's Printer, 2003), 6–8. This article does not mention Aldo Alviani by name

but refers to the influence of three coroner's inquests into deaths at Queen Street Mental Health Centre in 1981, of which Alviani's death was one, though he in fact died in 1980.

60. "Editorial: Campaign for the Prevention of Cruelty to Staff – An Update," *999: The Newsletter of OPSEU Local 531* 1:16 (26 July 1991). I would like to thank Josie, a former psychiatric patient and former nurse, for providing me with a copy of this newsletter shortly after it was issued in 1991.
61. Ibid.
62. *NOW Magazine*, Toronto, local news column, 26 September–2 October 1991 issue. The reference to Josie, a former patient and former nurse, who obtained a copy of this newsletter and demanded an apology from the union for it but was ignored, is based on my memory of this episode.
63. See, for example, two issues of *Phoenix Rising* for which housing was the cover theme for each issue: "Health begins at home....if you have one!" *Phoenix Rising*, 3:2 (1982); "Housing Options: Getting Walter out of Queen Street; Channon Court: A Boarding House Renewed," *Phoenix Rising*, 7:1 (1987).
64. *OPSEU* [Ontario Public Service Employees Union] *News*, 31 August 1994. I would like to thank Chava (Lilith) Finkler, a former member of OPSEU when she worked as a community legal worker at Parkdale Community Legal Services in Toronto, 1992–1999, for providing me with the *OPSEU News* sources in this article.
65. *OPSEU News*, 16 November 1994.
66. *OPSEU News*, 13 October 1993.
67. Douglas James Nesbitt, "Days of Action: Ontario's Extra-Parliamentary Opposition to the Common Sense Revolution, 1995–1998" (PhD Dissertation, Department of History, Queen's University, 2018). Accessed 10 August 2020 at: http://hdl.handle.net/1974/24271.
68. Fabris, *Tranquil Prisons*, 48–55.
69. Information about the 1 December 2000 protest is based on the author's recollection.

CHAPTER 16

Knowing Our Own Minds: Transforming the Knowledge Base of Madness and Distress

Alison Faulkner

The voices of people deemed mad or mentally ill are largely silenced by society and by mental health services, professionals and research intent on rendering us as 'other', on controlling and containing us. We are written about and talked about, treated, measured and counted, but mostly remain silent and silenced about our experiences of mental distress and of using services.

> historically, our experiences have been disbelieved or dismissed, while our distress has been reduced to symptoms of psychiatric conditions. (Sweeney 2013, p. 5)

In this chapter, I write from the perspective of a survivor researcher, someone who has been an ex-user and survivor of mental health services alongside having academic qualifications. I focus on the vital role that personal narratives play in the lives of people deemed mad and the value of the knowledge that emerges when people have safe spaces in which to share their stories. I outline the challenges that prevent people from

A. Faulkner (✉)
London, UK

R. Ellis et al. (eds.), *Voices in the History of Madness*, Mental Health in Historical Perspective,
https://doi.org/10.1007/978-3-030-69559-0_16

finding their voices and telling their stories without judgement and with credibility. These challenges come from within society and psychiatry, from the majority of researchers, clinicians and historians who seek to categorise, reframe and reinterpret voices of madness in the belief that their knowledge is better. Even historians who claim to be 'on our side' see us through the lens of their own and associated disciplines (Hayward 2014). As such, we rarely have the chance to give voice to our experiences *on our own terms*—without preconceived notions of what we can or cannot talk about constructed by others. And, as people deemed mad, we continue to face the ultimate challenge:

> the societal belief that people with psychiatric diagnoses or mental health challenges are not credible reporters or witnesses of our own experiences. When we speak we are not believed. (Wilda White, Vermont Psychiatric Survivors, 2018)

This issue and the challenges that face people deemed mad to be heard and taken seriously lie at the core of this chapter. It begins with a brief overview of the history of the UK service user/survivor movements: early accounts of people finding their voices in individual stories and collective action. I then outline the role and value of the experiential knowledge that emerges from shared experiences and how this can be developed and validated through peer support, activism and survivor research. I then outline the many challenges faced in the struggle to have our knowledge recognised as valid knowledge in its own right. Finally, I touch on the potential for Mad Studies to carry the baton into the future: through severing the links both with biomedical sciences and Patient and Public Involvement (PPI) and creating new connections across different disciplines.

Finding Our Voices: A Brief History

Finding our voices and telling our stories *on our own terms* has been central to the development of the service user/survivor movement(s), central to our shared history of organising for change (Costa et al. 2012). Many individual accounts of people's experiences of being deemed mad or incarcerated have surfaced over the years. One example in the UK is that of Margery Kempe, who wrote in 1436 of her experience of going 'out of her mind' after childbirth, which she understood as a spiritual journey (Staley 1996). In the US, Clifford Beers wrote an account in 1905 of his experiences of being incarcerated in 'A Mind that Found Itself' and is attributed with founding the mental hygiene movement (Beers 1981). In 1922, Rachel Grant-Smith (a pseudonym) wrote an account of her experiences of incarceration in five different asylums in England following the death of her husband. In 'Experiences of an Asylum Patient', she reflects on the impact of being certified mad:

> Once tainted with a certificate of madness, every statement made by the so-called lunatic can be characterised as a further sign of his or her unsoundness of mind. (Grant-Smith 1922, p. 50)

Throughout these early accounts, there is a persistent theme of people challenging treatments and incarceration, as well as challenging the validity of their own and others' supposed madness. This thread can be traced forward into the 1970s when a number of developments began what we might call the modern psychiatric survivor movements. In 1971, patients in the locked wards of a Scottish mental hospital established themselves as a 'union of mental patients' and began the Scottish Union of Mental Patients (SUMP). A related development in England, the Mental Patients' Union (MPU), came into being the following year. They and others were part of the movement that became the 'Federation of Mental Patients Unions' after a Manchester conference in April 1974 (Campbell and Roberts 2009). The mid-1980s in the UK became a particularly active period with the birth oforganisations like the Campaign Against Psychiatric Oppression, Survivors Speak Out, MINDLink (attached to mental health charity Mind), Nottingham Advocacy Group and, at the end of that decade and the beginning of the 1990s, the UK Advocacy Network, the National Self Harm Network and Hearing Voices Network. Many of these groups took a predominantly rights-based approach, seeking to assert their rights and the validity of their voice, about issues such as self-harm, self-advocacy, hearing voices or alternatives to hospitalisation and against forced medication (amongst other things) (Campbell and Rose 2011).

Most conventional accounts of the UK user/survivor movement exclude the contributions and activities of people from marginalised and racialised communities (Kalathil and Jones 2016; Kalathil 2013).There is some debate as to whether or not there is a single mental health user/survivor movement, or whether it is better to conceive of a plurality of movements. There is not a strong history of inclusion within what has been termed the 'user/survivor movement' in the UK (Wallcraft and

Bryant 2013; Kalathil and Jones 2016; Wallcraft et al. 2003).The voices of racialised groups and people marginalised by gender and sexual orientation (and those incarcerated for long periods, for example) have largely been excluded, with some people experiencing discrimination as much from within the user/survivor movement as from society at large (Carr 2013; Kalathil 2013).

In the 1980s and 1990s, there was a proliferation of service user groups, partly in response to the UK government policy directive to involve patients and carers in the design and delivery of health services, enshrined in the 1990 NHS and Community Care Act (Wallcraft et al. 2003). Funding for local groups brought with it the potential for the voices of service users to be heard both locally and nationally. Similar developments were occurring at the time in North America echoing this rise in consumerism, as referenced by Costa and others:

> In the 1980s and 1990s, psychiatric survivors began to insist that their perspectives represented real knowledge of how the psy-complex worked, and that this knowledge must be taken seriously in public decision-making. (Costa et al., p. 89)

This growth of self-organising service user groups was not without its challenges. With funding came the requirement for accountability to the state and to service providers (Campbell and Rose 2011). The 'user involvement' or consumer imperative could take over groups, to the exclusion of the mutual support and self-advocacy they started with (Wallcraft et al. 2003). Statutory services that funded the groups required service user representatives to sit on committees and attend meetings, with the result that 'involvement' in services could dominate a group's agenda. Involvement could easily segue into rubber-stamping: statutory funding inevitably compromises the degree to which a group can challenge the local service, potentially rendering involvement tokenistic (Campbell and Rose 2011; Wallcraft et al. 2003; Russo 2018).

In research too, UK government policy supported the involvement of 'patients and the public', resulting in a proliferation of Patient and Public Involvement (PPI) initiatives across the research platform. As with involvement in services, this can be a mixed blessing. Involvement in research also has the potential to neutralise and depoliticise the authentic voices of madness, with researchers approaching service users who are compliant with their ideology (Rose 2014b; Campbell and Rose 2011).

These mixed experiences of involvement, with the voices of madness diminished by incorporation into mainstream services, research and policy, have turned many activists away from participation towards leadership (Russo 2018; Yiannoullou and Faulkner 2018; McKinley and Yiannoullou 2012):

> So much depends on whether, despite all the hardship involved, we can start to turn the question of how much tokenism we can bear into how much leadership we can provide. (Russo 2018, p. 424)

It is all too easy in such a short space to give what appears to be a coherent yet far from accurate historical narrative. It is not my intention in this chapter to address service user involvement comprehensively, as my focus is on how voices of madness become heard and recognised as valid expressions of experiential knowledge. Suffice it to say that the history is far more complicated than I have outlined here; it is vitally important to read authentic accounts of service users and survivors (Campbell and Rose 2011; Campbell 2005; CAPS 2010; Kalathil 2013). Peter Campbell and Andrew Roberts (2009) write of the Survivors' History Group and the importance of survivors having the opportunity to put forward their (our) own versions of history:[1]

> ... to challenge inaccuracies and the interpretations that are placed on history. As in so many other contexts, when it comes to our history, it should be 'nothing about us without us'. (Campbell and Roberts 2009, p. 35)

Letting Stories Breathe: The Power of Personal Narratives

In this section, I aim to convey the potential power of personal narratives—not just as a route to tell an individual story, although that is important—but as a starting point for developing shared knowledge and expertise. As people who share the experience of distress, we take each other's stories seriously where often professionals do not (Morgan et al. 2016; Faulkner 2017). Telling our stories and listening to each other's stories is a political act and begins the process of creating and believing in individual and collective experiential knowledge, partly as a challenge to professional knowledge but also as knowledge in its own right (Noorani 2013; Morgan et al. 2016).

Sharing our stories with each other is a route through which we come to understand and recognise our experience and expertise (Seebohm et al. 2013), and to redefine or rebuild our identities (Morgan et al. 2016). There is a big difference between a psychiatric case history and a personal narrative (Costa et al. 2012; Morgan et al. 2016); not only is the owner and narrator of the story different but the story, too, takes a different course. The personal narrative is embedded within the political and social context of a person's life; it can document the different roles a person undertakes at different times in their lives and the story and the telling of it can change over time (Morgan et al. 2016; Faulkner 2010; Kalathil 2011b). Case studies, where a story is seen through a psychiatric lens, can fix an individual narrative both in time and in pathology.

Equally, the lack of continuity in mental health care means that people are often required to keep retelling the 'negative storyline' of their experiences (Brown 2008). Indeed, Morgan et al. (2016) suggest that telling our stories 'is both a routine experience and an impossibility' (p. 89) in mental health services. Within the context of a psychiatric interview, our stories can be (re)interpreted through the fixed technical framework of diagnostic categories where a symptom may be seen as the story (see Fig. 16.1). There is little space for 'letting stories breathe' (Frank 2010; Morgan et al. 2016).

Many narratives aim to challenge the dominant mental illness (or illness-recovery) narratives, or challenge the white, hetero-normative narratives that similarly dominate the Western mental health world. The Icarus Project, founded in the US in 2002, describes itself as 'a counter narrative for psychic diversity' (DuBrul 2014). One of the founders writes of creating a space, a new community and a new language for people experiencing mental distress to find and create meaning:

> when you are brave enough to tell your story, other people often feel compelled to tell you their story as well. I learned about the liberatory power of speaking our personal truths and about the power of personal narratives to challenge the power of the dominant narrative. (DuBrul 2014, p. 258)

Finding Safe Spaces

If service users and survivors are to make sense of our experiences on our own terms, we need safe spaces in which to find our voices and share our stories away from societal, conventional academic and psychiatric gazes.

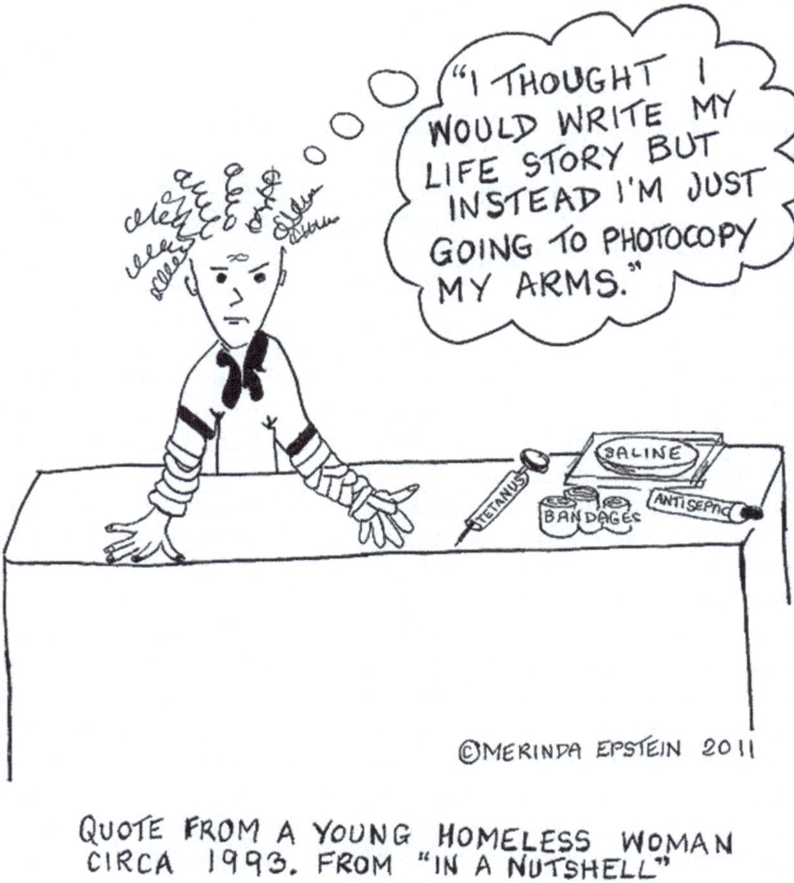
"I THOUGHT I WOULD WRITE MY LIFE STORY BUT INSTEAD I'M JUST GOING TO PHOTOCOPY MY ARMS."
SALINE
TETANUS
BANDAGES
ANTISEPTIC
©MERINDA EPSTEIN 2011
QUOTE FROM A YOUNG HOMELESS WOMAN CIRCA 1993. FROM "IN A NUTSHELL"

Fig. 16.1 Cartoon by Merinda Epstein: the symptom as story

Those spaces can be found within the many self-organised groups created by service users and survivors: service user groups, networks and forums, self-help and peer support spaces. At the turn of the century, Wallcraft et al. (2003) identified a total of 896 service user groups across England and found that 79 percent of them were engaged in self-help and mutual support; indeed, it was the most common activity reported. As Campbell (2005, p. 77) says:

> The successful existence of so many groups is witness to the way in which the activists' belief in the principles of self-organisation and self-help has been put into practical effect.

One such group is Launchpad in Newcastle, a group that has been running for over 14 years with the aim of improving local services through enabling the voice and experience of service users to be heard. They describe themselves as being 'by and for service users', and they run groups and engage in collaborative local initiatives with the aim of ensuring that people get heard and feel empowered (https://launchpadncl.org.uk/).

Many service users commonly find safe spaces wherever they come together and support each other in using mental health services—as inpatients, for example (Faulkner 2005; Jackson 2010; Walsh and Boyle 2009) or through user-controlled organisations and networks (such as Shaping Our Lives www.shapingourlives.org.uk and the National Survivor User Network www.nsun.org.uk).

A discussion about locating space for people to share their stories cannot take place without reference to the internet and social media. There are a number of user-led Facebook groups for particular service user or survivor dialogues and debates (e.g. Recovery in the Bin, Mad Studies, PD in the Bin) as well as a significant service user/survivor presence on Twitter. In addition to this, there are online communities and peer support sites where people can meet on virtual terms and support each other as well as share and create knowledge and activism. These, too, have become important, sometimes safe, spaces for people, providing a virtual alternative where physical spaces are unavailable, non-existent or inaccessible. The Icarus Project (https://theicarusproject.net/) is one such virtual community, where people can share their stories in online forums.

Some narratives go beyond the individual and incorporate community or collective narratives. Morgan et al. (2016) point out that it is often the voices from the margins that 'challenge conventions in first-person narratives' (p. 87)—the notion that a story comes from an individual 'self'. These shared narratives can more effectively incorporate and validate collective experiences of oppression, racism and marginalisation experienced by people who share particular social identities, experiences and backgrounds.

The key message from this section is to highlight the importance for people who experience mental distress to find safe spaces in which to share our stories with each other, for it is in these spaces that we can be heard, find meaning and begin to build confidence in our own (experiential) knowledge.

> Acknowledging that personal narratives offer their own theories and concepts of distress and madness is the first step towards deconstructing the dominance of psychiatric discourse and accepting that the psychiatric discourse is only one of many viable discourses about "problems of living" that we experience. (Morgan et al. 2016, p. 95)

Experiential Knowledge

The concept of experiential knowledge is explored. The freedom to share our narratives provides us with the opportunity to develop our individual and collective 'experiential' knowledge. Experiential knowledge is the knowledge that we gain through making sense of our experiences; it is 'specialised knowledge, grounded in an individual's lived experience' (Borkman 1990). It is the knowledge that we gain, not just from individual experience—although that is essential—but from the interactions and learning from each other as we make sense of our experiences. This process, at the heart of which is trust and belief, has the potential to be liberatory within a context that so often denies or dismisses our reality. Its roots lie in the civil rights movements of the 1960s and 1970s, where people came together to support and validate each other's experiences as a route to campaigning for their rights (Noorani 2013; Emerick 1996).

Experiential knowledge emerges from our relationship and connectedness: from within the peer support and self-help spaces that we find and create (Emerick 1996; Seebohm et al. 2013; Noorani 2013), whether it be through sharing our knowledge of distress and self-care/self-help, our experience of using (or not using) services, or of being subject to stigma, discrimination and abuse. Borkman (1990) refers to experiential knowledge as 'pragmatic' and holistic in nature with a focus on action in the here-and-now. Seebohm et al. (2010) document the significant role that self-organising groups play within racialised communities where historical, cultural and social factors are discussed to help account for the context for people's experiences of discrimination, marginalisation and abuse. Similarly, Gorman writes of situating our individual experience within its social context:

> As we discover how particular experiences are mediated through social relations, we can connect the 'immediate' experience we started with to the larger social organization. (Gorman 2013, p. 274)

Experiential knowledge is capable of questioning the adequacy and effectiveness of professional knowledge or practices. As we saw in the early accounts, the notion of madness or mental illness itself is contested—and not just by those so labelled. The experiential knowledge that people share and learn is vital to the process of challenging the treatments and services that people have found, and still find, harmful and controlling (Beresford 2003, 2013; Rose 2008; Emerick 1996; Faulkner 2017). Groups and networks have developed sophisticated strategies and campaigns based on the experiences and knowledge of their members. Some authors have referred to this as 'experiential authority' (Borkman 1990; Noorani 2013): the authority of the knowledge achieved through the active process of living with and working through mental distress within self-help and service user groups, passing down knowledge through the successive generations of group/space participants.

Examples of collective knowledge in mental health can be seen in the establishment of the Hearing Voices Network (HVN) and the early work on self-advocacy, self-harm and eating distress originating from the service user/survivor organisation Survivors Speak Out (SSO), the National Self-Harm Network and Harmless (Pembroke 1994, 1996; Harmless 2009). More recent examples can be found in the campaigning work of the National Survivor User Network and the development of their Members' Manifesto (see Fig. 16.2). But, every group has the potential to develop its own particular experiential knowledge and authority—enabling its members to learn from each other, not just about mental distress and self-help strategies, but about local services, applying for welfare benefits and other similar issues (Brown and Saini 2016).

Within these spaces too, the individual's story can develop and change over time:

> The centrality of storytelling within self-help and support practices enmeshes individual trajectories with understandings of similar ones, criss-crossing individual's narratives with those of others and using (parts of) others' to rework the individual's own. (Noorani 2013, p. 62)

The National Survivor User Network:

The National Survivor User Network (NSUN) is a network of people who have and do experience mental distress who want to change things for the better. NSUN connects people and influences policy, practice and perceptions by amplifying the experiences and aspirations of our members. Website: www.nsun.org.uk

NSUN Manifesto: We aim to:

1. *Campaign against the injustice and harm caused by cuts to public funding and welfare benefits.*
2. *Challenge the abuse and coercion that continues under mental health legislation and work to ensure that people understand and can enforce their rights under the UNCRPD.*
3. *Actively promote the need to work with us in decisions about strategy, commissioning and how services are provided, as well as the need for services to be user-led.*
4. *Challenge personal, institutional and structural inequalities, injustices, disadvantages and discrimination for everyone with experience of mental distress/trauma.*
5. *Promote people's right to informed choice so that people are in a position to understand their difficulties in whatever way they choose and to access the support that they find best.*
6. *Promote the validity and vital role of survivor knowledge and research.*

Fig. 16.2 The National Survivor User Network

The Role of Survivor Research

Survivor (or user-led) research is another route through which space can be created for developing and collectivising experiential knowledge. Founded in the emancipatory research of the Disabled People's Movement, survivor research has developed a presence in its own right for several decades (Beresford and Wallcraft 1997). Sweeney (2013) describes experiential knowledge as the bedrock of survivor research, a perspective shared by many other survivor researchers (Faulkner 2017; Russo 2012; Beresford 2005; Rose 2009; Sweeney 2013; Kalathil 2011b), in the collective move to challenge the exclusion of service user and survivor voices from mainstream research and knowledge production. The project of survivor research then is, at least in part, to hear people's narratives in meaningful ways, to enable silenced voices to speak from the margins and have the space to be heard (Kalathil 2011a; Carr 2013; Faulkner and Layzell 2000). As pointed out by Wallcraft (2009), mental health service users have:

> traditionally been excluded from creating the knowledge that is used to treat us, and many of us have suffered from the misunderstanding of our needs by people who have been taught to see us as by definition incapable of rational thought. (Wallcraft 2009, p. 133)

In other words, it is not just about being heard, it is about becoming believed as 'credible knowers' (Radden 2012) and producers of knowledge. Russo and Beresford (2014) and Costa et al. (2012) also emphasise the importance of service users and survivors ourselves becoming the 'knowers', rather than having the knowledge we have gained through our experiences appropriated, reframed and alienated from us in the academic arena just as it is within the psychiatric framework. They argue for a different means of doing research, incorporating emancipatory methods, to find ways for participants to retain power within the research process.

Research does not preclude the need for the 'experiential learning communities' of service user and peer support groups, although it can aid the process of achieving 'experiential authority'. As Rose (2008) describes, research is one way of 'systematically collecting user testimonies' to confront mainstream psychiatry with the 'flaws in its own research and practice' (p. 643). The value of survivor research lies in part in reducing the distance between direct experience and its interpretation, potentially leading to 'less distorted, inaccurate and damaging' knowledge (Beresford 2005, p. 7). Russo (2012) emphasises the importance of imparting an insider perspective to research; for her, too, closeness to the subject of the research is beneficial to the research quality.

It can be argued that experiential knowledge has a significant contribution to make where some of the basic tenets of professional knowledge are strongly contested, as is the case with mental health (Baillergeau and Duyvendak 2016; Thomas 2014; Carey and Pilgrim 2010). This, in theory at least, should open up the space for experiential knowledge. Glasby and Beresford (2006) challenge the nature of knowledge within the context of evidence-based medicine and practice. In their view, neglecting the views and experiences of people who use health and social care services gives a '*false and potentially dangerous view of the world*' (p. 271). They highlight the crucial contribution that 'experiential knowledge' has to bring to the evidence table, a theme taken up by many survivor researchers since (Sweeney 2013; Rose 2009; Russo 2012; Faulkner 2017). Survivor research that acts to foreground experiential knowledge also has the potential to enable and strengthen the inclusion and expression of diverse and marginalised voices (Carr 2013; Kalathil 2013; Kalathil and Jones 2016), even if it does not always realise that potential (Kalathil 2013).

The Challenges...

As outlined in the introduction, there are significant challenges facing those of us deemed mad or mentally ill wishing to tell our stories with credibility and without constraints or judgement, and to have our knowledge taken seriously by others.

Perhaps the most obvious challenge is the question of madness itself. Our voices are silenced by the assumptions that madness means irrationality—that we cannot be believed (Rose 2003)—and that madness is illness, meaning that what we say is heard through the filter of diagnosis (Russo 2012; Russo and Beresford 2014; Thomas 2013). Psychiatry's need to diagnose and treat often closes us down and prevents us from telling our stories from our own perspectives (Morgan et al. 2016). Stories or case studies may be used to illustrate a diagnosis or treatment effect in training, texts and conferences. However, the difficulty with individual narratives being incorporated through written or verbal accounts, lies in the potential this has to perpetuate the medical/psychological narrative of individual illness without social or political context.

> The unintentional effect can be to depoliticise madness and to minimise the structural barriers which might obstruct it, thus ironically preserving the status quo. (Woods et al. 2019, p. 17)

Russo (2012), in a review of the book *Agnes' Jacket* (Hornstein 2009), points out the 'massive barriers' service users and survivors face in seeking recognition in academic terms; the silencing of our voices continues when academics collate and (re)interpret stories of madness. Voronka (2019) similarly writes of the way in which our stories, told into spaces circumscribed by the psy disciplines, are constrained by current understandings of mental distress or madness as mental illness, to fulfill the requirements of another.

> The issue here is not which stories we share, but rather with how they are listened to and deployed within prevailing mental health metanarratives and the systems that work within them. (Voronka 2019, p. 9)

A further challenge to experiential knowledge ironically comes from the emergence of the Recovery approach in mental health. Recovery was reconceptualised by service users and survivors in the late twentieth century to mean the possibility of living a meaningful life, whether continuing to experience mental distress or not (Deegan 1988); it was an attempt to move away from seeking or expecting a cure and reintroduce hope. In this sense, recovery is often described as a journey, an individual and personal process focusing on people's skills, strengths and capabilities (see, for example, ImROC http://imroc.org/).Unfortunately, the concept of Recovery has been incorporated into services across the Global North and redefined and confused with medical understandings of recovery such that the original meaning has often been lost (Rose 2014a; McWade 2015). According to Rose (2014a), 'recovery is everywhere' (p. 217), having become the dominant approach in mental health services, invested with bringing hope and a renewed futurity to both individuals and services, but in reality:

> what began as a liberatory discourse has become instrumentalised and mainstreamed such that it is aligned perfectly with our neoliberal present. (Rose 2014a; p. 217)

Recovery (in partnership with social inclusion) has been used as a means and an excuse to close day services and discharge people from secondary care (Bryant et al. 2011; Beresford and Bryant 2008). For some, it has become colonised and is 'used to discipline and control those who are trying to find a place in the world, to live as they wish, trying to deal with the very real mental distress they encounter on a daily basis' (Recovery in the Bin n.d. https://recoveryinthebin.org/).

However, the Recovery approach did bring personal narratives to the fore: telling our stories became recognised as a stepping stone on the route to recovery—opening up a space for people to account for their own experiences (Dillon and May 2002; Thornhill et al. 2004; Brown 2008; Hutchinson and Lovell 2013). It is hard to argue with this notion, given that the value of personal narratives is the central theme of this chapter. The issue here, though, is the emerging dominance of the Recovery Narrative (Woods et al. 2019) as a *narrative genre*, one that involves a forward trajectory of moving from distress through overcoming adversity to recovery and leading a meaningful life. This genre then assumes the power to circumscribe the nature of individual stories such that they are obliged to conform with the Recovery narrative. Woods et al. (2019) suggest that this silences stories and storytellers who do comply with it:

frequently those voices who speak from the margins or refuse to be 'normalized' (Carr 2013; Morgan et al. 2016).

Another challenge to the credibility of experiential knowledge is the power of knowledge, or the knowledge that holds power within society. Experiential knowledge is inevitably devalued by embedded power dynamics, since professional knowledge is accorded a higher status and authority (Beresford and Boxall 2013; Jones et al. 2014; Rose 2014b; Russo 2012). Experiential knowledge does not sit comfortably within the tradition of positivist research methodology. First person experiences and small-scale qualitative studies are devalued in relation to the notion of 'objective' evidence produced through clinical trials (Beresford and Boxall 2013; Beresford 2016). Ultimately,

> the power to generate knowledge about particular phenomena is allotted ... to academics that have specifically been trained to 'treat' individual abnormality or pathology... mental health research in the US remains almost wholly dominated by clinically trained investigators. (Jones and Brown 2013, p. 7)

This results in little space being given to theories or ideas that challenge or conflict with the biomedical model (Russo 2012). To foreground experiential knowledge in research contradicts some of the basic tenets of traditional (scientific) research (Jones et al. 2014; Russo 2012; Beresford 2010; Rose 2013). In addition, the dominance of the biomedical model has resulted in an emphasis on technical expertise and reliance on an individualist framework which 'not only obscures people's social-material world in our understanding of people's experiences, behaviour and distress, it also *marginalises the lived experience and knowledge of those deemed mad*' (Coles et al. 2013, vii; my emphasis).

Another challenge to the credibility of experiential knowledge concerns the exclusion of voices that speak from the margins. As mentioned earlier in this chapter, historical accounts of service user/survivor knowledge often neglect the narratives and knowledge from marginalised and racialised communities. The marginalisation of voices extends to the marginalisation of knowledge and knowledge production; the work of survivor researchers from racialised communities rarely forms a part of the collective knowledge base:

> Where they do get mentioned or cited, it is often as part of a bid to accommodate 'diversity' or perform 'cultural competence' rather than to challenge and disrupt operative norms. (Kalathil and Jones 2016, p. 186)

This disrupts the credibility of the voices that are heard, and forces us to acknowledge the 'inconvenient complications' of madness and distress frequently ignored in much academic and activist discourse (Jones and Kelly 2015). It is imperative that when service users and survivors speak or write about survivor research or experiential knowledge, we are mindful of people creating knowledge within their own safe spaces and communities, even if we are not 'hearing' them (Seebohm et al. 2013; Faulkner and Kalathil 2012; Kalathil and Jones 2016). It is important to acknowledge the power of white privilege and move from thinking about inclusion towards thinking about partnership, from thinking about race and racism to thinking about white privilege—and recognise the contributions of black survivors as fellow knowledge-producers and 'knowers' (Kalathil and Jones 2016; LeFrancois 2013; King 2007).

Another challenge to experiential knowledge lies in the vulnerability of safe spaces, which are under threat from the dual forces of austerity and the co-option of peer support by mainstream services. A recent membership survey by the National Survivor User Network in England (NSUN 2019) found that over 50 user-led groups and organisations had closed in the previous year and a significant number were struggling to survive. An increasingly competitive environment with larger charities winning local contracts has led to more groups closing or trying to exist with sparse resources. Austerity crystallised the UK policy to 'modernise' day services in the name of Recovery in the early 2000s, a policy that led to the closure of many buildings-based day services. Although some such services were not inclusive and could become almost as institutionalised as the old asylums, many represented safe spaces for people to meet and support each other and form the core of peer support (Beresford and Bryant 2008; Malpas and Weekes 2001).

In recent years, the concept of 'peer support' has been redefined and developed as an intervention for use in mainstream mental health services, diverting it from its grass-roots self-help and user group context (Faulkner and Basset 2012). Peer support is the foundation stone upon which experiential knowledge rests. Through incorporating peer support as an intervention within mainstream services, the value of experiential knowledge is at risk of being compromised and depoliticised (Penney and Prescott

2016; Voronka 2017). Whilst an individual and personalised model of peer support as a means of supporting others has many strengths, there is a risk that, in supporting this model, commissioners will direct funding away from service user groups where community-based peer support takes place. Seen as a treatment intervention, 'peer support' will increasingly become time-limited, assessed and evaluated by measures inappropriate to the ethos of peer support (Penney and Prescott 2016; Voronka 2017). Together with an increasingly neoliberal approach to services in which the individual is the focus of understanding cause and care, this development has the potential to reduce the opportunities for people to meet together, support one another, develop collective knowledge and organise independently of mainstream services.

Looking to the Future

Despite these challenges, experiential knowledge has the potential to transform the knowledge base for mental health, even (perhaps especially) from within small self-help and peer support groups (Emerick 1996; Noorani 2013; Rose 2014b; Morgan et al. 2016). Research that enables us and our peers to reflect on our experiences and build and produce experiential knowledge as a means of both critique and empowerment is an essential development of our lived experience of mental distress (Faulkner 2017; Sweeney 2013). We need to (continue to) find more and better ways of being the 'creators of our own analysis and theory' (Beresford and Wallcraft 1997, p. 77), through building collective understandings of our experiences as well as acknowledging the 'inconvenient complications' (Jones and Kelly 2015) of our differences.

Recent years have seen the emergence of a field of enquiry called 'Mad Studies' (see, for example, LeFrancois et al. 2013), in which survivors and allies are talking about the connections between individual experience and collective, socially situated knowledge(s) about madness, oppression and discrimination. Mad Studies has been described by Lucy Costa (2014; no page no.) as 'an area of education, scholarship, and analysis about the experiences, history, culture, political organising, narratives, writings and most importantly, the PEOPLE'. The idea behind Mad Studies is to 'invoke a strand of human history that predates psychiatric discourse' (Church 2015, 7, p. 19). Thinking, writing and activism around these issues and ideas long pre-dates the seminal publication 'Mad Matters' and the coining of the term 'Mad Studies' (LeFrancois et al. 2013). Indeed, its very focus on historicising survivor/service user activism and survivor narratives demonstrates that it 'builds on a compelling tradition of critical activism and scholarship' (LeFrancois et al. 2013, p. 12).

The importance of Mad Studies lies in the space it is opening up for survivors to develop theories, models and ideas about how we understand ourselves, or our experiences in relationship to mental health system(s), research and politics (see Mad Studies Network website https://madstudies2014.wordpress.com/). Sweeney (2016) argues for fostering a strong relationship between survivor research and Mad Studies; that is, each needs the other in order to strengthen a 'radical counter-discourse to biomedical psychiatry and a model for conducting research beyond consumerist service user involvement arguments' (Sweeney 2016, p. 36).

'Mad Studies' itself faces some significant challenges. One of these is the need to remain true and connected to the grass-roots activism at the heart of our movements, to the shared narratives that inspire the creation of experiential knowledge(Faulkner 2017); those of us who write for academic publication need also to look towards the groups and communities where peer support and activism are happening now. 'Mad' people are beginning to infiltrate the academy, despite the fact that the bureaucracy and culture we find there do not lend themselves to collaborative or inclusive ways of working; indeed, they can be profoundly isolating (Carr 2019).

Conclusions

At the heart of this chapter is the fundamental significance of having the freedom to tell one's story without fear of judgement and with the expectation of being heard and believed. This is the cornerstone upon which people deemed mad or mentally ill can find meaning in our experiences and build our experiential knowledge. As we have seen in this chapter, there are many challenges to that freedom, particularly to people from marginalised communities. There are challenges, too, to the spaces in which we can create and develop our experiential knowledge. In the move towards the academy enshrined in both survivor research and Mad Studies, we need to retain contact with our variety of mad communities if we are to sustain credibility with those communities and maintain the trust that supports the development and maturity of our mad experiential knowledge. I finish with a plea to the reader to listen to the stories of people deemed mad or mentally ill without prior assumptions about rationality, insight or disease: to let their stories breathe.

Note

1. Further information about the history of the UK service user and survivor movements can be found on the Survivor History website: http://study-more.org.uk/MPU.HTM.

References

Baillergeau, E. and Duyvendak, J.W. (2016) Experiential knowledge as a resource for coping with uncertainty: evidence and examples from the Netherlands. *Health, Risk & Society*, 18:7–8, 407–426, DOI: https://doi.org/10.1080/13698575.2016.1269878.

Beers, C. (1981) *A Mind That Found Itself*, Pittsburgh and London: University of Pittsburgh Press, 1981 ISBN 0-8229-5324-2

Beresford, P. (2016) The Role of Survivor Knowledge in Creating Alternatives to Psychiatry. Chapter 4 (pp. 25–34) in *Searching for a Rose Garden: Challenging Psychiatry, Fostering Mad Studies.* edited by Russo and Sweeney (2016). Monmouth: PCCS Books.

Beresford, P. (2013) Experiential Knowledge and the Reconception of Madness. Chapter 11 in Coles S., Keenan S and Diamond B. (2013) *Madness Contested: Power and Practice.* Ross-on-Wye: PCCS Books.

Beresford, P. (2010) 'Re-examining Relationships between Experience, Knowledge, Ideas and Research: A Key Role for Recipients of State Welfare and Their Movements. *Social Work and Society International Online Journal,* 8 (1).

Beresford, P. (2005) Developing the theoretical basis for service user/survivor-led research and equal involvement in research. *Epidemiologia e Psichiatria Sociale, 14, 1, 4–9.*

Beresford, P. (2003) *It's Our Lives: A short theory of knowledge, distance and experience.* London: Citizen Press/Shaping Our Lives. www.shapingourlives.org.uk/documents/ItsOurLives.pdf.

Beresford, P. and Boxall, K. (2013) 'Where do service users' knowledges sit in relation to professional and academic understandings of knowledge?' Chapter Six in Staddon, P. (ed) *Service Users in Research.*

Beresford, P. and Bryant, W. (2008) Saving the day centre. *The Guardian*, 11 June 2008.

Beresford, P. and Wallcraft, J. (1997) Psychiatric System Survivors and Emancipatory research: Issues, overlaps and differences. Chapter 5 in Barnes and Mercer (Eds) *Doing Disability Research* http://disability-studies.leeds.ac.uk/files/library/Barnes-Chapter-5.pdf.

Borkman, T. J. (1990). Experiential, professional, and lay frames of reference. Chapter in *Working with Self-Help.* T. J. Powell. Silver Spring, Maryland, NASW Press: 3–30.

Brown, W. (2008) Narratives of Mental Health Recovery. *Social Alternatives* 27 (4), 42–48.

Brown, M. and Saini, G. (2016) A Day in the Life: What happens when you ask people who live with mental health difficulties to write about their everyday life? London: Social Spider cic/Centre for Mental Health. www.centreformentalhealth.org.uk/a-day-in-the-life.

Bryant, W., Tibbs, A. and Clark, J. (2011) Visualising a safe space: the perspective of people using mental health day services, Disability & Society, 26:5, 611–628, DOI: https://doi.org/10.1080/09687599.2011.589194.

Campbell, P. (2005), From Little Acorns: the mental health service user movement. Chapter 6 in *Beyond the Water Towers: The unfinished revolution in mental health services 1985–2005*, ed. Bell, A. and Lindley, P. Sainsbury Centre for Mental Health, London (pp73–82).

Campbell, P. and Roberts, A. (2009) Survivors' History. A life in the day Volume 13 Issue 3 August 2009.

Campbell, P. and Rose, D. (2011) Action for Change in the UK: Thirty Years of the User/Survivor Movement. Chapter 22 (pp. 452–470) in *The Sage Handbook of Mental Health and Illness*, ed. by Pilgrim, D., Rogers, A. and Pescosolido, B. Sage Publications Ltd.

Carey, T.A. and Pilgrim, D. (2010) Diagnosis and Formulation: What should we tell the students? *Clinical Psychology and Psychotherapy*, 17, 447–454.

CAPS (the Consultation and Advocacy Promotion Service) (2010) *Oor Mad History: A Community History of the Lothian Mental Health Service User Movement.* Edinburgh: CAPS. www.capsadvocacy.org/.

Carr, S. (2013) Individual Narratives and Collective Knowledge: capturing lesbian, gay and bisexual service user experiences. Chapter ten in Staddon, P. (ed) *Mental Health Service Users in Research*; Bristol: Policy Press.

Carr, S. (2019) 'I am not your nutter': a personal reflection on commodification and comradeship in service user and survivor research, Disability & Society, DOI:https://doi.org/10.1080/09687599.2019.1608424.

Church, K. (2015) *Making Mad Studies: Process, Practice and Contestations – Presentation to Ryerson University.* Toronto, Canada. https://ryecast.ryerson.ca/80/Watch/8844.aspx.

Coles, S., Keenan, S. and Diamond, B. (2013) *Madness Contested: Power and Practice.* Ross-on-Wye: PCCS Books.

Costa, L., Voronka, J., Landry D., Reid J., McFarlane B., Reville D. and Church K. (2012) Recovering our Stories: A Small Act of Resistance. *Studies in Social Justice* 6, (1) 85–101.

Costa, L. (2014) *Mad Studies – what it is and why you should care.* posted on the Mad Studies network website: https://madstudies2014.wordpress.com/2014/10/15/mad-studies-what-it-is-and-why-you-should-care-2/.

Deegan, P. (1988) Recovery: The Lived Experience of Rehabilitation. *Psychosocial Rehabilitation Journal.* 11(4):11–19. https://doi.org/10.1037/h0099565.

Dillon, J. & May, R. (2002) Reclaiming Experience, *Clinical Psychology*, 17, 25–77.

DuBrul, S.A. (2014) The Icarus Project: A Counter Narrative for Psychic Diversity. Journal of Medical Humanities, 35, 257–271.

Emerick, R.E. (1996) Mad Liberation: The Sociology of Knowledge and the Ultimate Civil Rights Movement. *The Journal of Mind and Behaviour*, Volume 17, No.2 pp.135–160.

Faulkner, A. and Layzell, S. (2000) *Strategies for Living: a report of user-led research into people's strategies for living with mental distress.* London: Mental Health Foundation.

Faulkner, A. (2005) Institutional Conflict: the state of play in adult acute psychiatric wards. *The Journal of Adult Protection7* (4), 6–12.

Faulkner, A. (2010) Measuring the Marigolds. Chapter 4 in Basset, T. and Stickley, T. (eds) *Voices of Experience: Narratives of Mental Health Survivors.* London: Wiley-Blackwell.

Faulkner, A. (2017) Survivor research and Mad Studies: the role and value of experiential knowledge in mental health research, Disability & Society. https://doi.org/10.1080/09687599.2017.1302320.

Faulkner, A. and Basset, T. (2012) *A Helping Hand: Consultations with Service Users about Peer Support.* London: Together for Mental Wellbeing.

Faulkner, A. and Kalathil, J. (2012) *The Freedom to be, the Chance to Dream: Preserving User-led Peer Support in Mental Health.* London: Together for Mental Wellbeing.

Frank, A.W. (2010) *Letting Stories Breathe: A Socio-Narratology.* Chicago: University of Chicago Press.

Glasby, J. and Beresford, P. (2006) 'Who knows best? Evidence-based practice and the service user contribution' *Critical Social Policy* 26(1): 268–284.

Gorman, R. (2013) Mad Nation? Thinking through Race, Class and Mad Identity Politics. Chapter 19 in LeFrancois et al, 2013. *Mad Matters: a Critical Reader in Canadian Mad Studies.*

Grant-Smith, R. (1922) *The Experiences of an Asylum Patient.* London: Allen and Unwin. http://mcgovern.library.tmc.edu/data/www/html/texascoll/Psych/EAP/EAPContents.htm.

Harmless (2009) In Our Own Words: Promoting insight and understanding of self harm. Harmless: www.harmless.org.uk/store/Merchandise-Books/In-Our-Own-Words-Electronic.

Hayward, R. (2014) *The Transformation of the Psyche in British Primary Care, 1870–1970.* A&C Black.

Hornstein, G.A. (2009/2012) *Agnes's Jacket: A Psychologist's Search for the Meanings of Madness.* Ross-on-Wye: PCCS Books.

Hutchinson, A. and Lovell, A. (2013) Participatory action research: moving beyond the mental health 'service user' identity. *Journal of Psychiatric and Mental Health Nursing*, 2013, 20, 641–649

Jackson, C. (2010), 'Critical friends', *Openmind*, Vol. 161, January/February, pp. 14–15.

Jones, N., Harrison, J., Aguiar, R. and Munro, L. (2014) 'Transforming Research for Transformative Change in Mental Health: Towards the Future'. Chapter 17 in *Community Psychology and Community Mental Health: Towards Transformative Change*. Edited by Nelson, G., Kloos, B. and Ornelas, J. Oxford University Press.

Jones, N. and Brown, R.L. (2013) The Absence of Psychiatric C/S/X Perspectives in Academic Discourse: Consequences and Implications. *Disability Studies Quarterly* 33 (1) http://dsq-sds.org/issue/view/100.

Jones, N. and Kelly, T. (2015) Inconvenient Complications: On the heterogeneities of madness and their relationship to disability. Chapter Three in *Madness, Distress and the Politics of Disablement*, ed. Spandler, Sapey and Anderson. London: Policy Press.

Kalathil, J. and Jones, N. (2016) Unsettling Disciplines: Madness, Identity, Research, Knowledge. *Philosophy, Psychiatry, & Psychology*, 23, 3/4, pp. 183–188.

Kalathil, J. (2013) 'Hard to Reach'? Racialised groups and mental health service user involvement. Chapter Nine in Staddon, P. (ed) *Mental Health Service Users in Research*. Bristol: Policy Press.

Kalathil, J. (2011a) *Dancing to Our Own Tunes: Reassessing black and minority ethnic mental health service user involvement*: Reprint of the 2008 report with a review of work undertaken to take the recommendations forward. London: NSUN.

Kalathil, J. (2011b) '*Recovery and Resilience: African, African-Caribbean and South Asian women's narratives of recovering from mental distress.*' London: Mental Health Foundation.

King, Colin (2007). "They diagnosed me a schizophrenic when I was just a Gemini. 'The other side of madness'". Chapter 2 in Man Cheung Chung, K. W. M. (Bill) Fulford, and George Graham, eds, *Reconceiving Schizophrenia,* Oxford University Press, Oxford, Pg 11–27.

LeFrancois, B.A., Menzies, R. and Reaume, G. (2013) *Mad Matters: A Critical Reader in Canadian Mad Studies.* Toronto: Canadian Scholars' Press Inc.

LeFrancois, B. (2015) *Acknowledging the Past and Challenging the Present, in Contemplation of the Future: Some (Un)Doings of Mad Studies.* Presentation at Mad Studies Conference, Durham University 2015.

McKinley, S. and Yiannoullou, S. (2012) Changing Minds: unleashing the potential of mental health service users – a critical perspective on current models of service user involvement and their impact on wellbeing and 'recovery'. Chapter

Nine in Barnes, M. and Cotterell, P. *Critical Perspectives on User Involvement.* Bristol: Policy Press.

McWade, B. (2015) The Neoliberal Politics of Recovery. Conference presentation, Making Sense of Mad Studies, Durham University.

Malpas, G. and Weekes, J. (2001) *An Investigation into Drop-Ins: Exploring the impact of peer support on mental health.* London: Mental Health Foundation.

Morgan, A., Felton, A., Fulford, B., Kalathil, J. and Stacey, G. (2016) *Values and Ethics in Mental Health: An exploration for practice.* London: Palgrave.

National Survivor User Movement. (2019) User-led groups continue to close. https://www.nsun.org.uk/news/user-led-groups-continue-to-close.

Noorani, T. (2013) Service user involvement, authority and the 'expert-by-experience' in mental health. *Journal of Political Power*, 6:1, 49–68.

Pembroke, L. (ed.) (1994) Eating Distress: Perspectives from personal experience. London: Survivors Speak Out. http://studymore.org.uk/edpfpe.pdf.

Pembroke, L. (ed.) (1996) *Self Harm: perspectives from personal experience.* London: Survivors Speak Out. http://studymore.org.uk/shpfpe.pdf.

Penney, D. and Prescott, L. (2016) The co-optation of survivor knowledge: the danger of substituted values and voice. In Russo & Sweeney (eds) *Searching for a Rose Garden: Challenging psychiatry, fostering mad studies.* Monmouth: PCCS Books.

Radden, J. (2012) Recognition rights, mental health consumers and reconstructive cultural semantics. *Philosophy, Ethics and Humanities in Medicine*, 7 (6) 1–8. http://peh-med.biomedcentral.com/articles/10.1186/1747-5341-7-6.

Recovery in the Bin. (n.d.): 20 Key Principles https://recoveryinthebin.org/recovery-in-the-bin-19-principless/ Accessed 28 September 2016.

Rose, D. (2003) Having a Diagnosis is a Qualification for the Job, *British Medical Journal*, 326(7402): 1331.

Rose, D. (2008) Commentary: Madness Strikes Back. *Journal of Community and Applied Social Psychology*, 18, 638–644.

Rose, D. (2009) Survivor-produced knowledge. Chapter 4 in Sweeney et al (eds) *This is Survivor Research.* Ross-on-Wye: PCCS Books.

Rose, D. (2014a) The mainstreaming of recovery. Editorial: *Journal of Mental Health*, 23(5); 217–218.

Rose, D. (2014b) Patient and public involvement in health research: Ethical imperative and/or radical challenge? *Journal of Health Psychology*, 19 (1), 149–158.

Russo, J. (2012) Survivor-Controlled Research: A New Foundation for Thinking About Psychiatry and Mental Health. *Forum: Qualitative Social Research* 13, No. 1, Art. 8 – January 2012

Russo, J. (2018) Experiential knowledge in mental health policy and legislation: can we ever change the agenda?. Chapter 50 in Beresford, P. and Carr, S. (eds) *Social Policy First Hand: An international introduction to participatory social welfare.* Bristol: Policy Press.

Russo, J. and Beresford, P. (2014) Between exclusion and colonisation: seeking a place for mad people's knowledge in academia. *Disability and Society.*

Seebohm, P., Chaudhary, S., Boyce, M., Elkan, R., Avis, M. and Munn-Giddings, C. (2013) The contribution of self-help/mutual aid groups to mental well-being. *Health and Social Care in the Community*, 21(4), 391–401.

Seebohm, P., Munn-Giddings, C. and Brewer, P. (2010) "What's in a name? A discussion paper on the labels and location of self-organising community groups, with particular reference to mental health and Black groups", *Mental Health and Social Inclusion*, Vol. 14 Iss: 3, pp. 23–29.

Staley, L. (ed.) (1996) The Book of Margery Kempe. Kalamazoo, Michigan: Medieval Institute Publications.

Sweeney, A. (2016) The Transformative Potential of Survivor Research. In Russo & Sweeney (eds) *Searching for a Rose Garden: Challenging psychiatry, fostering mad studies.* Monmouth: PCCS Books.

Sweeney, A. (2013) Sociology and survivor research: an introduction. Chapter One in: Staddon, P. (Ed.) Mental Health Service Users in Research.

Thomas, P. (2013) Pinball Wizards and the Doomed Project of Psychiatric Diagnosis. Mad in America Blog: www.madinamerica.com/2013/02/pinball-wizards-and-the-doomed-project-of-psychiatric-diagnosis/.

Thomas, P. (2014) *Psychiatry in Context: Experience, meaning and communities.* PCCS Books.

Thornhill, H, Clare, L. and May, R. (2004) Escape, enlightenment and endurance: Narratives of recovery from psychosis. *Anthropology & Medicine* Vol. 11, No. 2 August 2004, pp. 181–199.

Voronka, J. (2017) Turning Mad Knowledge into Affective Labor: The Case of the Peer Support Worker. *American Quarterly*, Volume 69, Number 2, June 2017, pp. 333–338.

Voronka, J. (2019) Storytelling Beyond the Psychiatric Gaze. *Canadian Journal of Disability Studies*,8, 4,pp.8–30.

Wallcraft, J. (2009) From activist to researcher and part-way back. In Sweeney et al (2009). *This is SurvivorResearch.* Ross-on-Wye: PCCS Books.

Wallcraft, J. with Read, J. and Sweeney, A. (2003) *On Our Own Terms: Users and survivors of mental health services working together for support and change.* London: Mental Health Foundation/User Survey Steering Group.

Wallcraft, J. and Bryant, M. (2013) The mental health service user movement in England. *Policy Paper 2*: The Sainsbury Centre for Mental Health. http://studymore.org.uk/policy_2.pdf.

Walsh, J. and Boyle, J. (2009) "Improving acute psychiatric hospital services according to inpatient experiences: a user-led piece of research as a means to empowerment", *Issues in Mental Health Nursing*, Vol. 30 No. 1, pp. 31–8.

White, W. (2018) Crazy Lives Matter Too: Imagining a World Where Everyone is Valued, Keynote speech at the Alternatives Conference, Catholic University of America, Washington DC, July 31, 2018. https://vimeo.com/286112464.

Woods, A., Hart, A. and Spandler, H. (2019) The Recovery Narrative: Politics and Possibilities of a Genre. Cult Med Psychiatry https://doi.org/10.1007/s11013-019-09623-y.

Yiannoullou, S. and Faulkner, A. (2018) Involvement for Influence: developing the 4Pi Involvement Standards. Chapter 44 in Beresford, P. and Carr, S. (eds) *Social Policy First Hand: An International introduction to participatory social welfare*. Bristol: Policy Press.

CHAPTER 17

Making Public Their Use of History: Reflections on the History of Collective Action by Psychiatric Patients, the Oor Mad History Project and Survivors History Group

Mark Gallagher

Introduction

At the beginning of the twenty-first century, two community history projects were established in the UK to recover the history of collective action by psychiatric patients. What is unusual about these historical inquiries is that they are conducted by people who are, or have been, at the receiving end of psychiatric diagnosis and treatment, some of whom have described themselves as survivors of mental distress and/or psychiatry, and many of whom have campaigned for changes to mental health services and social attitudes towards mental suffering. The first of these groups, the Survivors History Group (SHG), was formed in London in 2005, and, the second, Oor Mad History (OMH), started in Edinburgh in 2008. These projects

M. Gallagher (✉)
Scotland, UK

R. Ellis et al. (eds.), *Voices in the History of Madness*, Mental Health in Historical Perspective,
https://doi.org/10.1007/978-3-030-69559-0_17

have presented a challenge to professional historians and others conducting research in the history of psychiatry, including academics and medics based at universities, because they have opened the field of inquiry up to a range of sources and discourses about which most interested scholars had previously been unaware. Their subject is of particular interest to those concerned with the history of psychiatric patients (or sufferers of mental illness) and the post-war era of twentieth-century psychiatry. The study of history seeks an interpretive understanding of the past in terms of the ideas and practices through which human beings have experienced and acted in the world. Ideas structure experience differently, depending on where one stands and on the lenses through which one sees the world. The concepts and practices through which human beings have experienced and acted in history have been shaped and transformed in the context of changing circumstances over time. Research on the history of collective action by psychiatric patients must focus less on psychiatrists and the categories they have applied to their patients, and more on what psychiatric patients have done together as groups. Such 'histories from below' take account of and foreground the public discourses and social practices these groups were engaged in, the categories they brought to their experience of civil association and collective action, and their attempts to resist certain psychiatric and governmental practices (see Barnes 1999; Barnes and Bowl 2001; Brandon 1991; Campbell 1989, 1994, 1996, 1999, 2005, 2006; Campbell and Rose 2011; Claytor 1993; Davies 2001; Ferguson 2000, 2003; Gallagher 2017, 2018; Hervey 1986; Peterson 1982; Roberts 2009). For example, the term 'survivor' was employed by groups of activists to convey 'a definite criticism of services, emphasising the obstacles individuals have to overcome in their lives' (Campbell 2006). But this term was also disliked by other activists for being 'too negative and confrontational' (Campbell 2006). One member of a 1980s group, the Campaign Against Psychiatric Oppression, stated starkly that 'survivors of the mental health system are no more consumers of mental health services than cockroaches are consumers of Rentokil' (Barker and Peck 1987, p. 1). The empirical dimension of my inquiries into the history of collective action by psychiatric patients in Scotland has depended heavily on the research of SHG and OMH, both of which have collected and archived documents from various groups formed by psychiatric patients in the UK over the last half-century. These projects have shown that patients often see themselves and their predicament through a very different set of lenses from those perspectives which have been brought to bear on them by medics, policymakers, academics and others.

These community history projects have made it possible for almost anyone interested to access a vast wealth of primary source documentation (among other sources, including oral histories). These groups constituted forms of civil association, mutual aid and political campaigning. Anne O'Donnell (2008, p. 7) from OMH has suggested that psychiatric patients 'have long been the objects of social policy, of professional discourses and of the history of psychiatry' and 'have been constructed as people who are passive, rather than people who can act, however limiting the structural issues may be'. According to OMH:

> people with mental health problems have often been silenced and stigmatised by history and by society. As a whole, history related to mental health is dominated by the history of asylums, psychiatry or medicine. Little has been recorded of the histories of those who have experienced the system first hand or who have come together to change it. (CAPS 2010, p. 17)

For OMH, 'community history and oral history are powerful tools for reclaiming the histories of groups who have been marginalised by society and by mainstream history' (CAPS 2010, p. 8). 'Oral history', they say, 'is one way of democratising history, of putting history in the hands of those who have created it' (CAPS 2010, p. 8). The project asks, 'What is more relevant to a community than its own history?' (CAPS 2010, p. 8). Survivors History Group was founded in 2005 by 'veterans of the user-survivor movement [...] who believe that the history of individual and collective action by service users/survivors is both interesting and important, and worthy of preservation' (Campbell and Roberts 2009, p. 33). It seemed to me that some of the concerns of SHG and OMH converged on a series of issues relating to the historiography of patients/the sick/sufferers/service users/survivors which had been exercising others working in the history of medicine and related disciplines, such as medical sociology and the medical humanities. It is worth considering these issues by reviewing some academic perspectives on the history of patients before returning to SHG and OMH and the question of how they present a challenge to common attitudes towards the mentally ill. By bringing some of these different perspectives and voices into dialogue, the tensions between different approaches to the history of patients/the sick/sufferers/service users/

survivors emerge, and the implications for histories of collective action and social movements in mental health (or 'survivors history') are made visible.

The Disappearance of Patient Views and Voices in the History of Medicine

In 1985, British pioneer of the social history of medicine, Roy Porter, published a seminal paper which called for a reversal of perspective from historians, to see the history of medicine from 'the patient's view' by 'doing medical history from below'. Porter was not alone in shifting his attention to patients, in calling for inquiries which would bring the patient's experience into clearer focus, but he articulated better than anyone that it takes 'two to make a medical encounter—the sick person as well as the doctor' (Porter 1985, p. 175). He highlighted that

> indeed, it often takes more than two, because medical events have frequently been complex social rituals involving family and community as well as sufferers and physicians [...] In medicine's history, the initiatives have often come from, and power has frequently rested with, the sufferer, or with lay people in general. (Porter 1985, p. 175)

Two conflicting views of the patient's place in the medical encounter have been concerned, on the one hand with how the patient was constructed by discourses of medicine and, on the other, with how the patient exerted some degree of control, autonomy or choice over their medical treatment. David Armstrong has argued that in modern times the patient is an artefact of the 'medical gaze' (Armstrong 1995, p. 396). According to Armstrong (1984, p. 739), during the twentieth century 'the patient's view was not, in this sense, a discovery or the product of some humanistic enlightenment'. Instead, 'it was a technique demanded by medicine to illuminate the dark spaces of the mind and social relationships'(Armstrong 1984, p. 739). Conversely, Roy Porter (1985, p. 194) suggested that 'even under medical control patients have by no means been so passive as the various "medicalization" theories [...] might lead us to believe'. Alex Mold (2011, p. 512) has urged caution, warning that 'it should not be assumed that individual agency disappeared with the development of biomedicine, but nor is it the case that patients were either autonomous individuals or powerless subjects'. The concern expressed by Mold is suggestive of a possible middle way between the two very different perspectives of

Armstrong and Porter on 'the patient's view'. Other influential works on the relationship between the patient and medicine have emphasised the extent to which the balance of power in the medical encounter had shifted in favour of the doctor with the rise of 'hospital medicine' (Ackerknecht 1982, p. 146). In a seminal work, Nicholas Jewson (1976, p. 225) argued that the move from 'bedside medicine' to predominantly hospital-based medicine in the late eighteenth and early nineteenth centuries marked 'the disappearance of the sick man from medical cosmology' and established a doctor–patient relationship dominated by practitioners. For Jewson (1976, p. 225), medical cosmologies are 'conceptual structures which constitute the frame of reference within which all questions are posed and all answers are offered'. Malcolm Nicolson (2009, p. 640) noticed that what historians failed to appreciate in Jewson's analysis was 'that locus of epistemological authority had shifted—authoritative medical knowledge no longer flowed from the bedside encounter between an individual practitioner and the sick person as it had done earlier.' He underlines that previously medical knowledge was 'exoteric', where there had been 'a common medical culture, broadly shared between practitioner and the laity', but in the eras of hospital and laboratory medicine medical knowledge became 'esoteric', which meant that 'it was intelligible only to the expert physician' (Nicolson 2009, p. 641). The subtlety of Jewson's analysis for Nicolson lies in the fact that he 'gave new analytical utility' to the categorisations of 'bedside medicine' and 'hospital medicine' (borrowed from Erwin Ackerknecht), 'by tying them precisely to their material contexts and characterizing them as distinctive medical cosmologies', showing how an epistemic break was articulated through a locational and material shift (Nicolson 2009, p. 640).

Mary Fissell (1991, p. 99) argued that with the invention of hospital medicine during the eighteenth century, 'doctors begin to sound like doctors, and patients' voices disappear'. Similarly, in his controversial and influential study of the history of psychiatry, Michel Foucault averred that the mad were paradoxically excluded from discourse, and constituted as mentally ill by discourses which emerged with the rise of modern psychiatry and 'the great confinement' of the mad: 'The constitution of madness as mental illness [...] bears witness to a rupture in dialogue [...] The language of psychiatry which is a monologue of reason about madness has been established only on the basis of that silence' (Foucault 2006, p. xxviii). Sociologists influenced by Foucault, such as Armstrong and Nikolas Rose, have studied the way in which medical discourses and practices have, not simply silenced or excluded patients, but rather, formed and shaped subjects and objects from scientific knowledge, expertise and regulation. This follows Foucault's suggestion of 'depriving the subject (or its substitute) of its role as originator and analysing the subject as a variable and complex function of discourse' (Foucault 1991a, p. 118). But such a form of analysis seems to exclude the possibility of human agency, making the human subject the product of disciplinary practices and discourses, leaving little or no room for individual freedom. In response to the Foucaultian approaches of Armstrong and Rose, sociologist Nick Crossley (1998, p. 877) has claimed that 'power and dominant discourses have been the key focus of analysis, to the detriment of the proper consideration of resistance and counter-discourses'. In his research, Crossley sought to give proper consideration to groups of patients who contested psychiatric medicine in the second half of the twentieth century in Britain. Medical historians have tended to focus on the 'Foucaultian perspective which emphasises the patient as a construct of the medical sciences' (Condrau 2007, p. 536). The Foucaultian patient is seen as 'subjugated, submissive, docile, powerless [...] a symbol of medicalization gone wrong' and 'portrayed as characteristically voiceless' (Bacopoulos-Viau and Fauvel 2016, pp. 5, 7).

Flurin Condrau (2007, p. 527) suggested that 'the real minefield for the history of patients is to begin to make sense of Foucault'. He claims that 'a Porteresque history of the patient's view and a Foucaultian analysis of discourse and power leaves us with the paradoxical relation of a mainly empirical view "from below" and a theoretically informed account of how the patient gets constructed through discourse, knowledge and power'(Condrau 2007, pp. 527–528). For Condrau (2007, pp. 533–534), 'history from below implies power struggles, resistance and perhaps even a popular movement'. He thinks that 'if history from below has to do with power structures, then patients appear to be the least likely group to challenge medical power and influence', and he assumes that a 'political background for patients is not easy to unearth' (Condrau 2007, pp. 533–534). Similarly, writing in the 1950s on the prospects of patients organising themselves into collectives, sociologist Talcott Parsons articulated a normative conception of the 'sick role' in which

> the two most dangerous potentialities, namely group formation and successful establishment of the claim to legitimacy, are avoided. The sick are tied up, not with other deviants to form a sub-culture of the sick, but each with

> a group of the non-sick, his personal circle and, above all, physicians [...] deprived of the possibility of forming a solidary collective. (Parsons 1951, p. 477)

Nicolson (2009, p. 639) has pointed out that 'up until the 1960s, the history of medicine had been written almost entirely by doctors themselves, or by commentators who allied themselves closely with the values and interests of academic medicine'. He notes that the dominant theoretical schema of medical sociology in the mid-twentieth century was Parsonian functionalism. Parsons' 'normative conception of the "sick role" [...] urged upon the laity submission, cognitive as well as bodily, to the authority of the state-licensed physician' (Nicolson 2009, p. 640). But, Nicolson (2009, p. 640) observes that Foucault's (1973) *Birth of the Clinic*, along with the work of Jewson and others, such as Reiser (1978), represented 'the emergence of a more radical engagement with medical knowledge, the appearance of a discourse that was about medicine but not wholly of it'. For Nicolson (2009, p. 640), Foucault prescribed a method in which 'one should scrutinize medical knowledge as an archaeologist examines material artefacts'. In the context of the history of medicine and psychiatry, in his later work Foucault saw a place for the kind of research which required an 'archaeological excavation of subjugated knowledges', a digging up of discarded remnants which had hitherto been neglected (Philo 2007, p. 358). As if in recognition of the voices which had either been silenced or channelled through the psychiatric grid in his earlier work, he would come to see that something which was left out in that account had to be recovered.

A Twentieth-Century Turning Point: From Formal Systems and Functionalist Grids to the Insurrection of Subjugated Knowledges

Condrau (2007, p. 527) thinks the history of patients has not advanced methodologically since Porter's 1985 article 'The Patient's View', and he suggests that useful theoretical concepts for the history of patients might have come from 'a Parsonian tradition' in which 'medicine can be understood as a cultural system within which norms and behaviour as well as social structures and arenas are organised'. Such an approach would have been anathema to the Foucault working in the 1970s. Condrau (2007,

p. 527) remarks that 'the term "system" is the key because it suggests that all aspects of health care, medicine, health and illness are part of an integral system and contribute substantially to its functioning'. By the mid-1970s, Foucault (2003, p. 7) was speaking of 'the historical contents that have been buried and disguised in a functionalist coherence and formal systematisation'; of how 'historical contents alone allow us to rediscover the ruptural effects of conflict and struggle that the order imposed by functionalist or systematising thought is designed to mask'. Although there had been high-profile examples of patient advocacy organisations in the nineteenth and early-twentieth centuries, it was in the mid-twentieth century that asylums (by then renamed mental hospitals) and psychiatry became the focus of sustained criticism and resistance by patients and others. This was a time when the 'ruptural effects of conflict and struggle' become apparent, as psychiatric patients began to form civil associations, engaging in public deliberation and practical action for political change across many countries in North America and Western Europe. The moment of change when groups of patients came together to question and resist psychiatric knowledge and power, attempting to have their voices heard, and to recover a lost sense of agency, community and belonging, was just the kind of historical turning point that Foucault was interested in studying.

In an editorial of a 2016 special issue of Medical History, titled 'The Patient's Turn. Roy Porter and Psychiatry's Tales, Thirty Year's On', the authors refer to 'Foucault's and Porter's drastically different views on patient agency', remarking that 'manufactured through the ever-tyrannical "clinical gaze", the Foucauldian patient embodied victimising structures of "biopower", knowledge, discourse and control' (Bacopoulos-Viau and Fauvel 2016, p. 526). These remarks stand somewhat in contrast to the words of Foucault (2003, pp. 5–6) spoken in 1976, of 'the astonishing efficacy of discontinuous, particular and local critiques' and 'the strange efficacy, when it came to jamming the workings of the psychiatric institution, of the discourse, the discourses—and they really were very localised—of antipsychiatry'. Granted that Foucault was referring to a very recent period in time, and he was not referring to the discourses of resistant psychiatric patients alone, his Nietzschean turn to 'genealogy' in the 1970s involved the kind of reversal of perspective characteristic of a 'history from below' because it attended to counter-discourses and 'subjugated knowledges': 'let us give the term genealogy', said Foucault, 'to the union of erudite knowledge and local memories which allows us to establish a historical knowledge of struggles' (Foucault 2003, p. 8). Genealogy, he writes, is 'gray, meticulous and patiently documentary, [...] requires patience and knowledge of details, [...] depends on a vast accumulation of source material [and] demands relentless erudition' (Foucault 1991b, pp. 76–77).

Foucault referred to 'local' and 'subjugated' knowledges which, as Christopher Philo (2007, p. 346) points out, 'implicate the production of critiques—counterknowledges—emerging from particular people, settings, sites, points and maybe networks'. Foucault (2003, p. 8) remarks that these local knowledges 'have in a way been left to lie fallow, or even kept in the margins'. Place is important for Foucault because he sees an intimate connection and articulation of knowledge and location, of discourse and space, embodied in relationships, in the confluence of contingent social practices, local categories of understanding and material settings. As argued by Alison Faulkner in this volume, people engaged in collective action have recognised the importance of opening up spaces for the articulation of subjugated knowledges. Certainly the asylum space was seldom in the past a 'safe space' for such knowledge to come to fruition, but not without great difficulty, it was from just such unpromising places that the experiential knowledge of patients and survivors has grown and developed. The archaeology and genealogy of subjugated knowledges, Foucault thinks, allow us 'to decipher discourse through the use of spatial, strategic metaphors [which] enables one to grasp precisely the points at which discourses are transformed in, through and on the basis of relations of power'—echoing Jewson's analysis of the shifting loci of epistemic authority (Foucault 1980, pp. 69–70) . Opposition to the power of psychiatry over the mentally ill was, for Foucault (2002, p. 330), an 'immediate struggle' in which people 'criticise instances of power that are closest to them'. But he also saw it as a struggle against 'the privileges of knowledge' (Foucault 2002, p. 330). He spoke of an 'insurrection of subjugated knowledges', stating that he was referring to two things. On the one hand, he meant, by this, 'blocks of historical knowledges that were present in the functional and systematic ensembles, but which were masked, and the critique was able to reveal their existence by using, obviously enough, the tools of scholarship'. On the other hand, he believed that

> by subjugated knowledges one should understand something else, something which in a sense is altogether different, namely, a whole set of knowledges that have been disqualified as inadequate to their task or insufficiently elaborated: naive knowledges, located low down on the hierarchy, beneath

> the required level of cognition or scientificity [...]: the knowledge of the psychiatrized, the patient, the nurse, the doctor, that is parallel to, marginal to, medical knowledge. (Foucault 2003, p. 7)

The subjugated knowledges and counter-discourses were described by Foucault as

> what people know (and this is by no means the same thing as common knowledge or common sense but, on the contrary, a particular knowledge, a knowledge that is local, regional, or differential, incapable of unanimity and which derives its power solely from the fact that it is different from all the knowledges that surround it), it is the reappearance of what people know at a local level, of these disqualified knowledges, that made the critique [of the asylum] possible. (Foucault 2003, p. 8)

So here is a conception of local knowledge as something which grows out of the circumstances of specific places, which is not abstract and general, but concrete and particular. It could be described as descriptive, due to its being tied to the particular, as opposed to what can be explained (revealing causal connections) or universalised (the search for general and invariable laws). Condrau (2007, p. 536) suggested that 'the way forward' for the historiography of patients is 'to engage with debates that have raged elsewhere and to claim intellectual, empirical and theoretical importance in a field that has long enough been dominated by empirical, perhaps even descriptive, case studies'. The traces of debates that have raged elsewhere may lie in sources and places other than those traditionally sought by academic medical historians. Foucault (2003, p. 6) believes that 'the essentially local character of the critique in fact indicates something resembling a sort of autonomous and noncentralized theoretical production, or in other words a theoretical production that does not need a visa from some common regime to establish its validity'. 'What emerges out of this', says Foucault (2002, p. 14), is a 'genealogy' or 'a multiplicity of genealogical researches', concerned with the 'meticulous rediscovery of struggles and the raw memory of fights', and with the 'perspectival [...] polemical and strategic character of knowledge'.

A 'Question of Levels': Doing History from 'A Level Below Which You Cannot Sink'

When introducing his work on the social history of madness, Roy Porter (1996, pp. 1–2) remarked that he wished 'simply and quite literally to see what [patients] had to say'. He noted that 'it is curious how little this has been done; we have been preoccupied with explaining away what they said' (Porter 1996, p. 2). He wanted to see 'how the mad tried to explain their own behaviour to themselves and others in the language available to them' (Porter 1996, p. 2). 'But', he remarked, 'it would be foolish to fly to the other extreme and try to turn the mad *en bloc* into folk heroes, into radicals and rebels' (Porter 1996, p. 2). It must be noted that there are considerable difficulties in reaching the patient's voice, view or experience in recent history due to the paucity or inaccessibility of relevant primary sources. At this point we must turn our attention to SHG and OMH, to see what they had to say, to see how the foregoing historiographical reflections are closely connected to the concerns of these projects and how they might inform historical accounts of collective action by psychiatric patients and the methods used to explore this history. If Condrau found that 'a political background for patients is not easy to unearth', others, such as SHG and OMH, have had considerable success excavating such a background, particularly in the British context. According to Andrew Roberts, there have been two streams of research on the history of collective action by psychiatric patients, a 'survivor stream' and an 'academic stream' (Roberts 2010, p. 2). He believes that the academic stream has tended to take a 'theoretical approach external to the purpose of creating a history' and that 'until recently survivor historians knew and read the academic research, but academics appeared to be (and often were) ignorant of the survivor research' (Roberts 2010, pp. 1–2). Roberts (2010, p. 2) emphasises the importance of 'getting our empirical descriptions right and even avoiding theory'. SHG claim that their historical research is usually 'descriptive rather than theoretical' and that they aim to contribute to 'a fuller and more accurate description of the history of our movement', emphasising that their research has 'focused on the continuity of survivor action instead of considering it a by-product of intellectual trends, such as Laingian anti-psychiatry' (SHG 2011, p. 7). SHG (2011, p. 17) worry that 'the academic historian/sociologist may only be concerned to find some rough fit between theoretical models and data'. SHG (2011, p. 17) state that 'academics have suggested that in the broad sweep of history, the details we raise are trifling [...] whereas the detail of history matters to us because it bears on our lives and our heritage'. SHG see themselves as meeting the need to preserve the archives of their 'heritage' and 'the need to combine those archives with [...] memories' (Roberts 2010, p. 5). When SHG members Peter Campbell and Andrew Roberts (2009, p. 33) refer to John Perceval, member of the nineteenth-century Alleged Lunatics' Friend Society, as the energetic secretary at the centre of events, they, as the equally indefatigable secretaries of Survivors Speak Out and SHG in their time, see themselves more as the descendants of this long-dead son of an assassinated British prime minister, than the followers of the 'anti-psychiatry' intellectuals of the 1960s.

As a group founded and largely based in London, SHG has also identified the 'danger' of 'perpetuating the London-centric view of our history' (Campbell and Roberts 2009, p. 34). 'A way to guard against this', according to Campbell and Roberts (2009, p. 34), 'is to be aware that we are exploring a diversity of histories rather than one monolithic history'. 'Another way', they say, 'is to encourage the collating, preserving, and writing of history in different regions and localities' (Campbell and Roberts 2009, p. 34). Roberts (2009, p. 18) puts British anti-psychiatry of the 1960s and 1970s in its place, describing it as 'the cosmopolitan anti-psychiatry network in London's trendy Belsize Park'. He states that history is about 'more than a research method for survivors' (Roberts 2010, p. 3). The SHG manifesto refers to 'the construction of history to the exclusion of the patient' and 'the need for a space in which patients could make their own history' (Roberts 2010, p. 6). One of the stated aims of OMH, working in Edinburgh, was 'to enable [mental health] service users to see themselves and to be seen by others as active agents of change' (Maclean 2010, p. 8). Many of the people involved in these projects had themselves participated in histories of 'collective action', or in a 'movement' of mental health activists (known as the mental health service user, or survivor, movement) which emerged in the mid-twentieth century. They can be seen not only as local community history projects, but as politically self-conscious interventions in public debates around the place of the 'mad' or 'mentally ill' in contemporary society, as well as in the past. Roberts (2010, p. 3) argues that 'we must go back and reclaim our past so we can move forward; so we can understand why and how we came to be what we are today'. Part of what SHG are doing is 'attempting to build a positive and coherent self-identity' (Campbell and Roberts

2009, p. 33). The 'basic founding principle' of SHG is that 'service users own their history' (Roberts 2010, p. 6).

As Porter (1996, p. 25) has observed, psychiatric patients are often 'deeply conscious of having been made to feel different' with 'a sense of being rendered a non-person'. The 'walled and locked asylum [...] underscored the difference', thought Porter, and in response patients staked 'counter-claims, to shore up that sense of personhood and identity which they feel is eroded by psychiatry and society' (Porter 1996, p. 25). When the first mental patients' union in the UK was formed at Hartwood Hospital in Scotland, its members sent a strong message to the outside world. Thomas Ritchie, founder of the Scottish Union of Mental Patients (SUMP), was locked up in Hartwood for eight years before he joined with other patients to form a union and make their grievances known to the Mental Welfare Commission for Scotland, an independent body tasked with inspecting mental hospitals. Ritchie chose this name for two reasons, one of which, on the face of it, may appear more substantive than the other. The 'secondary reason' for choosing 'SUMP', instead of, say, National Union of Mental Patients ('NUMP'), was, according to Ritchie, 'to draw attention to the fact that there are variations between Scotland and England & Wales in respect of the mental health service' (Ritchie 1971, p. 1). The 'main reason for "Scottish" however', revealed Ritchie (1971, p. 1), was 'to contrive the abbreviation SUMP—a level below which you cannot sink'. Andrew Roberts has commented that

> a sump is a level below which one cannot go, it is the destruction of one's whole personality. That is where Tommy thought mental patients were, and what he wanted to change. As *Mental Patients News* wrote in February 1974: it was 'a question of levels', of rising up from the sump together. (Roberts 2018, personal communication/unpublished paper, 'Question of Levels')

Ritchie thought mental patients were regarded as 'the lowest form of life', that there was 'nothing lower' (Anonymous 1972, p. 2). Even for those psychiatric patients not detained in locked wards for an indefinite period of time, having their voices heard in the public sphere has been very difficult to achieve. OMH and SHG have managed to craft a place for themselves in the public sphere and their historical research is rooted in decades of social and political struggle, which in the UK can be traced to organisations like SUMP and the mental patients' unions which subsequently formed in the 1970s. The epistemic shift in which psychiatric subcultures rose to the surface and submerged knowledge was produced and transmitted by a marginalised group, owed much to material change and locational transition. Just as the shift from bedside to hospital medicine saw the disappearance of the sick person from medical cosmology, so too did the shift from asylum to post-asylum spaces and the cultural revolutions of the 1960s and 1970s afford more opportunities for psychiatric patients to enter into public discourse, whatever the merits or otherwise of deinstitutionalisation and the community care policies which transformed the social and geographical architecture of mental healthcare in the late twentieth century. These were grass-roots civil associations which emerged from the bottom-up, from particular people in local places, who, feeling stripped of individuality and agency, expressed solidarity with fellow patients and sought to recover their personhood and citizenship by joining with others in mutual aid.

Conclusion: Making Public Use of History Requires Embracing That Sinking Feeling of Difficulty and Conflict

Doing history from a level below which you cannot sink requires a public that is willing and able to act upon its shared situation. It is not without great difficulty that such an enterprise of community-based historical research, as opposed to academic history, can rise up to a space in social life which affords accessibility, visibility and dialogue between the various groups producing such knowledge and engaging in such action. Nonetheless, that is a problem often experienced in academic history too, particularly as the humanities have suffered in recent times from decisions made by political actors and the increasing emphasis placed on STEM subjects and 'useful' or 'practical' learning and knowledge. Although these projects have generated their own kind of internal order and exchange amongst their members, they sought to summon into being a public that did not yet exist, and in many respects they had no audience to begin with but themselves. They evidently do want to make public their use of history, and it is only through others paying attention to their work that it can occupy a public space and be transmitted to others interested in this field of work. They are seeking to 'give voice to an unheard class of people', but as Condrau points out, Porter's analogy from history from below is difficult because his patients 'stand against doctors' and 'there is not much room for social or local environment' (Condrau 2007, p. 533). Certainly OMH and SHG do not see themselves as merely 'contesting psychiatry', and they have emphasised the roots of their knowledge and action in solidarity and in local places. Andrew Roberts quotes survivor researcher and activist Peter Beresford (1998, pp. 11–12), who has suggested that 'if mental health service users/survivors are to take charge of our future, then we must also regain control of our past'. OMH and SHG raise questions about the nature of historical inquiry and of the authority of professional knowledge and expertise, but there are often tensions between the avowed aims of such groups to 'regain control of the past' and to 'make survivor history accessible to all who are interested in or studying mental health' (Campbell and Roberts 2009, p. 34). Whilst these groups have pioneered approaches to the history of psychiatry and mental health 'from below', often by contesting social identities imposed on them by others, there is a danger that history conceived as the possession, property or privileged perspective of one group, reinforces the existing boundaries and silences between academic and community history, and forecloses the possibility of boundary-crossing, fruitful exchange and knowledge sharing between those who identify as service users or survivors and others who do not. Likewise there is an obligation on those who do pay attention to the work of these groups to enter into a 'deep engagement' which is grounded in 'lived contradictions and dialogic relations with social movements themselves' (Cresswell and Spandler 2013, p. 139).

It cannot be assumed that historians have unmediated access to the historical past. It cannot be taken for granted that the historian re-enacts the past, or can reconstruct past events as they were experienced by those who participated in them. Condrau's distinction between an empirical view from below and a constructed, theory-laden perspective also encourages the assumption that there is the possibility of a pure description of data untouched by any interpretive viewpoint. Whilst it is appropriate for psychiatric patients or survivors to conduct historical inquiries, the attempt to create a distinct mode of inquiry such as 'survivor research', 'survivor history' and 'mad studies' appears to be predicated on the inquirer identifying as mad, or as a survivor, on the basis of their experience of being a psychiatric patient (Sweeney 2016; Sweeney et al. 2009). The differences of individual people who were involved in collective action must not be ignored, nor can we overlook the fact there are aspects of these historical events which were not known to participants. Of course, the historical research conducted by participants in the historical events under investigation is unique and important, but their indispensability should not preclude the possibility of those who did not participate in these historical events from also making valuable and critical contributions. History deals with individual and unique events, whereas science is a generalising mode of inquiry which seeks causal explanations, regularities and predictions. History, unlike science which often explains psychiatric patients' thought and action in terms of biochemical processes, natural necessities or deterministic causes, must account for the past in terms of the stuff of human conduct: intelligence, agency, shared ideas, discourses, practices and traditions, meanings and contexts. Accounts of the biochemistry of thinking cannot explain the meaning of what a person is thinking. The autonomy and importance of historical inquiry must involve a degree of detachment from present concerns to avoid the risks of anachronism and the smuggling of retrospective and presentist politics into accounts aimed at understanding what happened in the past. Nevertheless, it remains the case that historical knowledge is a construction and the past belongs to the present to the extent that our account of the past must be supported by the evidence available to us in the present. It is largely thanks to the research of groups like OMH and SHG that the primary sources necessary to interpret and construct an account of collective action by psychiatric patients in the past are preserved in an accessible form today, allowing for further reflection, inquiry and interpretation.

Conflict must be recognised by historians and neutral formal systems which impose neat frameworks and integrate the various parts into a comforting whole are inadequate to the task of investigating these histories. To do so belies the deeply fractured nature of society and the tensions between different groups, despite overlaps and the existence of people who straddle the boundaries between them. Only by acknowledging that tensions exist can a fruitful conversation between the academic historians and the community history projects proceed. No neutral perspective can be attained because these matters are deeply contested and value-laden. It is important to see social movements and community-history projects not merely as objects of research to be observed, described and explained, but as the work of intelligent agents who have the capacity to think and choose. There is also something valuable about the closeness of community history projects to communities of activists who have been part of recent historical waves of collective action. The attempt, as Faulkner puts it in this volume, to infiltrate the academy through the opening up of spaces within universities 'to develop theories, models and ideas about how we understand ourselves, or our experiences in relationship to mental health system(s), research and politics', is a helpful development, but it is not without its problems. Free inquiry is vital to gaining understanding of the history of psychiatry from the patient's view and investigating collective action by survivors of psychiatry, but as Geoffrey Reaume remarks elsewhere in this section, 'identity politics can work to exclude as well as include'. Reaume was part of similar projects in Canada which brought neglected community histories into the academy, directly inspiring OMH in the UK, where the purpose was not simply to centralise or universalise such local histories, but to bring them into the wider fold of historical research and to reveal a hidden past. Of course, people at the heart of the events and matters under investigation have something distinctive to offer that can't be found elsewhere, but it seems to me not to amount to the creation of a new method or subject matter, but rather it is unique individuals making their own original and valuable contributions to the wider body of knowledge. This does not require that we reduce people to single or group identities, nor does it entail that for historical research to be truly radical it must necessarily connect to present political struggles.

What is required is that we regard each person as different and worthy of respectful attention, and, as SHG advocates, we ought to be more attentive to the details that are sometimes neglected in over-intellectualised, over-theorised histories, which reduce the living, breathing stuff of historical change to desiccated abstractions. That said, theorising, debate, argument and alternative conceptualisations and interpretations are all part and parcel of free inquiry, and should not be dismissed out of hand. Whatever we call the inquiry, it is more about opening up possibilities for inquiring into neglected or hidden histories than dividing disciplines along lines of tribal group identity or politics. Whilst identity is part and parcel of making and studying history, genealogy, as advanced by Foucault, traces how social phenomena such as the mental health service user/survivor movement have grown out of foreign forms and antecedent events and are characterised by their own internal differences and divisions. By following the genealogical course of emergence and descent, we would then see the mental health service user/survivor movement as a 'massively differentiated entity', which speaks with many voices and is a sum of individual histories—'the purpose of history, guided by genealogy, is not to discover the roots of our identity, but to commit itself to its dissipation' (Foucault 1991b, p. 95). It is legitimate to say that collective action by psychiatric patients was not merely the product of 'anti-psychiatry' or intellectual trends, but still finds interesting links and connections with these movements. For example, in the Scottish context it is evident that there were strong affinities among patient activists with R.D. Laing's critical examination of psychiatric medicine, whilst not being reducible to an 'anti-psychiatry effect'. And perhaps it is worth considering the work of OMH and SHG not so much as against theory, but, like Foucault suggests, as an 'autonomous, non-centralised theoretical production' (Foucault 2003, p. 6). Rather than seeking, as Foucault puts it, a visa conferring validity from some common regime, the closeness to immediate struggles and the rootedness in settings both imposed and chosen—including those spaces created by people for the purpose of making this history public—offers something different, often something more directly drawn from primary sources, when compared with such inquiries undertaken in academic and university settings. Certainly there ought to be more collaboration between academic and community history on the history of mental health in order to make public use of this history. Without question, community history will require continuing support in the way of access to space and resources in order to sustain the valuable work they are doing, and it is vital that there are spaces outside of powerful and sometimes stifling institutions such as universities to do so.

There is no pure description or view from nowhere, and while the aims of historians are not the same as the theory constructors who seek universal knowledge at the expense of paying attention to particular people, actions and events, it must be recognised that historical knowledge is constructionist, interpretive and perspectival. The naïve realist or objectivist view sees the description of historical facts and the interpretive perspectives from which these are understood as neutral and unproblematic. Even those survivor historians and researchers, and particularly SHG, who want to subscribe to a model leaning more towards empirical research than abstract theory, must acknowledge that we are always organising our experience in ways that involve applying concepts and interpretations. What we see depends on how we look, and simply positing a 'direct experience' is inadequate to the task of making intelligible the situated and perspectival character of the knowledge drawn upon by community history projects such as OMH and SHG, those features which make them so distinctive and incapable of unanimity. As Allan Megill reminds us, 'historiography is a collective enterprise, and it is quite possible for an individual historian to forgo, in greater or lesser degree, the telling of a narrative that is already largely known' (Megill 1989, p. 651). When investigating a history that is largely unknown, or not well known, like the history of collective action by psychiatric patients, 'the question, "What was the case? is primal: it precedes the explanation-seeking question', a question which is concerned with theory production and discovering a cause that connects explanans and explanandum (Megill 1989, p. 648). Thanks to the likes of OMH and SHG, the history of collective action by psychiatric patients is becoming more widely known and better understood. A cultural heritage, like that which is explored by OMH and SHG, is never, as might be imagined, 'an acquisition, a possession that grows and solidifies; rather it is an unstable assemblage of faults, fissures and heterogeneous layers' (Foucault 1991b, p. 82). While we seek explanations, employ concepts and draw distinctions, we must also be aware of the motors of historical change in mobile social struggles and tensions, those complex forces of conflict and resistance which formed the backdrop for the emergence of collective action by psychiatric patients. The emergence of subjugated knowledge from the enclosed fortresses of the asylum and beyond has provided us with a greater appreciation of the demands by psychiatric patients for participation in civil society and the public sphere. It has also facilitated greater recognition of the echoes, resonances and reverberations between academic and survivor history. If the demand by OMH and SHG to recognise the individual agency and collective action of sufferers of mental illness and psychiatric survivors is to be met, they cannot simply be cast as people passively submissive to the interventions of medics and of social policy. Instead, a truly historical inquiry recognises the knowledge, agency and personhood of people who have often been objectified and subordinated by science and society. The nature of historical inquiry is such that it can preserve the dignity of persons sometimes denied by science, whilst recognising the vulnerability, the struggles and sufferings endured by those diagnosed with psychiatric conditions.

References

Ackerknecht, Erwin. 1982. *Short History of Medicine*. Baltimore, MD: Johns Hopkins University Press.

Anonymous. 1972. Special union to be formed for mental patients. *The Herald*, March 27.

Armstrong, David. 1984. The Patient's View. Social Science and Medicine 18: 737–744.

Armstrong, David. 1995. The Rise of Surveillance Medicine. Sociology of Health and Illness 17: 393–404.

Bacopoulos-Viau, Alexandra and Aude Fauvel. 2016. The Patient's Turn: Roy Porter and Psychiatry's Tales, Thirty Years On. Medical History 60: 1–18.

Barker, Ingrid and Edward Peck. 1987. Think it through: Theoretical perspectives. In *Power in Strange Places*, ed. Ingrid Barker and Edward Peck, 1–3. London: Good Practices in Mental Health.

Barnes, Marian. 1999. Users as Citizens: Collective Action and the Local Governance of Welfare. Social Policy and Administration 33: 73–90.

Barnes, Marian and Ric Bowl. 2001. *Taking Over the Asylum: Empowerment and Mental Health*. Hampshire: Palgrave.

Beresford, Peter. 1998. Past Tense. Peter Beresford on the need for a survivor-controlled museum of madness. *Openmind*, May/June: 11–12.

Brandon, David. 1991. *Innovation Without Change? Consumer Power in Psychiatric Services*. London: Macmillan.

Campbell, Peter. 1989. The Self-Advocacy Movement in the UK. In *Mental Health Care in Crisis*, ed. Anny Brackx and Catherine Grimshaw, 206–213. London: Pluto.

Campbell, Peter. 1994. The Contribution of Service Users in the Design and Implementation of Services. In *A Slow Train Coming: Bringing the Mental Health Revolution to Scotland*, ed. Christine Dean, 99–102. Glasgow: The Greater Glasgow Community and Mental Health Services Trust.

Campbell, Peter. 1996. The history of the user movement in the United Kingdom. In *Mental Health Matters: A Reader*, ed. Tom Heller, Jill Reynolds, Roger Gomm, Rosemary Muston and Stephen Pattison, 218–225. London: Palgrave.

Campbell, Peter. 1999. The service user/survivor movement. In *This is Madness: A Critical Look at Psychiatry and the Future of Mental Health Services*, ed. Craig Newnes, Guy Holmes and Cailzie Dunn, 195–210. Ross-on-Wye: PCCS Books.

Campbell, Peter. From Little Acorns: The mental health service user movement. In *Beyond the Water Towers: The unfinished revolution in mental health services 1985–2005*, ed. Andy Bell and Peter Lindley, 73–82. London: The Sainsbury Centre for Mental Health, 2005.

Campbell, Peter. 2006. *Some Things You Should Know About User/Survivor Action*. London: MIND.

Campbell, Peter and Andrew Roberts. 2009. Survivor's History Group. A Life in the Day 13 (3): 33–36.

Campbell, Peter and Diana Rose. 2011. Action for Change in the UK: Thirty Years of the User/Survivor Movement. In *The SAGE Handbook of Mental Health and Illness*, ed. David Pilgrim, Anne Rogers and Bernice Pescosolido, 452–470. London: SAGE.

CAPS (The Consultation and Advocacy Promotion Service). 2010. *Oor Mad History: A Community History of the Lothian Mental Health Service User Movement*. Edinburgh: Living Memory Association.

Claytor, Ann. 1993. A Changing Faith?: A History of Developments in Radical Critiques of Psychiatry Since the 1960s. Unpublished PhD thesis, University of Sheffield.

Condrau, Flurin. 2007. The Patient's View Meets the Clinical Gaze. Social History of Medicine 20: 525–540.

Cresswell, Mark and Helen Spandler. 2013. The Engaged Academic: Academic Intellectuals and the Psychiatric Survivor Movement. Social Movement Studies 12 2: 138–154.

Crossley, Nick. 1998. R.D. Laing and the British Anti-Psychiatry Movement: A Socio-Historical Analysis. Social Science and Medicine 47: 877–889.

Davies, Kerry. 2001. 'Silenced and Censured Travellers'? Patients' Narratives and Patients' Voices: Perspectives on the History of Mental Illness since 1948. Society for the Social History of Medicine 14: 267–292.

Ferguson, Iain. 2000. Identity politics or class struggle? The Case of the Mental Health Users' Movement. In *Class Struggle and Social Welfare*, ed. Michael Lavalette and Gerry Mooney, 228–249. London: Routledge.

Ferguson, Iain. 2003. Challenging a 'Spoiled Identity': Mental Health Service Users, Recognition and Redistribution. In *Disability, Culture and Identity*, ed. Sheila Riddell and Nick Watson, 67–87. Essex: Pearson Prentice Hall.

Fissell, Mary E. 1991. The Disappearance of the Patient's Narrative and the Invention of Hospital Medicine. In *British Medicine in an Age of Reform*, ed. Andrew Wear and Roger French, 92–109. London: Routledge.

Foucault, Michel. 1973. *The Birth of the Clinic*. London: Tavistock.

Foucault, Michel. 1980. Questions on Geography. In *Power/Knowledge: Selected Interviews and Other Writings, 1972–1977*, ed. Colin Gordon, 63–77. New York: Pantheon.

Foucault, Michel. 1991a. What is an Author? In *The Foucault Reader*, ed. Paul Rabinow, 101–120. Harmondsworth: Penguin.

Foucault, Michel. 1991b. Nietzsche, Genealogy, History. In *The Foucault Reader*, ed. Paul Rabinow, 76–100. Harmondsworth: Penguin.

Foucault, Michel. 2002a. Truth and Juridical Forms. In *Power: Essential Works of Foucault 1954–1984 Volume Three*, ed. James D. Faubion, 1–89. London: Penguin.

Foucault, Michel. 2002b. The Subject and Power. In *Power: Essential Works of Foucault 1954–1984 Volume Three*, ed. James D. Faubion, 326–348. London: Penguin.

Foucault, Michel. 2003. *Society Must Be Defended: Lectures at the College de France 1975–76*. Trans. David Macey. London: Penguin.

Foucault, Michel. 2006. *History of Madness*. London: Routledge.

Gallagher, Mark. 2017. From asylum to action in Scotland: the emergence of the Scottish Union of Mental Patients, 1971–2. History of Psychiatry 28(10): 101–114.

Gallagher, Mark. 2018. From associations to action: mental health and the patient politics of subsidiarity in Scotland. *Palgrave Communications* 4 34. https://doi.org/10.1057/s41599-018-0085-9.

Hervey, Nicholas. 1986. Advocacy or Folly: The Alleged Lunatics' Friends Society, 1845–63. Medical History 30: 245–275.

Jewson, Nicholas D. 1976. The disappearance of the sick-man from medical cosmology, 1770–1870. Sociology 10: 225–244.

Maclean, Kirsten. 2010. Introduction. In *Oor Mad History: A Community History of the Lothian Mental Health Service User Movement*, CAPS (The Consultation and Advocacy Promotion Service), 8–10. Edinburgh: Living Memory Association.

Megill, Allan. 1989. Recounting the Past: "Description," Explanation, and Narrative in' Historiography. The American Historical Review 94: 627–653.

Mold, Alex. 2011. Making the patient-consumer in Margaret Thatcher's Britain. The Historical Journal 54: 509–528.

Nicolson, Malcolm. 2009. Nicholas Jewson and the disappearance of the sick man from medical cosmology, 1770–1870. International Journal of Epidemiology 38: 639–642.

O'Donnell, Anne. 2008. Oor Mad History: Community history as a way of revitalising mental health collective advocacy. CONCEPT 18: 162–170.

Parsons, Talcott. 1951. *The Social System*. New York: Free Press.

Peterson, Dale. 1982. *A Mad People's History of Madness*. Pittsburgh: University of Pittsburgh Press.

Philo, Chris. 2007. 'Bellicose History' and 'Local Discursivities': An Archaeological Reading of Michel Foucault's Society Must Be Defended. In *Space, Knowledge and Power: Foucault and Geography*, ed. Stuart Elden and Jeremy W. Crampton, 341–365. Aldershot: Ashgate.

Porter, Roy. 1985. The Patient's View Doing Medical History from Below. Theory and Society 14: 175–98.

Porter, Roy. 1996. *A Social History of Madness: Stories of the Insane*. London: Phoenix Giants. (First published by Weidenfeld & Nicolson, 1987 with subtitle *The World Through the Eyes of the Insane*).

Reiser, Stanley Joel. 1978. *Medicine and the Reign of Technology*. Cambridge: Cambridge University Press.

Ritchie, Thomas. 1971. The Nature of the Association SUMP, Its Policy and Aims. The SUMP documents are held by Andrew Roberts of Survivors History Group (177 Glenarm Road, London, E50NB). Copies of the SUMP documents are held by Consultation and Advocacy Promotion Service (CAPS) (Old Stables, Eskmills Park, Station Road, Musselburgh, EH21 7PQ).

Roberts, Andrew. 2009. Scotland the Brave. Mental Health Today 9 6: 16–18.

Roberts, Andrew. 2010. History as research method: The Survivors History Group. Presentation at the Third Qualitative Research on Mental Health Conference, Nottingham, 25/8/2010, 1–12.

SHG (Survivors History Group). 2011. Survivors History Group take a critical look at historians. In *Critical Perspectives on User Involvement*, ed. Marian Barnes and Phil Cotterell, 7–18. Bristol: Policy Press.

Sweeney, Angela. 2016. Why Mad Studies Needs Survivor Research and Survivor Research Needs Mad Studies. Intersectionalities: A Global Journal of Social Work Analysis, Research, Polity, and Practice 5 3: 36–61.

Sweeney, Angela, Peter Beresford, Alison Faulkner, Mary Nettle and Diana Rose. 2009. *This is Survivor Research*. Ross-on-Wye: PCCS Books.

CHAPTER 18

Often, When I Am Using My Voice… It Does Not Go Well: Perspectives on the Service User Experience

Megan Alikhanizadeh, Corey Hartley, Sarah Kendal, Liz Neill, and Gemma Trainor

Introduction

This chapter aims to compare perspectives from the worlds of practice and lived experience, on using and hearing 'voice'. It explores some of the complexities and suggests what may happen next. It has been co-authored by young people who have personal experience of mental illness and by mental health professionals from the statutory and voluntary sectors.

M. Alikhanizadeh • C. Hartley • L. Neill (✉)
Common Room North Ltd, Leeds, UK
e-mail: liz.neill@commonroom.uk.com

S. Kendal
School of Healthcare, University of Leeds, Leeds, UK

G. Trainor
Liverpool John Moores University, Liverpool, UK

R. Ellis et al. (eds.), *Voices in the History of Madness*, Mental Health in Historical Perspective,
https://doi.org/10.1007/978-3-030-69559-0_18

Issues relating to youth mental health are discussed with the intention of encouraging readers to compare the political and social discourses of the twenty-first century with present-day predicaments and opportunities faced by young people who have mental health difficulties. We hear two voices: the first half of the chapter is built around the words of a mental health professional in the voluntary sector, who critiques the development of the youth service user movement. In the second half, a young mental health service user provides a contrasting commentary on her attempts to have her voice heard whilst carrying a label of 'mentally ill'. Their words are contextualised in wider discussions about voices of madness.

The Social and Political Background to Contemporary Models of Mental Health Care

It is perhaps inevitable that madness was within the reach of the new social movements that followed the Second World War. The second half of the twentieth century witnessed the questioning of deeply rooted concepts of 'other', feminist theory, for instance, permeating and disrupting gender and sexual politics in the US and beyond.[1] Kate Millet's passionate activism helped to push feminist critique into the sphere of mental health.[2] Similarly, in psychiatry, influential revolutionaries like Laing challenged the idea that madness was something that happened to other people, and validated patients' own accounts of their lived experience.[3] As Dyck and Russell put it, "the concept of 'mad pride' emerged in the 1960s and, like other pride movements, challenged the notion that madness, or gayness, or femaleness, was a disease to be treated rather than an identity to be celebrated."[4] Thus, we see a wide-ranging and energetic discourse about the language and importance of madness and other stigmatised human experience.

Goffman explored the meaning and impact of institutions during this period. He highlighted the problems created by separating individuals from the outside community and argued that a person who has spent a substantial period of time in any regulated and controlled environment will face potentially insurmountable challenges if they find themselves on the outside[5]. Long before Goffman, many such as John Langdon Down[6] had lobbied for places where people could be safe and adequately cared for, but Goffman pointed out the harmful effects of being institutionalised, even in a benign regime.

The work of Goffman and others questioned the long-standing practice of locking up children and adults who were perceived as having difficulties with their mental health or mental abilities.[7] Hence, when in the UK the 1959 Mental Health Act opened the way for a move towards community care, it was within a social narrative that was leaning away from asylums. Enoch Powell's 'water-tower' speech in 1961[8] made a case for the UK government's new direction of travel. By the 1980s, an NHS management review, 'The Griffiths Report', concluded with a recommendation to close the mental asylums and move the residents into facilities in the community.[9] This had already happened elsewhere, notably in Italy,[10] where the process was considerably quicker. The impetus was modernisation, though the argument put forward to the public emphasised a moral position.[11] 'Community Care' was implemented, but underfunded[12], and eventually recognised by the government as failed.[13] In the way that language for a stigmatised group keeps up with social trends, 'care in the community' became a new derogatory (if ungrammatical) collective noun for people who were struggling to cope outside mental institutions after decades of living within their walls.[14]

Many vulnerable groups, including children and young people in the care of the state, offenders, and people with learning disabilities, are in the care of institutions. Descriptions from Dickens and others[15] describe how certain types of children's institutions are inherently bad, and there are good reasons to have urgent concerns about children in institutions.[16] In the twenty-first century we have already seen many examples of abuse and stigmatisation.[17] Examples of abuse and neglect, of people largely deprived of a voice, continue to be exposed.[18,19]

There are, however, encouraging developments to mitigate this somewhat depressing picture. The idea of a beneficent institution for children has both historical[20] and current[21] credibility. The UK service user movement has had some success, though there are significant ongoing frustrations, as discussed for example by Elena Demke, Alison Faulkner, Mark Gallagher and Geoffrey Reaume's chapters in this volume. Activism in youth mental health seems increasingly relevant.

The first voice in this chapter consists of Liz Neill's personal reflections on the youth mental health service user movement. Liz is the director of 'Common Room North', an organisation in the UK voluntary (i.e. non-statutory) sector that connects the expertise of young people with researchers, policymakers and practitioners to ensure that lived experience influences research, policy and practice. Liz's words are italicised:

A PROFESSIONAL PERSPECTIVE ON THE RECENT HISTORY OF THE YOUTH SERVICE-USER MOVEMENT: LIZ NEILL, DIRECTOR OF COMMON ROOM NORTH

I have worked in the field of youth mental health for over 20 years, listening to and acting on young people's voices and enabling them to have an impact on mental health service provision, staff development and research.

During the 1990s, when I was first introduced to the term 'service user involvement', a prominent framework was Roger Hart's 'Ladder of Youth Participation'.[22] *This was a model that described positive engagement as moving from tokenism in the form of 'manipulation' and 'decoration', through to collaboration and shared decision-making alongside young people. At the time, however, there were few good examples of this happening in youth mental health. Those good practice examples which could be found tended to point towards consultation exercises or unambitious projects led by professionals, which fitted neatly into the current way of doing things. The idea of collaboration was little understood and not widely embraced.*

Resistance to listening to the voice of young service users

I witnessed some questionable models of practice, for example service users regularly re-telling traumatic events and disclosing personal stories in professional meetings, without a clearly defined purpose or aim. Professionals were unclear about how to respond and were often patronising, at times even clapped, and I imagine this was not a positive exercise for anyone in the room.

Some professionals were quite outspoken about their reservations about the 'service user movement' (e.g. see Femdal 2017[23]*). Some of their resistance, I'm sure, is rooted in the challenge that service user activism presents to mental health professionals who are used to believing they know best, possibly feel threatened personally, and are motivated to protect their professional discipline. But I think it is also about being frightened of change or being in systems that don't allow or encourage progression. It is risky to hand over power, and can also feel unfair when staff in large organisations have limited voice and influence. I believe that mental health staff often do not have the time or capacity to respond or grow in their professional roles, and that this is a major contributor to the resistance to enabling service user voice, that we find within the mental health professions.*

Enabling voice

I see more value in enabling young people's voice and influence, to challenge the status quo and ask people in positions of 'power' (by which I mean decision-makers and commissioners as well as practitioners and adults in general) to see things from a different perspective. I am also keen to explore the barriers to this, for example, when young people's experiences and views are too hard for us to hear, or do not fit with what seems feasible or reasonable. There is an opportunity here which often gets missed: for young people to learn how to play a part in decision-making processes and embrace the complexities; and to move beyond stating their opinions and views and onto participating in useful discussions, recognising challenges and helping to problem-solve.

In terms of individual care, there can often be a lack of autonomy or choice for young people about the support they receive in the mental health system. Furthermore, young people are still being sectioned (i.e. detained in hospital under the 1983 Mental Health Act)[24] *without understanding why or what will happen to them. Informing them properly is a great starting point but often gets missed.*

To give an example: Sophie, 15, sat on the strategic board of her local NHS Trust (mental health service provider), alongside representatives from the Royal College of Psychiatrists. She was invited to use this opportunity to comment on national publications and policy. While this was potentially a great opportunity, Sophie described to me meanwhile her struggles getting her voice heard regarding her own mental health care plan, and feeling totally compromised and frustrated in a recent meeting with her own psychiatrist, where information had not been shared properly with her and she was not able to have a say. The disconnect here is fairly common, as changes in operational systems are often easier to put into place than changes which involve personal relationships, and which may challenge clinical perspectives and approaches.

There is also a challenge to consider when young people become very ill, and their wishes and choices may not be in their best interests. In 1989, children's rights were enshrined in Article 12 of the UN Convention of the Rights of the Child,[25] *which states that 'every young person has the right to express their views, feelings and wishes in all matters affecting them and to have their views considered and taken seriously'. Here lies a real dilemma, in which young people may lack the capacity to make good decisions about their own care. Because of their illness, young people may not know at that time what is best for them. They may want to starve themselves or be adamant they want to die. Prioritising safety creates a grey area for promoting shared decision-making and is not straightforward. It can be easy to ignore what a young person is saying simply because they are inexperienced, but we need to be careful not to intensify the disempowerment that they are already experiencing because of their youth and mental health issues.*

Youth participation

Youth participation can be seen in various social trends throughout the 20th century,[26] *but as Rose et al.*[27] *shows, it is scarcely acknowledged in UK Mental Health Policy until the early years of the 21st century. The 1990 National Health Service and Community Care Act required a certain amount of local public consultation about mental health services, and promoted the idea of choice around service provider, but it did not bestow choice on individuals receiving compulsory treatment under the 1983 Mental Health Act. Subsequent policy did facilitate the involvement of (adult) mental health service users in some levels of discussion about service design and delivery. Tensions between how to offer service users choice while managing risk were evident in a government policy document published in 1999.*[28] *This may have been linked with the apparently declining interest in understanding collective opinion, in favour of providing a range of choices for individuals regarding their personal health and social care arrangements. However, the terms 'shared vision and commitment' were highlighted in proposals to transform services (in adult social care)*[29] *suggesting that the service user perspective was seen as important in policy development.*

First published in May 2005, National Youth Agency's Hear by Right framework[30] *provided a good practical basis for participation and coined the phrase 'built in not bolted on'—arguably asking for a cultural shift in which service provision would be steered by the voices of service users rather than clinicians. This seemed to reflect the impact of youth activism in the mental health service user movement. The cultural shift, however, was somewhat alien to statutory services. It was much easier to achieve from within a progressive third sector environment, where the provision is person-centred in its nature, and the needs of young people themselves have directly instigated the creation of a grassroots project to support them, rather than within an institution responding to government policy or statutory duty of care, such as the NHS. Furthermore, specialist provision tends to rest on sophisticated professional discipline and clinical expertise. Conversely, service users do not tend to distinguish between a psychiatrist, psychologist or psychotherapist, despite the emphasis placed on the distinction by the three professions. Service users are much more concerned with how comfortable a relationship feels, and simply experience a person helping or not helping.*

In the last two decades, the case for youth participation has been made persuasively, and is now seen in NHS-backed initiatives. For example, some sensible content was presented in the 'You're Welcome' framework[31] *which was supported by the Department of Health and first published in 2007. 'You're Welcome' required organisations to be better at considering young people's perspectives and how they access and experience service provision, rather than supporting them to navigate the inflexible operational systems which have been designed around staff and professional structures.*

In more recent years, the concept of participation and collaboration has featured increasingly in good practice guidelines and government policy. Despite Sophie's evidence, it does feel as though there is broad acceptance across service providers that this is generally the right thing to do and a useful approach. However, as a mental health professional working in the voluntary sector, my perspectives may well be different from those of professionals who work in the statutory services.

In September 2014, the UK Coalition government established the Children and Young People's Mental Health and Well-being Taskforce, which ultimately produced a key document: Future in Mind.[32] *The purpose of the Taskforce was to improve the state of child and adolescent mental health services in the UK. Amidst rising concerns about the state of children and young people's mental health, the Taskforce highlighted the importance of local action as opposed to centralised planning, underpinned by a philosophy suggesting that if young people feel good about themselves and are confident and optimistic about their future, they may become more resilient and better able to manage their mental health. Therefore, there was a certain confidence in young people's ability to find their own solutions. This reflects wider interest in models of healthcare that acknowledge the value of lived experience,*[33] *and contrasts with the doctor-patient power imbalances documented elsewhere in this volume. Future in Mind has young people's voice and influence embedded throughout. Whether practitioners have the resources or the capacity to do this well is another issue.*

Social media

A major issue for youth mental health is the role of social media, for better or worse.[34,35] *Social media may mean that young people's voices in relation to mental health are becoming louder. Furthermore, to some extent stigma is being tackled through an openness to share personal experiences of mental ill-health. Via online platforms, particularly twitter, there is—on the face of it—an equal playing field where anyone, regardless of age or status, can share their opinions and claim airtime; though it is questionable whether expressing a view on social media has much meaning or impact. Online groups lend themselves to peer support, which can grow organically and be there for people in a way that traditional support services cannot. This is a fantastic opportunity, has its own complexity and worrying implications; and like everything else that happens on line, no-one can fully control it or stop it happening. However, we need to embrace the positive elements of social media, and so do what we can to safeguard vulnerable young people.*

Facilitating voice?

There is now a real need to move on from basic consultation to more detailed meaningful conversations with young people. Nowadays, we can claim that we have consulted young people over many years about what they want and need, but consultation alone is not enough as has been clearly documented in the 'How many times do we have to tell you?' report.[36] *The themes found in that report back in 2011 are simple, yet disappointingly they are still relevant today: young people continue to ask for friendly, confidential, accessible services which communicate with them in relevant ways and are flexible and designed with young people in mind.*

Facilitating the voice of young people who are experiencing mental health difficulties is about respecting and supporting them, in a way that safely challenges them, where they are one part of the jigsaw in the decision-making scenario, one part of the solution, where everybody involved is learning from each other. We need to form partnerships where these relationships are mutually beneficial. It takes time, patience and investment. It requires a level of honesty and transparency and being ready with contingency plans, especially when young people have ongoing, fluctuating support needs and may dip in and out of being engaged and being well. Mental health professionals are still a long way off doing away with 'us and 'them', and we need to be better at listening to and learning from the voices of young people we are going to provide support in ways that best help them.

Liz Neill.

Liz's perspective highlights a narrative around ethical practice in relation to working with mental health service users. There is ongoing discussion around what empowerment means in mental health,[37] for instance whether mental health service users find it empowering or disempowering to relate their stories. Using mental health services is associated with powerful feelings of shame.[38] An important issue for mental health professionals is how to balance a mental health services user's right to participation (in anything and everything), with concerns around protecting them while they are vulnerable. Under-protection risks exposure to exploitation, yet overprotection risks undermining autonomy, recovery and growth. The problem is knotty, and for mental health professionals, it is not academic; they also have to work towards practical, accountable, decision-making on the ground.

There are parallels between professional and academic responsibilities. Chapter 1 of this volume refers to a debate between the editors, around naming individuals whose stories are presented within the chapters: whether revealing someone's full name and personal background shows respect or exposes a potentially shaming personal history. As Coleborne argues,[39] mental health historians need to retain a sharp awareness of the present whilst exploring the past.

The Policy Context

Liz's professional practice can be considered in the context of current policy around supporting young people's mental health in an era of social media. The responsibilities of schools and colleges to support student wellbeing have been expanding steadily since the UK coalition government came to power in 2010. In December 2018, the UK government consulted on proposals for further increase in the remit of the education sector to provide mental health support for young people. This was partly a response to the recommendations of 'Future in Mind',[40] which was unusual in the extent to which it incorporated the views of young people. The vision was that children and young people should be able to access good-quality mental health support, either via the National Health Service or via school- or college-based mental health services [41].

Making schools a main provider of mental health care could in theory tackle some of the pernicious and lasting stigma attached to mental illness and potentially make it easier for young people to find their voice and get help with their mental health. Yet these undoubtedly welcome developments were counterbalanced by the burden they placed on schools. Educators must extend their traditional pastoral roles to become mental health workers, and schools themselves did not appear to have choices about the new arrangements.

Already in 2017, the media had been reporting on the effect of budget cuts on schools[42]; by 2020, the struggles of schools to meet these expectations have been well documented. That vision of a new era in which young people would have a voice, and be enabled to access mental health support, via new non-stigmatising venues in the education systems, seemed to have become lost amongst the financial restraints.

Is Social Media the Future for Youth Mental Health Support?

One way to manage the costs of mental health services for young people and reduce the burden on schools is to harness the potential of social media platforms to deliver mental health support to young people. As pointed out earlier in this chapter, young people who want to talk about mental health and illness may find that social media gives them a platform. Social media is an obvious way in which young people with mental health difficulties can break through centuries of silence, sharing their ideas and experiences, accessing expertise and support and getting messages out to the wider world. For example, there are digital mental health resources such as 'KOOTH', which offer safe and supportive online spaces where young people can express their concerns and find guidance and treatments that have been proven to work. In the future, it is likely that such platforms will be providing new forms of mental health care to a large number of young people, at reduced cost compared with both the traditional models of mental health care, which are structured around face-to-face appointments with specialists in clinics and hospitals, and also the newer ideas that involve the participation of the education sector.

Yet these innovations bring their own costs. We have seen throughout this book that historical attitudes to madness frequently involved institutionalisation together with close supervision. (It is worth noting that there are many examples worldwide of oppressive cultures in modern children's institutions, including cases that are close to home,[43] alongside formal, albeit imperfect,[44] channels for complaint.[45]) Whether an institution is experienced as therapeutic or punitive, those on the receiving end may have limited opportunities to make their own decisions.

Outside institutional settings, many young people are growing up in environments where pressures such as 'impression management', often via their social media profiles, are intense influences on how they express themselves and conduct their lives, alongside the new pressures of a global pandemic. Thus, regardless of differences between the life of a modern child and their eighteenth-century peer, they too can be in distress, unheard and vulnerable to tragedy. Therefore, new developments in helping young people to improve their mental health require new ways of thinking about what the risks are and how to manage them—the familiar discourses around autonomy, safety, power, agency and voice.

Mitigating the Risks of Social Media

The risks of social media to mental health are well rehearsed in public discourse, though it seems that the public's concerns may be more anecdotal than evidence-based.[46] One cause of great anxiety, much discussed in the media and borne out by tragic events, is the idea that young people who use the internet put their mental health at risk. High suicide rates among young people in the trans community have also been linked with social media.[47] Internet use has been associated with suicide, self-harm and eating disorders in young people. In the UK, a national inquiry into suicide-related internet use found that almost a quarter of the children and young people who had died by suicide in the UK between 2014 and 2016 had searched the internet for information on suicide methods.[48]

User-generated online content and communities can be filtered by the use of social media moderation. Regulation and moderation initiatives have created a patchwork of rules and cultural norms but these have not been consistent or potent enough to address the challenges. Illegal and unacceptable content is widespread. However, in the recent UK government policy statement 'Online Harms',[49] plans are proposed for a new system of accountability and oversight for tech companies to keep UK users safe online. The document sets out the government's intention to establish a new, statutory duty of care to make companies take more responsibility for the safety of their users, which will be overseen and enforced by independent regulation. This is the first time that a westernised government has set out to regulate the companies that dominate the online world and potentially improves the potential of social media to be a reliable space for young people to have helpful conversations about mental health.

The Voice of Lived Experience

The second voice in this chapter belongs to Megan Alikhanizadeh, a young adult with lived experience of mental illness and accessing mental health services. Megan's account resonates closely with the glimpse of Sophie's experiences that Liz Neill described above. She reflects on voice through her experiences of attempting to contribute to mental health services development, the impact of celebrity mental illness on public attitudes to madness, and what happens to the right to a voice when a person is actively unwell. Megan's words are italicised:

MEGAN ALIKHANIZADEH: BEING UNHEARD AND UNDER-VALUED

Today, there is a narrative about mental health recovery in society, not institutionalisation. Across the UK, there are some new care models for youth mental health that illustrate how things are continuing to move further away from the asylum model, and towards the community instead. The general aim of these models is usually to keep young people out of hospital, provide intensive personal treatment with as few restrictions as possible, and to give people (and their families) as normal a life as possible.

Many of these newer models, their values and their aims, are guided by direct discussions with young people and their families. However, despite the positive intentions, some important issues have not been resolved. There are still very real, ongoing, themes of disempowerment for young people. We feel patronised and misunderstood, as though we are not taken seriously, and that our struggles are not valid, especially if we are not in hospital. Over time, I have come to recognise that feelings of being unheard and under-valued are still a big feature of the adult service user's experience, but yet young people do feel we would be treated better in this respect if we were not so… young.

Furthermore, keeping people in the community and out of hospital is not as simple as it may sound. Some people do need to be in hospital, and some people want to be in hospital. This "want" often comes from a need for validation. It is complex, and there is still a great need for a cultural shift in both service users and services. People should not have to feel as though, in order for their illness to be valid, they have to hurt themselves or prove that they are "ill enough". It is crucial that people's struggles are taken seriously, especially in the community, if young people's mental health care is going to work properly.

As a service user, I have first-hand experience of resistance to my voice. I received a clear message about tokenistic service user involvement when I was invited onto a panel to interview for a consultant psychiatrist. The reality was that I had to ask readily prepared questions, in a room separate to the rest of the panel. What does that say about the relevance of my voice, or how far we have climbed up Hart's ladder of participation[22]*?*

The value of the mental health service user voice is supposedly recognised in policies that require us to be paid for our time and reimbursed for our expenses. However, my experience is that payments and reimbursements do not happen unless they are chased up. This concerns me, both because I feel that some vulnerable people, who aren't aware of the availability of payments or able to follow this up; and also because it makes me, the service user, feel even less worthy, less valued, less confident, and less likely to engage in the future, that ultimately, my voice means nothing.

Money and privilege: The problem with celebrity mental illness

The mental health struggles of Amy Winehouse, among notable others, were somehow glamorised in the press, making her into a tragic (but attractive) figure. The popular view that our society is more open, more accepting and the stigma around mental health has been dramatically reduced, is arguably evidenced by many celebrities disclosing their own struggles. This is often quoted as positive, and good for breaking down stigma, because ultimately celebrities are role models in our society, and they often set an example for others to follow, particularly young people. Unfortunately, if you unpick this it is actually problematic.

When someone, such as a celebrity, takes their own life, people get upset. Often in the aftermath people say they are strongly in favour of raising mental health awareness, improving support, etc., just as they do on World Mental Health Day and similar occasions. However, this is generally as far as it goes, and it feels superficial. In reality these same people still squirm, turn away or respond negatively when people do display symptoms of mental health struggles. People say they want to help make things better, but there's still an inability to view others with open-mindedness, compassion and sensitivity, particularly in the digital age of internet and media.

Headlines are presented and worded in a way that tells us people are 'admitting' to their struggles with mental illness, as if they are something to be ashamed of. We might suspect that this something gives the celebrity some more credentials. But what kind of illnesses are we are talking about? It seems that this admission comes from a place of luxury and privilege. It is sugar coating some of the real issues for many (ordinary) people around isolation, poverty etc. Wealthy celebrities can pay to access specialist therapies when they feel they need it, whereas the general public, especially those in hospital, do not have that luxury of having resources at our fingertips. For example, celebrities may talk about "deciding" to have (private) therapy during a period of poor mental health. This type of opinion implies that not accessing therapy when you need it is just a matter of choice, and it makes painful reading for those of us who cannot afford such luxury.

The privileges of celebrity do not necessarily prevent severe mental health difficulties but, in some cases, can a personal story of mental illness actually be used to help with promoting a product, a tour, a career? As the magazine Marie Claire said,[50] *"Here are a few celebrities who have bravely admitted their struggles with mental health"; and yet, if you tell people that you have a mental illness, but it is not the right kind, you will not be categorised as "bravely admitting" to your problem. Many of the more severe illnesses are only spoken about in connection with chaos and danger.*[51] *It seems to be romantic to be emotionally unwell, provided that you do not cross a certain line. It can feel to me as though only people with certain experiences and backgrounds are 'allowed' to have a voice. Despite all social change, we are faced with a culture of toxic masculinity, where we act tough, show no weakness and do not easily talk about emotional wellbeing. If we do talk about our mental illness experiences, we have to tidy them up so that they do not make anyone feel uneasy. We have to be 'other', i.e. so different from you, that you do not, for one second, feel as though what is happening to us could ever happen to you. I think this is a version of censorship, a way to silence us. Suicide is the biggest killer in men under the age of 45, and all genders under 35. We can mention cancer or heart disease anywhere, any time. But, there are many young people who look around at how comfortable society is with talking about (and funding) certain other health conditions, and conclude that from society's point of view, we do not really matter. We are only young people, it is only mental illness, we do not have anything useful to say. Since no one listens to us, no one actually has to do very much about it.*

Voices that people don't want to hear

It is no secret that there is an abundance of stigma surrounding mental health. In our current society it seems that a lot of people think we have removed much of the stigma and yes, people are talking more; but in reality, this is only scratching the surface. The conversations are only really about the more 'palatable' parts of mental ill health, such as mild depression or anxiety, and when people talk about their experience of mental illness it is generally when they are seen to be in their "right mind", rather when they are experiencing symptoms strongly. In my opinion, stigma is still a massive issue. One of the hardest things, still, about having a mental illness, is people expecting you to behave as if you do not.

Often, when I am using my voice to explain how I'm feeling and ask for help, it does not go well. I meet so many professionals who confuse my ability to be articulate with an ability to cope, telling me that despite what I am saying, the very fact that I am saying it at all means that I am okay, job done. This is incredibly dismissive and damaging. The idea that 'mentally ill' must equal 'non-communicative' also puts me (and others) into a neat category, that means our voice is not ever considered in the first place anyway. However, when I am functioning in a way that signifies to these professionals that I am more "well", I am not classed as being in that "mentally ill" category, so I do not have a useful voice here, either.

Maybe these people are viewed as less stable and people are less inclined to listen to what they have to say. People detained under sections of the Mental Health Act for example, do not get to make decisions about their treatment. Often, when unwell, people are unable to articulate their thoughts, feelings and needs clearly. Yet, they still have valid, useful and REAL feedback. They may just need some support in communicating it—but this is not something that is readily facilitated. When a person is unwell, their concern is not necessarily on campaigning to reduce stigma. But still then why, when they are doing well, are the people with more severe mental illnesses not being allowed a voice?

With diagnoses like depression and anxiety, which seem to be spoken about most often, there is a variety of symptoms, but generally the experiences are fairly similar between sufferers. Yet in more severe illnesses, the symptoms, presentations and experiences can vary so greatly that perhaps people looking on do not know where to start when summing these up—and in fact, often jump to old stereotypes, i.e. people with severe mental illnesses are dangerous criminals, addicts, homeless etc—sweeping generalisations that preserve the comforting illusion of distance between themselves and a "mad" person.

I have argued here that only those people who are out of their 'dark depths', who are well enough to function as a regular part of society, are allowed a voice. And I suspect that this is the reason: such people will be able to represent mental illness in a way that does not cause fear, discomfort, or present issues that are just too difficult for society to digest. Maybe people are still scared, even in modern times. They fear what they do not understand. In the more traditional models that paired insanity with asylums, people were outcasts from society. Like Foucault, I think society finds it uncomfortable to accept these people, who have been outcast from society for a long time.[52]

Megan Alikhanizadeh

Conclusion

This chapter draws on lived experience to portray a complex picture of shifting spaces and places in the treatment (in both senses) of mental illness. This is a world which might seem to be growing generally inclusive and open-minded, and to mental health service users specifically. Yet Megan and Liz's narratives tell us something different. Megan still feels voiceless and vulnerable, and Foucault's reflections on power relations seem as pertinent as ever.

We have aimed to highlight different positions regarding how voice is interpreted when its owner is deemed to be 'mad'. There is an alliance between service user and professional, although they might appear to have discordant agendas: one grapples with the labyrinthine task of balancing competing ethical arguments and professional responsibilities, and the other is embroiled in the preposterous riddle of trying to articulate madness to people who think you are too mad to be worth listening to. Though the agendas do differ, they are also synergetic.

We emphasise the disconnect between the casual assumption that a 'mad' voice is welcomed in contemporary settings and the reality of being silenced. Mental health historians argue that it is naïve to suggest the past was really so bad as to have little in common with the present. Megan argues that it would be naïve to believe the rhetoric that tells us society feels comfortable around mental illness. What the legislation and guidelines say may bear no relation to how that feels to the person on the receiving end. Aims, resources and expectations change over time and distance, yet the facilitation and hearing of 'voice' is consistently unreliable.

As Megan says: *It is important for young people that adults who are in positions of influence take a more realistic, less reactive view of mental illness, one that allows for things to be difficult and complicated. This would help those with mental health difficulties to break through centuries of silence, sharing their ideas and experiences, accessing expertise and support and getting messages out to the wider world.*

Acknowledgement Grateful thanks to Dr Andrew Clifton, Associate Nursing Professor at de Montfort University, for his helpful comments on this chapter.

Notes

1. Ceballos, Jacqueline; Greer, Germaine; Johnston, Jill; Trilling, Diana; Mailer, Norman. 1979. *Town Bloody Hall.*
   Hegedus, Chris and Pennebaker, D.A. (Directors). Pennebaker Hegedus Films, Inc. United States.
2. Millet, Kate. 1969. *Sexual Politics.* Illinois: University of Illinois Press. See also: Shulevitz, Judith. 2017. *Kate Millett: 'Sexual Politics' and Family Values.* The New York Review. Available at: https://www.nybooks.com/daily/2017/09/29/kate-millett-sexual-politics-and-family-values/. Accessed 07 April 2020.
3. Laing, R.D., *The Divided Self: An Existential Study in Sanity and Madness.* 1960, Harmondsworth: Penguin.
4. Dyck, E. and G. Russell, *Challenging Psychiatric Classification: Healthy Autistic Diversity and the Neurodiversity Movement*, in *Healthy Minds in the Twentieth Century: In and Beyond the Asylum. Mental Health in Historical Perspective Series.* 2020. pp. 167–187. (p168).
5. Goffman, *Asylums: Essays on the Social Situation of Mental Patients and Other Inmates.* 1961, New York: Anchor Books.
6. Ward, O. (1999) John Langdon Down: The Man and the Message. *Down Syndrome Research and Practice*, 6(1), 19–24. doi:10.3104/perspectives.94.
7. Bentall, R.P., *Madness explained : psychosis and human nature.* 2004, London: Penguin.
8. Powell, E.J. 1961. *The Rt. Hon. J. Enoch Powell Minister of Health Address to the National Association of Mental Health Annual Conference, 9 March 1961.* Available a*t* http://www.nhshistory.net/watertower.html. Accessed 07 April 2020.
9. Davidmann, M.M., *Reorganising the National Health Service: An evaluation of the Griffiths report.* Reorganising the National Health Service : An evaluation of the Griffiths report, 1985.
10. Micheli, G.A., *Not just a one-man revolution: The multifaceted anti-asylum watershed in Italy.* History of Psychiatry, 2019. **30**: pp. 133–149.
11. Tomlinson, D.R., *Utopia, community care and the retreat from the asylums.* 1991.
12. Brandon, S., G. Hemmings, and C.R. Tomson, *Asylums in an age of community psychiatry.* The Lancet, 1985. 326(8460): pp. 894–894.
13. Rose, D., et al., *How do managers and leaders in the National Health Service and social care respond to service user involvement in mental health services in both its traditional and emergent forms? The ENSUE study.* Health Services and Delivery Research, 2014. **2**: pp. 1–94.

14. Ramon, S., *The impact of the Italian psychiatric reforms on North American and British professionals.* International Journal of Social Psychiatry, 1989. **35**: pp. 120–127.
15. *Dickens, Charles. 2015. Oliver Twist. New York, New York: Open Road Media Integrated Media.*
    Dickens, Charles. 1907. Nicholas Nickleby. London: Dent.
    Brontë, Charlotte. 2014. Jane Eyre. Minneapolis: Lerner Publishing Group.
16. Julian, M.M., et al., *Young Children in Institutional Care: Characteristics of Institutions, Children's Development, and Interventions in Institutions BT—Children's Social Worlds in Cultural Context*, T. Tulviste, D.L. Best, and J.L. Gibbons, Editors. 2019, Springer International Publishing: Cham. pp. 217–229.
17. Multiple signatories. 2019. *Open letter to the Secretary of State for Health and Social Care 12 June 2019* Available at https://www.vodg.org.uk/wp-content/uploads/20190612-VCSE-sector-Hancock.pdf Accessed 07 April 2020.
18. Bessant, J., R. Hil, and R. Watts, *Violations of trust: how social and welfare institutions fail children and young people.* 2005.
19. The scope of this chapter does not allow a broader discussion about institutional abuse of children, though we recognise it as another urgent topic.
20. For example, see chapters by Hutchison and Junghans in this volume.
21. Holmes, Lisa, Cath Connolly, Emily Mortimer, and Rowan Hevesi. 2018. "Residential Group Care as a Last Resort: Challenging the Rhetoric." *Residential Treatment for Children & Youth* 35 (3): 209–224. See also: Gearing, R.E., et al., *Prevalence of Mental Health and Behavioral Problems Among Adolescents in Institutional Care in Jordan.* Psychiatric Services, 2013. **64**(2): pp. 196–200.
22. Hart, R.A., *Stepping Back from 'The Ladder': Reflections on a Model of Participatory Work with Children*, in *Participation and Learning: Perspectives on Education and the Environment, Health and Sustainability*, A. Reid, et al., Editors. 2008, Springer Netherlands: Dordrecht. pp. 19–31.
23. Femdal, I. and I.R. Knutsen, Dependence and resistance in community mental health care—Negotiations of user participation between staff and users. *J Psychiatr Ment Health Nurs*, 2017. **24**: pp. 600–609.
24. Mind, *Sectioning.* mind.org.uk, 2020.
25. UNICEF. *United Nations Convention on the Rights of the Child.* United Nations. 1989.
26. Loncle, P., *Youth participation in Europe: beyond discourses, practices and realities.* 2012.
27. Rose, D., et al., *How do managers and leaders in the National Health Service and social care respond to service user involvement in mental health*

services in both its traditional and emergent forms? The ENSUE study. Health Services and Delivery Research, 2014. **2**: pp. 1–94.

28. Britain, G., *Modernising Mental Health Services: Safe, Sound and Supportive.* 1999, The Stationery Office: London.
29. Department of Health, *Putting People First: A Shared Vision and Commitment to the Transformation of Adult Social Care.* 2007, HM Government: London.
30. Wade, H., et al., *Hear by right: Standards for the active involvement of children and young people.* 2003, National Youth Agency: Leicester.
31. Department of Health England. *You're Welcome: Quality Criteria for Young People Friendly Health Services.* 2011. London, England.
32. Department of Health and NHS England. *Future in mind: Promoting, protecting and improving our children and young people's mental health and wellbeing.* 2015. Department of Health and NHS England.
33. NHS Improvement. 2018. *Valued care in mental health: Improving for excellence: Experts by experience.* Department of Health. Available from: https://improvement.nhs.uk/documents/3450/NHS_Mental_Health_Improvement_Chpter_1.pdf
34. Department for Digital Culture Media and Sport, *Online Harms White Paper—CP 57.* 2019: pp. 1–102.
35. *Dickson K, Richardson M, Kwan I, MacDowall W, Burchett H, Stansfield C, Brunton G, Sutcliffe K, Thomas J (2018) Screen-based activities and children and young people's mental health: A Systematic Map of Reviews, London: EPPI-Centre, Social Science Research Unit, UCL Institute of Education, University College London.*
36. Lavis, P. and L. Hewson. *How Many Times Do We Have To Tell You? A Briefing From The National Advisory Council About What Young People Think About Mental Health And Mental Health Services.* 2011.
37. See for example Allison, R., *Power to the people: practitioners, patients and power*, in The Mental Elf, 2017. Blog. Accessed 03 August 2020 from https://www.nationalelfservice.net/populations-and-settings/service-user-involvement/power-to-the-people-practitioners-patients-and-power/
38. Jones A, Crossley D., In the mind of another shame and acute psychiatric inpatient care: An exploratory study. A report on phase one: Service users. *J Psychiatr Ment Health Nurs.* 2008;15(9):749–757. doi:10.1111/j.1365-2850.2008.01316.x.
39. See volume Coda:- Coleborne, C: Speaking Madness: Word, Image, Action.
40. Department of Health and NHS England. *Future in mind: Promoting, protecting and improving our children and young people's mental health and wellbeing.* 2015. Department of Health and NHS England.

41. Parkin, E., R. Long, and M. Gheera, *Children and young people's mental health—policy, services, funding and education*, 2019. House of Commons Briefing Paper 07196 , House of Commons: London.
42. Ratcliffe, R., *Cuts, cuts, cuts. Headteachers tell of school system 'that could implode'*, in *The Guardian*. 2017, Guardian News & Media Limited online.
43. Amongst other UK examples, see: Challenging Behaviour Foundation, Positive Active Behaviour Support Scotland, 2019. *Reducing restrictive intervention of children and young people: Case study and survey results.* RRISC group.
44. Prisons & Probation Ombudsman. *Young people in custody make few formal complaints but some are serious, says Ombudsman* | Prisons & Probation Ombudsman: Prisons and Probation Ombudsman; 2017 [Accessed 03 August 2020 from: https://www.ppo.gov.uk/news/young-people-in-custody-make-few-formal-complaints-but-some-are-serious-says-ombudsman].
45. Kmieciak B, Gmitrowicz A. The dignity of the child in a psychiatric hospital. [Polish, English]. *Psychiatr Psychol Klin.* 2012;12(4):273–82.
46. *Dickson K, Richardson M, Kwan I, MacDowall W, Burchett H, Stansfield C, Brunton G, Sutcliffe K, Thomas J (2018) Screen-based activities and children and young people's mental health: A Systematic Map of Reviews, London: EPPI-Centre, Social Science Research Unit, UCL Institute of Education, University College London.*
47. For example, see: Chang, Brie and Kathleen Delaney. 2019. "A Heuristic Inquiry on the Role of person-environment Interaction in Suicide Risk among Transgender Youth." *Journal of Child and Adolescent Psychiatric Nursing* 32 (2): 47–50. and Ortiz, Patricia and Eindra Khin Khin. 2018. "Traditional and New Media's Influence on Suicidal Behavior and Contagion." *Behavioral Sciences & the Law* 36 (2): 245–256.
48. NCISH, *Suicide by children and young people in England*. in *National Confidential Inquiry into Suicide and Safety in Mental Health (NCISH)*. 2016. Manchester.
49. Department for Digital Culture Media and Sport, *Online Harms White Paper—CP 57*. 2019: pp. 1–102.
50. Proudfoot, J., *For World Mental Health Day 20 celebrities speak honestly about their mental health battles*, in *Marie Claire*. 2019, TI Media Limited: London.
51. Parry, R. and S. Moyes, *1,200 killed by mental patients*, in *The Sun*. 2013, updated 2016, News Group Newspapers Limited: UK.
52. Jones, C. and R. Porter, *Reassessing Foucault: Power, medicine and the body* 1994, Routledge: London & New York.

CHAPTER 19

Coda: Speaking Madness: Word, Image, Action

Catharine Coleborne

Writing about the history of madness through the lives of former inmates of institutions has taken me to many physical spaces—both imagined and real—and has introduced me to hundreds of individual stories of mental breakdown and confinement. Over time I have come to understand this as an enormous privilege: I recognise that my ability to enter into the world of the past through the archive of written accounts, and sometimes oral recordings, has given me an insight into the experiences of people struggling for affirmation, support, care and understanding at different historical moments. These experiences were voiced at one time or another by people who found themselves confined, or by people close to them who had cared for them at home, or by institutional staff who watched and listened to the 'mad' and recounted what they saw and heard. My attempts to understand the language of madness means that I have scrutinised words and sounds in detail, collecting and analysing the way madness presented itself in the past.[1] The voices of madness are often mediated and

C. Coleborne (✉)
School of Humanities and Social Science, University of Newcastle, Callaghan, NSW, Australia
e-mail: Catharine.Coleborne@newcastle.edu.au

R. Ellis et al. (eds.), *Voices in the History of Madness*, Mental Health in Historical Perspective,
https://doi.org/10.1007/978-3-030-69559-0_19

refracted in this way, and historians have been attentive to the problem of 'voice' in their discipline.

The contents of this new volume originated at the 'Voices of Madness' conference held at Huddersfield in 2016. These sophisticated pieces of history are testament to the success of that event, which signalled that a new generation of histories of mental health was about to come of age. The chapters here advance our thinking and appreciation of what the volume editors argue in their Introduction is a broader understanding of 'the multiplicity of voices in mental ill-health'. Through their conference, Robert Ellis, Sarah Kendal and Steve Taylor wanted to reflect on the way that historians had 'sought to place voices of previously silent marginalised, disenfranchised individuals at the heart of their analyses'. Their aim was to explore and reveal the voices of not only those with mental illness but also those treating mental illness.

These voices tumble out of what the editors describe as the 'industry of madness', with all of its professionals, carers, helpers, families, commentators and the patients themselves. The idea of the 'industry' hints at a deeper engagement with the ideas of a number of scholars, including Andrew Scull and Jonathan Andrew, who documented the 'trade' of mad doctors as part of a new economic and social ordering of peoples in Britain and Europe over time.[2] The exciting idea here is that the 'voices' we start to listen for and hear suggest more complex relationships and readings of institutional care and patient experience, sometimes also challenging our expectations of the voices we hoped to hear. This is especially true when we think about the role of advocates: those people who took up the causes of children, or patients who had no opportunity to voice their own stories or accounts. In this way, we are pushed beyond the perhaps simplistic engagement with the idea of 'the patient voice' and find significant meaning in the work of scholarly historians who can locate and interpret this source material. In doing this work, these historians also inhabit the worlds of the speakers, the interlocuters of the past, including carers and practitioners.

As a scholar who has been part of the wider scholarly milieu of asylum histories for over twenty years, my own sense of the future for the history of madness as a field of inquiry has been changing since the first decade of the new century. From the mid-2000s, histories about mental health care, institutions and post-institutional communities, including patient, survivor and consumer movements, have been jostling for position in the hierarchy of historiographical explanations of mental health. By then, as I have argued elsewhere, it was no longer possible to write about insanity, mental breakdown or madness without reference to the experiences of those confined as mad.[3] It has been something of a challenge to historians that the valency of historical arguments about the nineteenth-century institution using patient records retrieved from archives was contested as institutional closures gave rise to new ideas and ways of thinking about historical renditions of madness, largely driven by the mad themselves.[4]

The conference was, in my experience, a vital conversation across the table with colleagues involved in mental health activism and advocacy, as well as multidisciplinary approaches to talking about mental health. It was at times an uncomfortable space to be in, but in a productive way. I was listening to academic papers in a different way, or with new skills of 'hearing' about the history of madness. Highlights of the conference programme included poetry, theatre and the introduction to the radical work of *Asylum Magazine* in historical perspective by practitioners and academics active in radical mental health politics.[5] I found myself reflecting that it was not satisfactory to write about the case notes and files of the mad in the manner of 'writing about patients' without a deep understanding of the impact of that act on readers, or listeners in the room, or whole communities of people who have experienced the mental health system. This message had been continually delivered to me over the previous decade, not with hostility, but with strength; it was stated at public events around the history of mental health as witnessed through art, at public talks promoting museum exhibitions, and through the community and network of mental health practitioners and those with lived experience of institutional care.[6]

The scope of these understandings is also important. In my keynote address for the conference, I wanted to take the audience through my periodisation of mental health history in a transnational context, referring to this as 'talk, dissent, and silence'. As this book also spotlights in its discrete section focused on madness and activism, I also wanted to privilege the importance of a collective identity for the mad. There has always been talk by the mad themselves, but it has not always been heard or easy to access, a theme I pursue in my book *Why Talk About Madness*.[7] There has been plenty of talk about madness, which at various points in the past has created dissent: forms of dialogue, debate, disagreement. Dissent, then, should be seen as a historical process in the long history of mental health care and treatment regimes, and not confined to one period in the latter part of the twentieth century. Silence has also always been present—for the mad, labouring inside institutions that did not listen to them; for those trying to advocate for people will mental illness conditions; and sometimes as a response from policymakers, governments and whole societies trying to understand the meaning of madness in their own places and communities.

Part of my argument was to suggest that the history of madness can now be seen as having new potential as a scholarly field. This follows widespread institutional closures from the 1970s in Western countries, opening up the possibility of talk, dissent and a reckoning with the silences of previous eras. The question of where it all started, where the intellectual debate and revisionist histories began, is important. Ellis, Kendal and Taylor remind us that the field of the history of insanity was 'impoverished' until social historians made their entry in the early 1990s. This also chimes with my suggestion that it was deinstitutionalisation that made it possible for new voices to be heard, and for different forms of history to appear using images, material objects, oral accounts and testimony, as well as political interventions such as national inquiries and commissions. Among my questions for the conference audience were how do psychiatric patients 'speak out'? How is their speech enabled or enacted? What's the collective impact of their speech? What forms does it take?

'Speaking madness' is the focus of this short Coda, a piece designed to help situate this book for readers, including students and general audiences. It is the flipside to the important work of 'Hearing Voices' communities through the Mental Health Foundation in the United Kingdom, itself a play on words that points to the way we hear madness in our communities, as well as fostering a special kind of listening to the voices some people experience as part of their own mental health conditions.[8] In the reflection that follows, I explore the way the contributions to this book highlight the roles played by words, actions and images as part of this act of 'speech'. This Coda is not a review, nor is it designed to be a comprehensive overview of the book; instead, it offers ways to make sense of the worlds of madness explored by these authors.

Making Sense of Madness

This volume *Voices of Madness* offers us further evidence of the shift that has taken place in the writing of the history of madness, prompted by both positive changes in how societies now tackle mental health itself, and the inadequacies of psychiatric treatment and care.[9] In his recent thinking about the historiography of institutions and psychiatry, David Wright has commented that new areas for the history of mental health include consideration of the emotions.[10] There is high emotional content in this volume, even though the authors do not all pursue questions of the emotions from a methodological standpoint.[11] The emotional quotient of the book is important because it reminds us of the people who are part of these stories of madness, of those who spoke, and of those who were the subjects of speech over time and in a range of places covered in the chapter contributions here. Emotional responses by readers also invited readers who might identify with the lived experience of madness, activism, disability, caring for the mad, spaces and work communities, violence and aggression inside institutional walls, or the sorrow in discovering case records highlighting 'delusions', or the silencing of people confined in still other settings where little to no trace of their speech or words can be found.

These writers all point to the politics of madness, to the attenuated identities of the mad and their profound separation from others, as well as to the need for advocacy and action. There's a long history of first-person accounts of madness and also protest, as this book reminds us.[12] This volume started with a satirical poem written by a patient at an asylum in Northampton in 1906, inviting the reader to enter the rarefied world of the institution and experience its community as a 'guest'. Voices are heard, not heard or 'distant' in all kinds of places here: through the work of psychiatrists in France between the world wars, where disagreement about institution care regimes dominated; through the observations of the clinical record of children in Denmark from the 1930s to the 1970s; or through admission records in Scotland at an earlier period of history.

Thinking about the emotional landscape this book evokes, the 'distant voices' of the children in the 1930s offer us a stark reminder of the periodisation of madness. This era saw widespread classification of peoples and was the high point of mental hygiene policies in many countries. The silencing of voices at various historical moments tells us more about the power and possibility inside the old 'madhouse' or asylum described in the second section of this book, where the 'reconstruction' of patient experiences, building on the patient case files and records, offers an example of the scholarship that now reorients our thinking about the patient identity of the past.[13]

Evidences of patient work, human rights and activism remind us of the powerful shifts that took place in the lives of people experiencing mental illness over the twentieth century and into our present time. This book offers a vibrant set of accounts of the enormous potential of the patient voice through word, action and political participation. In most cases, the historian becomes the mediator in these stories and accounts, unable to fully occupy the status of a lived identity in order to describe these worlds of experience. The question of why historians are drawn to this material in the first place is important and needs to be considered as part of a much larger pattern of historical thinking about social change, different social groups and marginalisation or oppression.

Word, Image, Action

Stories by the mad, whether in traces of their own words, in letters or in more detailed lengthy written or oral accounts of mental breakdown and hospitalisation, bring us into contact with what the editors describe as peoples' 'preferences, hopes and losses'; that is to say, in touch with people and their lives. I like the idea that we can access 'what people had to say' about their own hospitalisation, bearing in mind our evidence of these matters is patchy, coloured by power relations and also the serendipity of the historical record.

Several contributions here share patient narratives: a patient-produced newsletter of the late twentieth century in Indiana in the United States, rich with reflections about imminent institutional closure, what might lie ahead and fears about change. Oral interview testimony about planned institutional closures in Nottingham in the United Kingdom likewise points to ambivalence about deinstitutionalisation, with the spectre of community care that provoked uncertainty in many in the psychiatric community, but also challenges the idea that a psychiatric institution was monolithic in its power over its community.

Different narratives, less immediate than those found in oral testimony, remind us of how far the worlds of mental health have come in practical terms, but also tell us something about the resilience of people in conditions of hospitals of the past. The life stories of patients in the casebooks of the Grahamstown Asylum in South Africa, like the records of the early modern 'madhouse', tend to exemplify the way institutional inmates found ways to be heard, despite their obvious lack of power. We can find 'personality', as well as examples of resistance, or strategic compliance, and expressions of dissatisfaction about the limited provision of clothes or space. Although these words are sometimes only traces of the past, they live in the bigger story of mental health institutions and in the lives of those who uttered them or wrote about madness.

The editors offer the insightful comment that visual creations can take us to new places of interpretation and push us beyond the 'traditional bounded walls of the archive', in the words of one of the authors, Cheryl McGeachan. There are differences, too, between forms of creative representations of madness or image—say from artworks to official asylum photography—sometimes meaning that sources strain against each other, or even signal contrary histories. The places where images are made also tell us about the possibilities for creative practices of caring as we move into the future for mental health care. The 'Art Extraordinary' collection in Scotland suggests that by combining perspectives from medical humanities, history and historical geography might offer us more dynamic understandings of madness in place and context, sensibilities which move with people and help to break down a sense of isolation or division between people experiencing mental illness.

Photographs of patients could also be considered as traces, hints of the story of madness in their early days: photographic techniques and representations were sometimes oblique or surprising. Photographic accounts of the lives of people inside institutions could offer disarming truths about the experience of madness: suggestive of histories that cannot be found in written accounts. These communications are vital, both rounding out the textual sources and connecting us with the emotions and places of the past in more material and physical ways.

Perceptions of institutions to house the mad are also images. How communities pictured, saw and remembered former asylums depends on the visual knowledge about places over time. Heritage interpretations highlight again the role played by material things and spaces in the experiences of madness. These discussions about former asylums open up the final and most powerful aspect of this volume's approaches: the engagement with the politics of madness, or action and activism.

What did it mean to 'survive' the institution, to come out the other side of the experience of confinement and speak about it? Institutional confinement and its aftermath, fashioned in the form of community psychiatry, both engendered ways for mental health service users and former patients to use their voices. The contributions of patient movements, such as the Oor Mad History Project, challenge our conceptions of the narrative of mental health and knowledge about it. In Ontario, Canada, the 'mad activists' of the 1970s did their best to engage a broad base but discovered that diversity was important to their success and coherence. In both examples, mad movements reveal the locus of power, the use of language in the politics of madness, as well as the need for inclusion: these were all new problems outside of institutions, because inside institutional spaces inmates tended to be herded together as one group, despite multiple differences between them. In a very divergent context, Soviet Lithuania from the 1940s' institutional violence produced 'purposeful acts of communication' by patients in the form of letters of complaint, reminding us again of the longer history of the patient as complainant, also evoked elsewhere in this book.

A very strong thread that runs through this collection of chapters considers the continuity of past and present. As historians note, the asylum is a 'symbolic and protean space, [and] it has allowed for complex variations of experience', and yet the shared accounts of what it means to voice madness also signal a collective experience defined by the common humanity of people confronting their mental illness, as well as the humanity of those people who hoped, cared and tried to help.[14] Historians offer valuable expertise in the way they can plot the very dynamic shifts in the potential for mental health care to respond to social and political change in specific places and historical moments: they can break into the silences and offer ways to create a 'meaningful dialogue among historians, patients and psychiatrists'.[15]

There is more research to undertake at this juncture in history about the mental health service user movements around the world, within a global narrative of mental health activism. This history is uneven precisely because it has had an 'uncertain rise and impact', as Ellis, Kendal and Taylor say, and yet it might tell us so much more about the way voices in madness are active and always at the forefront of political and social change.

This Coda ends appropriately with this reflection on the importance of the mental health, madness and activism focus of this volume. We should all embrace the notion that, as the editors conclude, 'when we listen to patient voices, we hear new and different ideas'.

Acknowledgements Thanks to Robert Ellis and Sarah Kendal for the invitation to present a keynote at the Voices of Madness conference in Huddersfield in 2016, and to colleagues at the conference for their feedback and contributions.

Notes

1. Catharine Coleborne, "His Brain Was Wrong, His Mind Astray: Families and the Language of Insanity in New South Wales, Queensland and New Zealand, 1880s-1910," *Journal of Family History* 31, no.1 (January 2006): 45–65. See also Catharine Coleborne, *Madness in the Family: Insanity and Institutions in the Australasian Colonial World 1860s–1914* (Basingstoke and New York: Palgrave Macmillan, 2010), Appendix: Indications of Insanity, 154–55.
2. See, for instance, Andrew Scull, Charlotte MacKenzie and Nicholas Hervey, *Masters of Bedlam: The Transformation of the Mad-Doctoring Trade* (Princeton: Princeton University Press, 1996); Jonathan Andrews and Andrew Scull, *Customers and Patrons of the Mad-Trade: The Management of Lunacy in Eighteenth-Century London* (Berkeley and Los Angeles: University of California Press, 2003).
3. Catharine Coleborne, "An End to Bedlam? The Enduring Subject of Madness in Social and Cultural History," *Social History* 42, no. 3 (2017): 420–29.
4. See, for instance, Brenda LeFrançois, Robert Menzies and Geoffrey Reaume, eds., *Mad Matters: A Critical Reader in Canadian Mad Studies* (Toronto: Toronto Canadian Scholars' Press Inc., 2013).
5. One participant was Helen Spandler. See Spandler, "Asylum Magazine: 30 Years of Speaking Out and What's Changed?" Voices of Madness Conference, University of Huddersfield, UK, 15–16 September 2016; See also Helen Spandler, "From Psychiatric Abuse to Psychiatric Neglect?" *Asylum Magazine* 23, no. 2 (2016) https://asylummagazine.org/2017/09/from-psychiatric-abuse-to-psychiatric-neglect-by-helen-spandler-2/. Accessed July 2019.
6. See Catharine Coleborne, *Why Talk About Madness? Bringing History into the Conversation* (Cham, Switzerland: Springer Palgrave, 2020), 35–6.
7. Coleborne, *Why Talk About Madness?*
8. See the website for the Hearing Voices: Mental Health Foundation UK, https://www.mentalhealth.org.uk/a-to-z/h/hearing-voices. Accessed 30 March 2020.
9. Alexandra Bacopoulos-Viau and Aude Fauvel, "The Patient's Turn: Roy Porter and Psychiatry's Tales, Thirty Years On," *Medical History* 60, no. 1 (2016): 1–18.
10. David Wright, "The Great Confinement Revisited: What Have We Learned After 40 Years of Asylum Studies?' Unpublished paper, Society for the Social History of Medicine Conference, Liverpool, UK, 11–13 July 2018.
11. See Catharine Coleborne and Peter N. Stearns, "Institutional records: A Comment," in Katie Barclay, Sharon Crozier-De Rosa and Peter N. Stearns,

eds., *Sources for the History of Emotions: A Guide* (London and New York: Routledge, 2020), 92–8.
12. Rab A. Houston, "Asylums: The Historical Perspective Before, During and After," *Lancet Psychiatry* Epub 17 December 2019: 1–9, https://doi.org/10.1016/S2215-0366(19)30395-5.
13. Angela McCarthy et al., "Lives in the Asylum Record, 1864 to 1910: Utilising Large Data Collections for Histories of Psychiatry and Mental Health," *Medical History* 61, no. 3 (2017): 358–79.
14. Bacopoulos-Viau and Fauvel, "The Patient's Turn," 17.
15. Ibid.

Correction to: Mental Health in the Vernacular: Print and Counter-Hegemonic Approaches to Madness in Colonial Bengal

Pradipto Roy

Correction to:

Chapter 3 in: R. Ellis et al. (eds.), *Voices in the History of Madness*, Mental Health in Historical Perspective, https://doi.org/10.1007/978-3-030-69559-0_3

The book was inadvertently published without the funding acknowledgement in the footnote of the first page of chapter 3. This has been updated in the book.

The updated version of the chapter can be found at https://doi.org/10.1007/978-3-030-69559-0_3

R. Ellis et al. (eds.), *Voices in the History of Madness*, Mental Health in Historical Perspective,
https://doi.org/10.1007/978-3-030-69559-0_20

Name Index[1]

A

Ackerknecht, Erwin, 363
Advocacy Resource Centre for the Handicapped (ARCH), 314, 323
Alleged Lunatics' Friend Society, 370
Alviani, Aldo, 321
Anderson, Gordon, 221
Anderson, Rev George, 33
Andrews, Jonathan, 118
Annales Médico-psychologique, 77, 79, 90n14
Annual International Conference on Human Rights and Psychiatric Oppression, 317
Anubiksan, 59
Armstrong, David, 362–364
Associated Patient Services (APS), 175, 177, 179, 180, 182, 183
Asylum Magazine, 405

B

Balmer, Thomas, 36
Bangstad, Tongeir. R., 274
Battie, William, 5
Bauer, Fritz, 294
Beaudouin, Henri, 75
Beeby, June, 323, 324
Beers, Clifford, 334, 335
Beresford, Peter, 343–349, 373
Berrios, German, 4
Bhattacharya, Kunjabehari, 56
Bleuler, Eugen, 76, 91n23
Blind Organization of Ontario with Self-Help Tactics (BOOST), 315
Bly, Nellie, 9, 10
Boussion, Samuel, 96
Bovet, Theodor, 295, 296
Boyatzis, Richard, E, 266
Boyle, Jimmy, 228, 229, 340
Breaugh, Mike, 321

[1] Note: Page numbers followed by 'n' refer to notes.

R. Ellis et al. (eds.), *Voices in the History of Madness*, Mental Health in Historical Perspective,
https://doi.org/10.1007/978-3-030-69559-0

Bressey, Caroline, 242
Brink, Cornelia, 289
British East India Company, 50, 57
British Journal of Psychiatry, 55
Brodie, Bob, 48n91, 226–228
Bronte, Charlotte, 16
Brookes, Barbara, 242, 253, 254, 258
Brothers, Richard, 122, 129, 130
Bruce, Alexander, 33
Brückner, Burkhart, 289
Bruckshaw, Samuel, 120, 121, 123, 125, 126, 129
Buck, Dorothea, 14, 287–302, 311
Bundesverband Psychiatrie-Erfahrener (BPE e V), *see* German association of psychiatric survivors
Bynum, William. F., 18n19, 275

C

Cairns, Stephen, 273
Campaign Against Psychiatric Oppression, 335, 360
Campbell, Peter, 335–337, 339, 360, 361, 370, 373
Capponi, Diana, 325
Capponi, Pat, 319
Carey, William, 53, 344
Carkesse, James, 123
Carmichael, James, 35
Checkland, Olive, 26
Chekhov, Anton, 162
Children and Young People's Mental Health and Well-being Taskforce, 388
Christie, Adam, 221, 229–231
Club 70, Hamburg, Germany, 298
Coalition of Provincial Organizations of the Handicapped (COPOH), 314
Coffin, Jean-Christophe, 82, 96
Cole, Vickie, 183–185, 186n2
Colin, Henri, 75, 77
Collins, Hugh, 228
Common Room North, 385–390
Condrau, Flurin, 364, 365, 368, 369, 372, 373
Conolly, John, 80, 244
Cooper, David, 5, 310
Costa, Lucy, 334, 336, 338, 344, 349
Courbon, Paul, 79, 80, 85, 87
Cowper, William, 128, 130
Crandell, Doug, 184
Crossley, Nick, 364
Cruden, Alexander, 120, 124–126, 128, 129
Cuckoo's Nest, 319

D

Das, Radhaballabh, 56
Dausset, Louis, 82
Davies, Kerry, 160, 299, 360
Davis, Lennard J., 126, 309, 310
DDU Review, 174, 178–181, 183, 186n1
Demay, Georges, 76–78, 84–87
Dendron, 307
Department of Health, U.K. Government, 388
Descartes, Rene, 50
Diamond, Hugh Welch, 240, 244, 259, 261n26
Dickens, Charles, 385
DIE ZEIT, 296
Doerner, Klaus, 4
Dörner, Klaus, 292
Dostoyevsky, Fyodor, 16
Down, John Langdon, 384
du Plessis, Rory, 10, 118, 137–150, 195, 242
Dubuffet, Jean, 231
Duston, Northants, 1
Dyck, Ericka, 384

E
Eastlake, Lady Elizabeth, 240, 258
Edensor, Timothy, 274
Edgar Hill, Rev., 35
Edwards, Elizabeth, 241, 258
Egsgaard, Jens, 103
Eichmann, Adolf, 294, 295
Ellis, Rev. Norman, 319
Elphinstone, Mountstuart, 52
Ernst, Waltraud, 7, 58, 73
Esdaile, James, 57, 58
Esquirol, Jean-Étienne Dominique, 74

F
Facebook, 340
Fair Labour Standards Act (U.S.)(FLSA), 176
Falret, Jean-Pierre, 74
Federation of Mental Patients Unions, 335
Fellowes, Dorothea, 126
Finkler, Lilith, 318, 320
Fissell, Mary E., 159, 363
Fitch, A. J., 33
Flores, Mike, 182, 186n1
Foart Simmons, Samuel, 122, 127, 129
Foucault, Michel, 4, 5, 9, 15, 39, 159, 363–368, 375–377, 396, 397
  Foucauldian, 159, 366
Franklin, Bridget, 271
Fraser, John (Commissioner in Lunacy), 27
Friends of India, 53
Future in Mind, 388–390

G
German association of psychiatric survivors, 288, 292
Ghosh, Gopalchandra, 56
Giddens, Anthony, 159
Gilman, Charlotte Perkins, 8
Gittins, Diane, 268, 275, 276
Goffman, Erving, 4, 193, 196, 206, 384
Goldney, Edward, 120, 125, 126
Goodwill Industries, 179
Grant-Smith, Rachel, 335
Greenlees, Thomas Duncan, 138–140, 142–147
Green-Lewis, Jennifer, 241
Grier, Ruth, 323
Griesinger, Wilhelm, 80
Griffiths Report, 385
Guardian (U.S.), The, 309, 310
Gutersloh Asylum, Westphalia, Germany, 78

H
Hack Tuke, Daniel, 4
Hall, Rev. Robert, 124, 125, 129
Hamlett, Jane, 12
Hansen, Niels, 106
Harper, Vern, 316
Harris, Michael, 324
Harrison, Rodney, 272, 274
Hart, Roger, 386, 394
Hayward, Rhodri, 50, 334
Hear by Right framework, 388
Hearing Voices Network (HVN), 335, 342
Heyde, Werner, 294, 295
Hobbs, John, 2, 10, 12
Hodgkin, Katharine, 119
Holochuck, Steve, 309
How many times do we have to tell you? Report, 389
Human Rights for the Handicapped (org), 313
Hunter, Richard, 4, 9, 117

I
Icarus Project, The, 338, 340
Imperial Fireworks, 180
ImROC, 346
Indian Health Periodicals
Bhisaka-darpana, 55, 62, 65
Svyastha Samacara, 62
Indian Medical Service (IMS), 62–64
Ingram, Allan, 118, 119
Ireland, W. W., 26, 34, 35
Irrenoffensive, Berlin, 289

J
Jabloner, Antonia, 230, 231
Jackson, Mark, 12, 26
Jacobs, Jane M, 273
Jewson, Nicholas, 363, 365, 367
Jones, Kathleen, 4
Journal of Mental Science, 4, 55, 64

K
Kanners, Leo, 100
Kar, Radhagobinda, 62
Karmakar, Panchanan, 53
Keddie, Kenneth, 230, 231
Kelly, Brendan, 223
Kempe, Margery, 334
Kennedy, J. F., 8
Kenny, Michael, 268
Klee, Ernst, 297, 298
KOOTH, 391
Kraepelin, Emil, 79
Krieger, Hans, 296, 297

L
Ladame, Charles, 76–78
Laing, Joyce, 219, 220, 226, 227, 230, 231, 310
Laing, R.D., 5, 376, 384
L'Aliéniste français, 84
Lamb, Mary, 124
Lanark District Asylum, Hartwood, Scotland, 40
Lapon, Lenny, 309
Larbert, Sterling, 25, 27, 33, 40
Launchpad, Newcastle, 340
Lavigne, Ron, 323
Le Mans, France, 72, 88
Leverndale Hospital, Glasgow, Scotland, 220
L'Hygiène Mentale, 78, 79
Lithuanian Ministry of Health, 155, 157
Long, James, 55
Loughran, Tracey, 11
Low, David, 35
Lynch, Kevin, 273

M
Macalpine, Ida, 4, 9, 17n9, 117
Mackenzie, Charlotte, 118
MacKenzie, Mavis, 320
Macmillan, Duncan, 199
Mad Studies Network, 350
Marie Claire, 395
Marland, Hilary, 138
McKague, Carla, 314, 323
Medicaid, 185
Medical Times and Gazette, The, 244
Megill, Allan, 376, 377
Mental Health Foundation, 406
Mental Patients Association (Canada), 313
Ontario Mental Patients Association (OMPA), 319
Mental Patients News, 371
Mental Patients' Union (MPU), 335, 371
Mental Welfare Commission for Scotland, 371
Meux jnr, Richard, 121, 127
Miller, Sanderson, 121, 122

Millet, Kate, 384
Mills, Jim, 60
Mills, Mrs, 123
Mind (Mental Health Charity), 335
MINDLink, 335
Mold, Alex, 362
Monro, John, 5, 126
Moons, Graham, 270, 275
More Active Therapy (MAT), 7, 78–89
Morel, Bénédict-Augustin, 74, 76, 91n23
Morrock, Richard, 309
Moses, Sarah, 271
Mulroney, Brian, 315

N

Nahwegahbow, Bobbi, 316
National Anti-Klan Coalition (U.S.), 316
National Self Harm Network, 335, 342
National Survivor User Members' Manifesto, 342
National Survivor User Network, The (NSUN), 340, 342, 343, 348
Naumburg, Saxony-Anhalt, 291
Nazi Party (Nazism), 290, 297
New Democratic Party (Canada), 315, 321, 325
New York Times, 289
NHS Management Inquiry, Report (1983), *see* Griffiths Report
Nicolson, Malcolm, 20n33, 327n8, 363, 365
Noble Industries, 180
Nottingham Advocacy Group, 335

O

Oaks, David, 307
O'Donnell, Anne, 361
Ogborn, Miles, 224, 232, 235n20
Online Harms Report, 392
On Our Own (Activist Group), 314, 319, 331n59, 334, 338
Ontario Advocacy Commission, 324
Ontario Coalition Against Poverty, 324
Ontario Coalition to Stop Electroshock, 315
Ontario Friends of Schizophrenics (OFOS), 323, 324
Ontario Public Sector Employees Union (OPSEU), 319–321, 323, 332n60, 332n64
Oor Mad History (OMH), 15, 359–377
Owen, Wilfrid, 11, 21n50

P

Parchappe, Maximien, 74
Parker, Dorothy, 16, 22n68
Parry-Jones, William, 30, 45n19, 117, 131n3, 132n6, 136n63
Parsons, Talcott, 171n14, 364, 365
Paul, Harry, 82
Pavlov, Ivan, 158
Pendlebury, John, 269, 270, 280n40, 280n47
Perceval, John, 370
Philo, Chris, 131n5, 132n6, 132n7, 132n9, 209n6, 209n7, 233n3, 236n40, 277n2, 277n5, 365, 367
Phoenix Rising, 313, 318, 320, 328n11, 329n23, 329n24, 329n27, 329n30, 331n42, 331n43, 331n44, 331n46, 332n63
Pinel, Philippe, 73, 80
Pitt, William, 122
Plath, Sylvia, 8, 16
Porot, A., 79, 80, 82, 85, 92n48

Porter, Roy, 3, 5, 9, 17n9, 18n14, 18n16, 18n19, 19–20n33, 20n41, 21n52, 90n4, 111n3, 117, 118, 131n1, 131n2, 131n4, 132n10, 132n13, 133n17, 134n30, 134n39, 135n60, 137, 150n1, 157, 170n8, 188n22, 191, 208n1, 211n27, 223, 234n12, 262n52, 280n43, 283n92, 284n94, 327n8, 362, 363, 365, 366, 369, 371, 372
Powell, Enoch, 385

Q
Queen Street Patients Council, Toronto, Canada, 317, 330n41

R
Raynier, Julien, 75, 90n12
Reijnders, Stijn, 271, 278n13, 280n45, 281n52
Reil, Johann Christian, 80
Reville, David, 314, 328n14, 329n31
Rhys, Jean, 16, 22n64
Richardson, Ruth, 264, 278n15
Richter, Horst-Eberhard, 297
Ritchie, Thomas, 371
Roberts, Andrew, 337, 360, 361, 369–371, 373
Rogers, William, 121, 123
Rose, Diana, 213n44, 335–337, 342–347, 349, 360
Rose, Nikolas, 171n13, 363, 364
Rothman, David, 4
Russell, Ginny, 384

S
Said, Edward, 51, 149
Sargent, William, 9
Sassoon, Siegfried, 11
Saxe-Coburg and Gotha, Albert Edward (Prince of Wales), 59
Schmitt, Sandra, 290
Scottish Mental Health Arts and Film Festival (SMHAFF), 220
Scottish National Institution, The, 25–43
Scottish Union of Mental Patients (SUMP), 335, 371
Scull, Andrew, 4, 5, 118, 271, 272, 281n55, 281n56, 281n58, 404
Sekula, Allan, 240, 241
Shaping Our Lives, 340
Shephard, Ben, 11
Simmons, Harvey, 312
Simon, Hermann, 78
Skinner, Quentin, 65
Smith, Laurajane, 274
Smith, Leonard, 9, 117–131, 147, 195, 223, 268, 269, 274
Sniekers, Maloe, 271
Sontag, Susan, 254
Standen, Thomas, 266, 267
Steele, Eliza, 39, 40
Stromberg, Per, 274
Sturdy, Harriet, 30, 45n19
Survivors History Group (SHG), 15, 359–377
Survivors Speak Out (SSO), 335, 342, 370
Suzuki, Akihito, 18n19, 118
Swartz, Sally, 2, 238, 254
Szasz, Thomas, 5, 309, 310

T
Taylor, Barbara, 210n20, 271, 281n57
Taylor, Steven, 1–16, 18n24, 19n29, 96, 111n4, 139
Thomas, Warren, 323
Thompson, Edward Palmer, 58

Tiesa, 165
Tolstrup, Kai, 98, 103, 105
Trevor, Edward, 125, 126
Trigg, Dylan, 268, 279n33
Trosse, Rev. George, 119, 125, 127, 128, 130
Tuke, John Batty, 33
Twitter, 340, 389

U
UK Advocacy Network, 335
UN Convention of the Rights of the Child, 387
United Nations Convention on Rights of Persons with Disabilities (UNCRPD), 343
Urban Alliance on Race Relations, Toronto, 317

V
Van der Veer, Peter, 58
Vermette, Lionel, 316
Vié, Jacques, 84
Voronka, Jijian, 345, 349

W
Wakefield, Edward, 5, 44n5
Walk, Alexander, 4, 17n7
Walker, Marylène, 219
Wallcraft, Jan, 335, 336, 339, 343, 349
Walton, John K., 270
Waugh, Jim, 231
Weitz, Don, 316, 329n22
Wilkins, Charles, 53
Willoughby, Lady Honoria, 126, 129
Wilson, Bp. William, 33
Wimmer, August, 98, 110
Winehouse, Amy, 394
Wood, Mary Elene, 299
Wright, David, 265, 277n7, 278n18, 279n37, 280n44, 281n64, 283n90, 284n94, 284n97, 407
Wylie, Beth, 230
Wynter, Rebecca, 223, 234n14, 261n24

Y
Yale, Mike, 313
York Courant, 5
You're Welcome framework, 388

Z
Zerchin, Sophie, 288, 304n18

Place Index[1]

A
Aix les Baines, Savoie, France, 31
Alexandria, Egypt, 291
Asile Clinique, Paris, France, 72, 81, 83–87, 92n59
Asile de la Sarthe (ADLS/AD), Le Mans, France, 72, 81, 83, 84
Auschwitz concentration camp, 294
Ayr District Asylum (ADA), Ayrshire, Scotland, 34

B
Baldovan Asylum, Dundee, Soctland (Baldovan Institution), 25
Barlinnie Prison, Glasgow, Scotland (Barlinnie), 222, 224–229
Bellsdyke Hospital, Stirling, Scotland, 39
Belsize Park, London, England, 370
Bengal, India (Bengali), 49–66
Berrywood Asylum, Northants., England (Berrywood), 2
Bethel Hospital, Bielefeld, North Rhine-Westphalia, Germany, 300
Bethlem Hospital, London, England (Bethlem Asylum), 5
Bispebjerg Hospital, Copenhagen, Denmark, 99
Blackwell Asylum, New York, U.S.A., 9
British Raj, The, 52
Burntisland, Fife, Scotland (Burntisland), 35

C
Calcutta, 53–55, 57, 64
Cardiff, Wales, 291
Central State Hospital (CSH), Indiana, U.S.A (Central State), 174–181, 183–185

[1] Note: Page numbers followed by 'n' refer to notes.

R. Ellis et al. (eds.), *Voices in the History of Madness*, Mental Health in Historical Perspective,
https://doi.org/10.1007/978-3-030-69559-0

Charlestown, Fife, Scotland, 32
Coll, Inner Hebrides, Scotland, 31
Copenhagen, Denmark, 96, 97, 103, 111
Copenhagen University Hospital, Denmark, 8, 95–111

D
Dingleton Hospital, Melrose, Scotland, 198
Dumbarton Poorhouse, West Dumbartonshire, Scotland, 30
Dundee, Scotland, 25, 32

E
Earlswood Asylum, Surrey, England (Earlswood), 39
Edinburgh, Scotland, 15, 33, 36, 359, 370
Ely Mental Hospital, Cardiff, Wales, 11

F
Fort William College, Kolkata, India, 53
Friern Hospital, Barnet, England, 271

G
Glasgow Museums Resource Centre (GMRC), Glasgow, Scotland, 11, 220
Goosnargh, Lancashire, England, 267
Govan District Asylum, Scotland, 220
Gowrie House, Liff/Dundee Royal Asylum, 32
Grahamstown Lunatic Asylum (GLA)/Grahamstown Asylum, South Africa, 137–150

H
Hartwood Hospital, N. Lanarkshire, Scotland, 371
Heidelberg, Baden-Württemberg, 289
Hessen, Germany, 294
Holloway Sanatorium, Surrey, England, 39, 238, 244, 248, 254
Hooghly, West Bengal, India, 53
Huddersfield, W. Yorks., England, 404

I
Indiana Central State Hospital, Indiana, U.S.A., 10
Indianapolis, Indiana, U.S.A., 176, 184
Islay, Inner Hebrides, Scotland, 31, 37
Isle of Cumbrae, Buteshire, Scotland, 34

K
Kirkliston, West Lothian, Scotland, 38
Kirkwall, Orkney, Scotland, 39
Kolkata, West Bengal, *see* Calcutta

L
Lakeshore Psychiatric Hospital, Toronto, Canada, 320
Lithuanian Central State Archive, Vilnius, Lithuania, 157
London, England, 5, 10, 15, 36, 97, 118, 120–122, 125, 370

M
Mapperley Hospital/Mapperley, Nottingham, England, 197–199, 202–205, 209n6
Maudsley Hospital, London, England, 97

Montrose Asylum, Scotland, 229, 230
Moor Hospital, Lancaster, England, 266, 276
Mumbai, Maharashtra, India (Bombay), 52

N

Nazareth House, Aberdeen, Scotland, 37
Newcastle-upon-Tyne City Lunatic Asylum, 238, 243
New York, U.S.A, 9, 16, 289, 316
North Sea, The, 291
North Uist, Outer Hebrides, Scotland, 31
Nottingham, Notts., England, 118, 196–201, 204, 207, 208, 408

O

Oldenburg, Lower Saxony, Germany, 291
Ontario, Canada, 15, 307–326, 409
Open Museum (Glasgow), The, 221, 225, 226
Orkney, Scotland, 39
Ottawa, Canada, 315

P

Painswick, Gloucestershire, England, 39
Pažaislis Hospital, Kaunas, Lithuania, 161
Port Alfred Asylum, South Africa, 146, 147

Q

Queen Street Mental Health Centre, Toronto, Canada, 321

R

Recovery College, Nottingham, England, 204, 205, 214n49
Retreat, The, York, England, 5
Royal Infirmary of Edinburgh, Scotland, 33

S

St Luke's, London, 5, 129
St. Thomas' Hospital, Ontario, Canada, 320
Santpoort Asylum, Holland (Santpoort), 78–81, 87
Saxondale Hospital, Notts., England, 200, 203, 204
Scarborough Centenary Hospital, Toronto, Canada, 320
Seine Asylum, Paris, France, 84
Shanghai, China, 31, 34
Sleepyhillock Cemetery, Montrose, Scotland, 222, 224, 229–232
Smyllum Orphanage, Lanark, Scotland, 37
Stirling District Asylum, Scotland (SDA), 38, 39
Stracathro Hospital, Angus, Scotland, 32
Surrey County Asylum, Hooley, England (Netherne), 240

T

Thornhill, Dumfriesshire, Scotland, 37, 346
Toronto, Canada, 311, 314, 316–321, 323, 325

U

University Hospital, Copenhagen, Denmark (Copenhagen University Hospital), 8, 95–111
University Hospital, Oslo, Norway, 97

V

Villejuif Asylum, Paris, France, 75, 77

W

Watson's School, Edinburgh, Scotland, 36
Weglaufhaus, Berlin, Germany, 289
Westmains Private Asylum, Kirkintilloch, Scotland, 29
Whittingham Hospital, Lancashire, England (Whittingham), 264–269, 271, 272, 274–276
Winterbourne View, Gloucs., England, 11
Woodilee Hospital, Lenzie, Glasgow, Scotland, 29

Y

York, England, 5, 9, 16, 316
York Lunatic Asylum, England, 5

Z

Žiegždriai Psychiatric Hospital, Šlienava, Lithuania, 155, 164

Subject Index[1]

A
Autism, 105

B
Binet-Simon test, 106, 113n20
Biopower, 366
Brain scans, 106, 107

C
Causation of mental disorder, theories of, 72
  organicist, 73
Celebrities and mental health, 395
Children/child, 7, 8, 11, 25–43, 44n2, 74, 80, 95–111, 111n2, 112n9, 128, 139, 176, 187n10, 195, 270, 291, 300, 384, 385, 387, 388, 390, 392, 399n19, 404, 407
  childhood, 26, 96
Class, 7, 9, 11, 26, 28, 40, 50, 53, 57, 58, 60, 74, 87, 118, 119, 141, 226, 227, 229, 239, 258, 318–325, 372
Coercion
  confined, 125
  use of restraints, 126
Community care
  care in the community, 192, 193, 196, 205, 206, 208, 385
  deinstitutionalisation, 192, 193, 372, 408
Community Treatment Orders (CTO) (Canada), 324
Complaint letter, 156, 157, 161, 162, 164, 166, 168, 169, 178
  letters of complaint, 118, 410
Co-production, 192, 194
Counselling, 128
  counsel, 146

[1] Note: Page numbers followed by 'n' refer to notes.

R. Ellis et al. (eds.), *Voices in the History of Madness*, Mental Health in Historical Perspective,
https://doi.org/10.1007/978-3-030-69559-0

Crafts/Craft
pottery, 292
wood carving, 292
Culture or acts of violence
abuse, 10, 110, 165, 193, 196, 267, 300, 320–322, 341, 385, 399n19
violence, 156, 161, 163
violent, 77, 78, 104, 108, 125, 129, 140, 163, 225, 226, 228

D
Degeneration theory, 74
Developmental psychology, 101, 107
Disability (as a social construct), 175–176
Doctor-patient relationship, 257, 363

E
Elderly, the, 210n15, 254
Enlightenment, the, 50, 73
Ethnicity, 9, 15
Experiential knowledge (value of), 334, 348

F
Family, 3, 6, 7, 9, 12, 30–35, 37, 38, 40–43, 60, 64, 73, 100, 101, 107, 119–121, 127–129, 157, 160, 161, 180, 181, 206, 221, 230, 241, 251, 266, 269, 291, 292, 300, 307, 324, 362, 393, 404
First World War/World War I, 8, 11, 71, 73, 75, 82, 85, 87, 89
Functionalism, 365

G
Gender, 9, 15, 16, 137, 138, 141, 212n33, 258, 291, 309, 316–318, 336, 384, 395
masculinity, 395

H
Heritage sector, 274
uncomfortable heritage, 269, 270
History methodologies and subjects
emotions (history of), 50
historiography of illness, 168
mental health history, 4, 6, 7, 15, 65, 191, 222–224, 229, 232, 233, 376, 404, 405, 407, 410
psychiatry and medicine, history of, 361, 365
social history, 269, 275, 362, 369

I
Indian Medical Concepts
Ayurveda, 51, 52, 62
ayurvedic medicine, 7
bot-tala books, 54
dharma, 52
Dharmasastra, 51
dhat-syndrome, 62
dhatu-dourbalya, 62–65
kathakata, 53
Manasik Rog, 57
Nitisastra, 51
Siddha medicine, 52
Unani medicine, 52
Institutionalisation, 11, 13, 39, 40, 138, 146–150, 193, 207, 392, 393

L

Law of June 30, 1838 (France), 74
Legal Aid, 314
Lethal injection, 291
  "euthanasia," 291
Local Government
  Parish Councils, 29
  parochial boards, 25, 30, 31

M

Madhouse Proprietor, 128
Mad Studies
  Mad History, 288
  mad wisdom, 301
Magistrate, 1, 123
Medical discourse, 7, 10, 64, 157–169, 363
Medicalisation, 158, 362, 364
Medical or Hospital Personnel
  administrators, 320
  alienist, 138–150, 240
  chief medical officer, 74, 76, 81, 83–89
  doctor, 7, 9, 26, 31–33, 37, 54–56, 58–60, 62, 64, 74–78, 80, 83–85, 88, 89, 128, 139–143, 148, 159, 162, 164, 193, 238, 241, 245, 247, 251, 257, 258, 271, 289, 293, 294, 296, 301, 362, 363, 365, 368, 404
  hospital administrators, 3, 321
  medical man, 28
  medical Officer, 35, 141, 245, 247, 248, 250, 251
  medical orderly, 163
  medical Superintendent, 2, 26, 34, 35, 138
  mental health staff, 386
  nurses, 9, 73, 77, 80, 84, 87–89, 108, 148, 162, 163, 167, 177, 193, 195, 197–200, 202, 207, 254, 267, 301, 320, 368
  nursing, 26, 82, 87, 88, 100, 165, 185, 269, 313, 319, 320
  orderly, 80, 155, 161, 165, 167
  psychiatric specialists, 165
  psychiatrist, 4, 5, 9, 33, 50, 71–89, 98–102, 105–107, 158, 177, 197, 201, 207, 230, 270, 292–296, 318, 360, 387, 388, 394, 407, 410
  psychologist, 83, 104, 110, 177, 292, 388
  psychotherapist, 388
  psychotherapy, 79, 80, 106, 107
  speech pathologist, 178
Medical Records
  application folios, 26
  casebooks, 2, 10, 118, 137–150, 238, 239, 242–245, 248, 250, 253, 254, 408
  case histories, 138, 157, 243, 244, 338
  case notes, 34, 38, 39, 42, 97, 100, 101, 106–108, 110
  medical case-notes, 100, 106–108
  medical certificates, 31, 139–144, 149, 243
  medical history, 65, 100, 101, 109–110, 290, 362, 366
  medical notes, 3, 12, 39
  patient casefiles, 12
Medical textbooks, 96, 105, 249
Medication
  aminazine, 162
  chlorpromazine, 104
  chlorprothixene, 104
  lithium, 104
  neuroleptics, 289, 290, 293, 312
Mesmerism, 56–58
Migrants, 14

Mind, concept of/ mind, 3, 9, 33, 49, 50, 52, 55–57, 59, 73, 80, 98, 106, 124, 128, 139, 143, 147, 149, 161, 166, 223, 228, 232, 271, 333–350, 362, 389, 408
Models of care, 8

N

Neurological Disorders
- dementia, 16, 62, 63, 76, 77
- epilepsy, 26, 30, 32, 35, 42, 57, 62, 63, 104, 176
- epileptic, 32, 36

Neurology, 59, 63, 82, 83, 88
- neurological, 65, 83, 107

New social movements, 15, 308, 310, 384
Nursing home, 185, 313, 319, 320

O

Occupational therapy, 60, 73, 83, 84, 89, 138
Oral history/oral histories, 3, 10, 174, 179, 185, 191, 192, 194–196, 200, 203, 206–208, 299, 361

P

Parents, 7, 26–28, 30–35, 37, 40, 42, 99–104, 107–109, 291
Participatory action research (PAR), 192, 194–196
Patient Accounts (savings account), 180, 181, 265, 288
Patient and Public Involvement (PPI, UK Government Policy), 334, 336
Patient work
- work, 7, 71–89, 174, 178, 407
- work program, 174, 182

Patriotism, 11
Pauper lunatic asylums, 12, 139
Peer support (concept), 201–203, 334, 339–341, 344, 348–350, 389
Photography
- photographic equipment, 12
- photographic images, 238, 240, 241
- photographs, 12, 13, 97, 106, 107, 223, 237–259, 409

Physical illness/disease
- bronchitis, 37
- bronchopneumonia, 39
- diphtheria, 37
- phthisis, 37
- scarlet fever, 37
- syphilis, 77, 148
- tuberculosis, 34

Physical impairment or condition
- blindness, 32, 168, 187n10, 313
- deaf and dumb, 32
- hydrocephalus, 33
- sensory impairment, 42

Police, 14, 317, 325
Psychiatric disorders, conditions or symptoms
- anxiety, 16, 197, 228, 272, 273, 392, 395, 396
- Attention Deficit Hyperactivity Disorder (ADHD), 105
- delusions, 76, 119, 125, 137–150, 301, 407
- delusions of grandeur, 142
- delusions of persecution, 76, 142, 146
- depression, 52, 228, 395, 396
- hallucinations, 2, 119
- mania, 76, 142, 243, 246
- monomania, 62, 63
- schizophrenia, 52, 76, 288, 290

Psychiatric Survivor Pride Day (Canada), 316, 318

Psychiatric survivors liberation movement, 307
Psychiatry
child psychiatry, 96–98, 100, 102, 105, 107, 110, 111, 112n9
community-oriented psychiatry, 193
social psychiatry, 193, 199
soviet psychiatry, 156–158
Psychoanalysis, 8, 9, 96, 107, 158, 296

R
Racial discrimination and/or bias
racism, 316, 317, 340, 348
racists, 317
Recovery (concept), 127, 128, 145, 160, 161, 166, 194, 196–202, 204–207, 237, 288, 293, 295, 345, 346, 348, 390, 393
recovery in the Bin, 340, 346
Recreation therapist, 178
rehabilitation therapists, 177, 178
Rehabilitation programs, 177
Religion
Anglicanism, 319
clergy, 43
confirmation, 102, 108, 296
evangelical christians, 26
Protestant Church, 43, 290
quakers, 5
Scottish Episcopal Church, 33
Sisters of Nazareth, 37
Rights movements
civil rights movement, 341
Disabled People's Movement, 343
gay and lesbian rights movement, 308, 310, 318, 325
human rights, 14, 160, 307, 315, 316, 325, 407
mad pride, 316, 384
patients' rights, 160, 169, 195, 314, 319, 322, 324
Royal College of Psychiatrists, 4, 387

S
Safe spaces (importance of), 11, 302, 333, 338–341, 348, 367
Schools (as providers of mental health care), 27, 34–37, 40, 42, 53, 87, 99, 102, 108, 176, 181, 292, 293, 390, 391
Second World War (World War II), 73, 89, 107, 384
Self-sufficiency (American ideal of), 175, 181
self-help, 10, 197, 204, 289, 292, 298, 339–342, 348, 349
Service user movement/ or survivor movement
service user activism, 350, 386
user, 3, 13, 15, 194, 195, 200, 202–208, 334–340, 342–345, 347–349, 361–362, 370, 371, 373, 375, 409
Sheltered employment
semi-independent living programs, 185
sheltered workshops, 10, 174–179, 182–184
supported employment, 174, 175, 178, 183, 184
Social inclusion, 312, 346
Social media, 340, 389–393
Social worker(s), 14, 177, 293
Souder v. Brennan (U.S), 176
Sterilization, 291, 292, 298, 300, 301, 306n61
Suicide, 145, 206, 230, 294, 392, 395
Survivor narratives, 350
narratives, 350

T
Theosophy, 57
Therapeutic community (TC) movement, 192, 193, 197–199, 225
Therapeutic relationships (loss of), 196, 199–202, 204, 206–208
Transgender, 318

U
U.K. Government Acts
  County Asylums Act (1808), 266
  Lunacy (Amendment) Act (1862), U.K., 27
  Lunacy (Scotland) Act) (1857), U.K., 30
  Mental Health Act (1959), U.K., 384
  Mental Health Act (1983), U.K., 200, 387
  Mental Treatment Act (1930), U.K., 268
  Murder (Abolition of Death Penalty) Act (1965), U.K., 225
  National Health Service and Community Care Act (1990), U.K., 387
  NHS and Community Care Act (1990), 336
  Poor Law (Scotland) Act (1845), 26
Urban decay, 273

W
Welfare, 141, 316, 321, 342
  welfare systems, 2
Wellbeing, 30, 76, 194, 200, 207, 390, 395

The manufacturer's authorised representative in the EU is Springer Nature Customer Service Centre GmbH, Europaplatz 3, 69115 Heidelberg, Germany. If you have any concerns regarding our products, please contact ProductSafety@springernature.com

Printed and bound by CPI Group (UK) Ltd, Croydon, CR0 4YY

30/09/2026

02225434-0010